NURSING CONCEPT
ANALYSIS

Joyce J. Fitzpatrick, PhD, MBA, RN, FAAN, is an Elizabeth Brooks Ford professor of nursing, Frances Payne Bolton School of Nursing, Case Western Reserve University (CWRU) in Cleveland, Ohio, where she was dean from 1982 to 1997. She is an adjunct professor in the department of geriatrics at Mount Sinai School of Medicine in New York, New York. She earned her BSN from Georgetown University, Washington, DC, an MS in psychiatric-mental health nursing from the Ohio State University, Columbus, Ohio, a PhD in nursing from New York University, and an MBA from CWRU in 1992. She has received numerous honors and awards, and was elected as a fellow to the American Academy of Nursing in 1981 and to the National Academies of Practice in 1996. She has received the *American Journal of Nursing* Book of the Year Award 18 times. Dr. Fitzpatrick is widely published in nursing and health care literature. She served as co-editor of the *Annual Review of Nursing Research* series, Volumes 1 to 26. She edits the journals *Applied Nursing Research, Archives in Psychiatric Nursing,* and *Nursing Education Perspectives* (the official journal of the National League for Nursing). She has published several books with Springer Publishing Company, including three editions of the classic *Encyclopedia of Nursing Research (ENR).*

Geraldine McCarthy, PhD, MSN, MEd, DipN, RNT, RGN, Fellow RCSI, is emeritus professor of nursing at the Catherine McAuley School of Nursing and Midwifery at University College Cork (UCC) and Chair of the South/South West Acute Hospital Group, which comprises nine hospitals in the south of Ireland. Prior to this, she was founding professor and dean of the nursing school at UCC, and held the post of head of the UCC College of Medicine and Health, providing strategic leadership in research and educational programs in medicine, dentistry, therapies, pharmacy, nursing, and midwifery. She has also held a variety of other positions in Ireland, the United Kingdom, the United States, and Canada. She holds an MEd from Trinity College Dublin, and MSN and PhD degrees in nursing from Case Western Reserve University, Cleveland, Ohio. She has been a member of a number of national and European bodies and her ministerial appointments include one to the Fulbright Commission. She has been the editor/author of a number of books and continually contributes to nursing publications.

NURSING CONCEPT ANALYSIS
APPLICATIONS TO RESEARCH
AND PRACTICE

Joyce J. Fitzpatrick, PhD, MBA, RN, FAAN
Geraldine McCarthy, PhD, MSN, MEd, DipN, RNT, RGN, Fellow RCSI

Editors

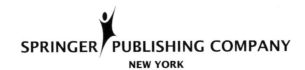

SPRINGER PUBLISHING COMPANY
NEW YORK

Springer Publishing Company, LLC
11 West 42nd Street
New York, NY 10036
www.springerpub.com

Acquisitions Editor: Margaret Zuccarini
Production Editor: Kris Parrish
Composition: diacriTech

ISBN: 978-0-8261-2677-1
e-book ISBN: 978-0-8261-2682-5

16 17 18 19/ 5 4 3 2 1

The author and the publisher of this Work have made every effort to use sources believed to be reliable to provide information that is accurate and compatible with the standards generally accepted at the time of publication. The author and publisher shall not be liable for any special, consequential, or exemplary damages resulting, in whole or in part, from the readers' use of, or reliance on, the information contained in this book. The publisher has no responsibility for the persistence or accuracy of URLs for external or third-party Internet websites referred to in this publication and does not guarantee that any content on such websites is, or will remain, accurate or appropriate.

Library of Congress Cataloging-in-Publication Data
Fitzpatrick, Joyce J., 1944- , editor. | McCarthy, Geraldine, 1950- , editor.
 Nursing concept analysis : applications to research and practice / Joyce J. Fitzpatrick, Geraldine McCarthy, editors.
 New York, NY : Springer Publishing Company, LLC, [2016] | Includes bibliographical references and index.
 LCCN 2015041029 | ISBN 9780826126771 | ISBN 9780826126825 (e-book)
 | MESH: Concept Formation. | Nursing Theory. | Nursing Research. | Philosophy, Nursing.
 LCC RT81.5 | NLM WY 86 | DDC 610.73072—dc23 LC record available at http://lccn.loc.gov/2015041029

Special discounts on bulk quantities of our books are available to corporations, professional associations, pharmaceutical companies, health care organizations, and other qualifying groups. If you are interested in a custom book, including chapters from more than one of our titles, we can provide that service as well.

For details, please contact:
Special Sales Department, Springer Publishing Company, LLC
11 West 42nd Street, 15th Floor, New York, NY 10036-8002
Phone: 877-687-7476 or 212-431-4370; Fax: 212-941-7842
E-mail: sales@springerpub.com

Printed in the United States of America by McNaughton & Gunn.

CONTENTS

PART III: ORGANIZATION-FOCUSED CONCEPTS

CONTRIBUTORS

Linda Ahn, MSN, RN, ANP-BC, Nurse Practitioner, Memorial Sloan Kettering Cancer Center, New York, New York

Karen Bauce, DNP, MPA, RN, NEA-BC, Adjunct Professor, School of Nursing, Sacred Heart University, Fairfield, Connecticut

Miriam Bell, MSc, RGN, Interim Director, Nursing and Midwifery Planning and Development Unit, Office of the Nursing and Midwifery Services Directorate, Health Service Executive, Dublin, Ireland

Aliza Bitton Ben-Zacharia, DNP, RN, ANP, Neurology Teaching Assistant, The Icahn School of Medicine, Mount Sinai Hospital System, New York, New York

Corazon B. Cajulis, DNP, RN, ANP-BC, NEA-BC, Nurse Practitioner, Mount Sinai Hospital, New York, New York

Alice Corbett, MS, RN, FNP, CPEN, NEA-BC, Vice President, Patient Care Services, Chief Nursing Officer, New York Presbyterian/Hudson Valley Hospital, Cortlandt Manor, New York

Patrick Cotter, DN, RGN, RM, RNP, RANP, Advanced Nurse Practitioner, Emergency Department, Cork University Hospital; Adjunct Senior Lecturer, Catherine McAuley School of Nursing and Midwifery, University College Cork, Cork, Ireland

Mary Rose Day, DN, RGN, RM, RPHN, College Lecturer, Catherine McAuley School of Nursing and Midwifery, University College Cork, Cork, Ireland

Colleen DeBoer, MSN, RN, ANP-BC, Nurse Practitioner, New York-Presbyterian Weill Cornell Medical Center, New York, New York

Serena M. Fitzgerald, PhD, RGN, College Lecturer, Catherine McAuley School of Nursing and Midwifery, University College Cork, Cork, Ireland

Joyce J. Fitzpatrick, PhD, MBA, RN, FAAN, Elizabeth Brooks Ford Professor of Nursing, Frances Payne Bolton School of Nursing, Case Western Reserve University, Cleveland, Ohio

Kari Gali, DNP, RN, CPNP, Be Well Kids, Cleveland Clinic Children's Hospital, VA Quality Scholars Fellow, Louis Stokes Veteran's Hospital, Cleveland, Ohio

Mary Joy Garcia-Dia, DNP, RN, Director Clinical Applications, Mount Sinai Health System, New York, New York

Donald Gardenier, DNP, RN, FNP-BC, FAANP, FAAN, Assistant Professor and Clinical Program Director, The Icahn School of Medicine, Mount Sinai Medical Center, New York, New York

Irene Hartigan, PhD, RGN, RNT, College Lecturer, Catherine McAuley School of Nursing and Midwifery, University College Cork, Cork, Ireland

Margaret A. Harris, PhD, RN, Associate Professor, School of Nursing, Oakland University, Rochester, Michigan

Catrina Heffernan, MSc, RGN, Lecturer, Department of Nursing and Health Care Sciences, Institute of Tralee, Tralee, County Kerry, Ireland

Janet H. Johnson, DNP, RN, ANP-BC, ACNP, FAANP, Cardiology Nurse Practitioner, Mount Sinai Hospital, New York, New York

Bernadette Khan, MSN, RN, NEA-BC, Vice President Nursing and Patient Care Services, New York-Presbyterian Lower Manhattan Hospital, New York, New York

Sapina Kirpalani, MSN, RN, GNP, ANP-BC, Nurse Practitioner, Mount Sinai Hospital, New York, New York

Bertha Ku, MPH, RN, Corporate Nursing Program Director, New York-Presbyterian Hospital, New York, New York

Margaret G. Landers, PhD, RGN, College Lecturer, Catherine McAuley School of Nursing and Midwifery, University College Cork, Cork, Ireland

Patricia Leahy-Warren, PhD, RGN, RM, RPHN, Senior Lecturer, Catherine McAuley School of Nursing and Midwifery, University College Cork, Cork, Ireland

Elaine Lehane, PhD, RGN, College Lecturer, Catherine McAuley School of Nursing and Midwifery, University College Cork, Cork, Ireland

Jill Matthes, MSN, RN, CHSE, Instructor, Lorain County Community College, Lorain, Ohio

Geraldine McCarthy, PhD, MSN, MEd, DipN, RNT, RGN, Fellow RCSI, Emeritus Professor, Catherine McAuley School of Nursing and Midwifery, University College Cork, Cork, Ireland

Ernesto P. Mir, MSN, RN, CCRN, Director of Nursing Cardiac Services, New York-Presbyterian Hospital, New York, New York

Helen Mulcahy, DN, RGN, RM, RPHN, College Lecturer, Catherine McAuley School of Nursing and Midwifery, University College Cork, Cork, Ireland

Zamzaliza A. Mulud, PhD, RN, Lecturer, Faculty of Health Sciences, University Teknologi Mara, Puncak Alam, Malaysia

Joan Murphy, MSc, RPN, RGN, RM, Lecturer, Department of Nursing and Health Care Sciences, Institute of Tralee, Tralee, County Kerry, Ireland

Germaine Nelson, MSN, MBA, RN, NEA-BC, Independent Consultant, New York, New York

Denise O'Dea, MSN, RN, ANP-BC, OCN, Nurse Practitioner, Mount Sinai Hospital, New York, New York

Moira O'Donovan, MSc, RPN, RGN, College Lecturer, Catherine McAuley School of Nursing and Midwifery, University College Cork, Cork, Ireland

Deirdre O'Flaherty, DNP, RN, APRN-BC, NE-BC, ONC, Senior Administrative Director, Patient Care Services, Lenox Hill Hospital, New York, New York

Máirín O'Mahony, PhD, RNT, RGN, RM, College Lecturer, Catherine McAuley School of Nursing and Midwifery, University College Cork, Cork, Ireland

Patricia Prufeta, DNP, RN, NEA-BC, Director of Surgical Nursing, New York-Presbyterian Hospital, New York, New York

Mary E. Quinn, MSN, RN, Director of Quality and Nursing Improvement Initiatives, New York-Presbyterian Hospital, New York, New York

Mary T. Quinn Griffin, PhD, RN, FAAN, ANEF, Professor, Frances Payne Bolton School of Nursing, Case Western Reserve University, Cleveland, Ohio

Jennifer Siller, DNP, RN, ACNP-BC, Nurse Practitioner, New York, New York

Lauraine Spano-Szekely, DNP, RN, MBA, Senior Vice President Patient Care Services, Chief Nursing Officer, Northern Westchester Hospital, Westchester, New York

Deborah J. Stilgenbauer, MA, RN, NEA-BC, Director of Nursing Finance, New York-Presbyterian Hospital, New York, New York

Siobhan Sundel, DNP, RN, GNP-BC, ANP, Nurse Practitioner, Mount Sinai Hospital, New York, New York

Rosemary Ventura, MA, RN, Director of Nursing Informatics, New York-Presbyterian Hospital, New York, New York

Elizabeth Weathers, PhD, RGN, Postdoctoral Researcher, Catherine McAuley School of Nursing and Midwifery, University College Cork, Cork, Ireland

Teresa Wills, DN, RGN, College Lecturer, Catherine McAuley School of Nursing and Midwifery, University College Cork, Cork, Ireland

PREFACE

Nursing science, theory, and research are in the early stages of development. As the number of nurse scientists increases, there is a concomitant advancement in the scientific basis that guides professional nursing practice.

As the science develops, there is a need to name the core concepts that define the disciplinary perspective. Many of those concepts have been named here, by authors who are expert clinicians and researchers. Because the discipline of nursing includes both the content and the process of nursing, the concepts chosen are grouped into categories that reflect the core of nursing, the nurse–patient relationship. These categories are patient/client-focused concepts, caregiver (nurse)-focused concepts, and organizational concepts. The organizational category reflects the reality that the majority of nursing practice takes place within health systems.

Each concept analysis chapter in the book follows the same structured format. This allows for comparison across concepts, particularly those that are closely related within a category. Each chapter also includes a diagrammatic representation of the concept attributes, antecedents, and consequences. This visual representation of characteristics across concepts allows the reader to make comparisons and, ultimately, to build on the knowledge base available in this book.

It is expected that the concepts included in this book will lead nurse scholars to further develop and critique existing nursing knowledge. While a number of concept analyses have been published in nursing journals in the past decade, this book includes the largest collection of concept analyses that are presented together, thus facilitating further disciplinary development.

We encourage the reader to expand the concept analyses and build on this work, both in theory development and research. We believe that, together with the chapter authors, we have set an important direction for the future. We are indebted to all of the chapter authors for their contributions to this seminal work and look forward to their future contributions.

Joyce J. Fitzpatrick
Geraldine McCarthy

Part I   Patient/Client-Focused Concepts

JOYCE J. FITZPATRICK AND GERALDINE McCARTHY 1

CONCEPT ANALYSIS

The basis of theoretical thinking in nursing lies in delineation of the concepts that are relevant to the discipline. While the metaparadigm concepts of persons, environment, health, and nursing are central to the disciplinary perspective, it is important for nurse scholars and clinicians to draw from these four basic concepts and thus further explicate nursing knowledge to guide research and professional practice.

The concepts that are chosen for further explication and refinement are often the result of the background of the nurse scholar, whether in direct patient care with specific patient populations or in nursing administration, attending to system designs and processes. The challenge of the broad disciplinary perspective of nursing is in further refining the knowledge base so that it can practically guide research and practice. While concept labels may be the same across disciplines, it is important to distinguish any specific disciplinary perspective on the concept. Once this disciplinary perspective is made explicit, it will guide further development of nursing research and professional practice. In the chapters that follow, it is apparent that some of the concepts could be used in a range of disciplines. As an example, *anxiety* is a concept that has relevance to a wide range of disciplines, perhaps all of the biobehavioral disciplines. In the explication within the discipline of nursing, each of the concepts is considered within one of the key concepts in the metaparadigm of nursing (persons, environment, health, nursing) or the interrelationships among these concepts. In the case of anxiety in the concept analysis included here, the defined cases serve to embed the concept within the nursing discipline through the relationship to the metaparadigm concepts. Several of the chapters also can be used to illustrate this disciplinary perspective.

The basic purpose of concept analysis methodology is to distinguish between concepts, and thus to clarify the relationships and the distinguishing characteristics between concepts. For example, *anxiety* and *fear* are often used interchangeably within general discourse, and in fact some of the consequences of both anxiety and fear may be the same (e.g., increased blood pressure due to vasoconstriction). Yet, the essential characteristics of anxiety and fear are not the same, and the two concepts are defined differently both in the scientific literature and in general use. For both scientific and professional practice interventions, it is important to more precisely define the concepts that are important for understanding and interventions.

Concept analysis provides the methodology for this evaluation. Concept analysis serves to clarify overused concepts, and provides a standard language for mutual understanding within a discipline. Furthermore, concept analysis leads to a specific measurable definition of a concept and/or identifies the gaps in knowledge and in measurement that should be undertaken in future theoretical work.

METHODS OF CONCEPT ANALYSIS

A number of different concept analysis methodologies are described in the scientific literature. The methodology for concept analysis can be traced to the work of Wilson (1963), who delineated the methodology as an important step to gain scientific and conceptual clarity to guide research. Within the nursing discipline, concept analysis began in the early 1990s, and included the models developed by Rodgers and Knafl (1993), Walker and Avant (1994), Morse (1995), and Chinn and Kramer (1995). All of these methods of concept analysis appear in the nursing science literature, as do a wide range of nursing concept analysis papers.

The Walker and Avant (1994) method of concept analysis is the most frequently used method in nursing and was chosen as the basis for analyzing the core concepts selected for analysis. The Walker and Avant method includes several steps, each of which is described here. The first step is to select a concept. This is followed by a review of the recent literature to determine all of the uses of the concept. An important next step is to identify the defining attributes of the concept: those characteristics that are essential to the concept. A definition of the concept is derived from the critical defining attributes. This definition includes all of the defining attributes and specifically excludes other elements related to the concept. Then, a number of cases are constructed to illustrate how the concept is used. Within this book, it was deemed important for the cases to be explicitly related to nursing professional practice. The additional types of cases that are included in each of the chapters include related cases, borderline cases, and contrary cases. Following the description of the various types of cases, both the antecedents and the consequences of the concept are delineated. *Antecedents* are those factors, derived from the literature, that precede the occurrence of the concept. The consequences also are derived from the literature and represent those factors that result from the concept. The last step in the process of concept analysis is the identification of empirical referents, or ways to measure the concept.

It is important to further describe the types of cases that are used in the concept analysis process. The model case describes a real-life example of the use of the concept that includes all of the critical attributes of the concept. In the model cases described in each of the chapters, there is specific notation of each of the defining attributes within the case. That is, in the specific component of the case that illustrates each of the defining attributes, a notation of that defining attribute is made in parentheses. The related cases are cases that are related to the concept but do not necessarily include the defining attributes. Related cases may include some of the defining attributes, but also may include some attributes that are commonly mistaken for the defining attributes of the concept. The borderline case includes some, but not all, of the defining attributes. In the examples in the chapters that follow, in each borderline case each of the defining attributes that is present is identified in parentheses. One or more of the defining attributes is missing. In each case, this is identified by the term *failed* for each of the attributes that is not present. Contrary cases do not include any of the defining attributes of the concept. In related and contrary cases described in each of the chapters, the authors have noted the defining attributes that are present. The defining attributes that are not present are indicated as failed attributes.

In this book, each of the cases described in the concept analyses are embedded in nursing science development (research) or professional nursing practice. Further, the concepts are categorized as to whether they are presented with specific reference to the recipient of care, the individual patient/ client, the carer (nurse), or the organization in which the nurse works. The specific categorization is reflected most explicitly in the cases provided.

SUMMARY

The concept analysis process is an important stage in theory development. It helps the scientist refine the concepts under study and thus further refine the disciplinary content. Such deliberative analysis of nursing content helps to move both the science and professional practice to a new stage of development.

REFERENCES

Chinn, P. L., & Kramer, M. K. (1995). *Theory and nursing: A systematic approach.* St. Louis, MO: Mosby.

Morse, J. M. (1995). Exploring the theoretical basis of nursing using advanced techniques of concept analysis. *Advances in Nursing Science, 17,* 31–46.

Rodgers, B. L., & Knafl, K. A. (Eds.). (1993). *Concept development in nursing: Foundations, techniques, and applications.* Philadelphia, PA: Saunders.

Walker, L., & Avant, K. C. (1994). *Strategies for theory construction in nursing* (3rd ed.). Norwalk, CT: Appleton & Lange.

Wilson, J. (1963). *Thinking with concepts.* Cambridge, UK: Cambridge University Press.

2

ELDER SELF-NEGLECT

Self-neglect is a complex multidimensional concept that was first identified in the 1950s. Historically, terminologies used to describe self-neglect have included: Senile Squalor Syndrome (Clark, Mankikar, & Gray, 1975), Diogenes syndrome (Reyes-Ortiz, Burnett, Flores, Halphen, & Dyer, 2014), and "domestic squalor" (Snowdon, Halliday, & Banerjee, 2012). There are many definitions of self-neglect, yet no consensus has emerged. Self-neglect is described as a behavioral condition, whereby an individual is unable or unwilling to provide care for himself or herself and consequently the individual's health and safety are threatened; this can extend to the wider community (National Center on Elder Abuse, 2005). A multiplicity of factors are associated with self-neglect, such as old age, living alone, poor social networks, alcohol and substance abuse, impaired physical and cognitive function, depression, dementia, executive dysfunction (ED), economic decline, poor coping, hoarding, and animal hoarding (Braye, Orr, & Preston-Shoot, 2011; Day, Leahy-Warren, & McCarthy, 2013; Pickens et al., 2013).

Growth in aging populations, associated burden of chronic diseases, declining economic resources, and migration all have the potential to increase substantially the risk for self-neglect (Dong, Simon, & Evans, 2010). Adult protective services (APSs) in the United States investigate approximately 1.2 million self-neglect cases annually (Dong et al., 2010; National Center on Elder Abuse, 2005). Self-neglect reports to APS varied from 37.2% (Teaster et al., 2006) to 87% of all alleged neglect reports (Pavlik, Hyman, Festa, & Bitondo Dyer, 2001). A population-based U.S. study reported prevalence of self-neglect at 9%, and noted higher prevalence for men (10.1%) compared to women (7.5%) in people aged over 85 years (Dong, Simon, & Evans, 2012a). Self-neglect accounts for 18% to 21% of referrals to senior case workers (SCWs) in Ireland (Health Service Executive, 2013). In 2013 (Health Service Executive, 2014), there were 463 absolute self-neglect referrals and in addition 87 self-neglect cases that involved elements of elder abuse. At year-end 2013, 191 cases were still open, highlighting the ongoing nature of self-neglect (Health Service Executive, 2014). Some countries have no data on self-neglect

(Braye, Orr, & Preston-Shoot, 2011). Multiple factors make it very difficult to precisely ascertain the incidence and prevalence of self-neglect.

There is consensus within the literature that, globally, self-neglect is a serious and understudied issue. A growing number of research teams (Chicago Health and Aging Project [CHAP], the Consortium for Research of Elder Self-Neglect in Texas and Schanfield Research Institute, Chicago), nurses (Day, 2014; Gibbons, 2009; Lauder, Roxburg, Harris, & Law, 2009), and social workers (Braye, Orr, & Preston-Shoot, 2013; McDermott, 2008) are making important contributions to the understanding of self-neglect. Self-neglect cases present many ethical challenges in practice for health and social care professionals (Braye et al., 2013; Day et al., 2012, 2013; Gunstone, 2003). Self-neglect is conceptualized in many different ways by health and social care professionals and by individuals across communities and populations. Gibbons, Lauder, and Ludwick (2006) developed a nursing diagnosis and definition of self-neglect which is included in the North American Nursing Diagnosis Association (NANDA) lexicon. According to nurse researchers, self-neglect is socially constructed and is the product of a series of social judgments that are influenced by social, cultural, and professional values (Day et al., 2013; Lauder, Anne Scott, & Whyte, 2001). Assessment of self-neglect, professional judgments, and decisions can be influenced by professional philosophy (Day et al., 2012), organizational background (McDermott, 2010), and knowledge (Day & McCarthy, 2015; Doron, Band-Winterstein, & Naim, 2013; Dulick, 2010). A concept analysis of self-neglect can establish essential components and provide guidance to both research and clinical practice.

DEFINING ATTRIBUTES

The defining attributes of self-neglect are *environmental neglect* and *cumulative behaviors and deficits* (intentional or unintentional).

Environmental neglect is a significant and defining factor in self-neglect. Environmental neglect can include lack of equipment; unmaintained or non-functioning appliances; unsafe environment; observed home/physical living environment that is very unclean, unsafe, and unhygienic; presence of vermin; animal hoarding; accumulation of items; and failure to pay bills or replace equipment despite having adequate income—any or all of these raise serious health, and safety concerns (Day, 2014; Day et al., 2013; Dong & Simon, 2015; Dong, Simon, & Evans, 2012b; Gibbons et al., 2006; Hurley, Scallan, Johnson, & De La Harpe, 2000; Iris, Ridings, & Conrad, 2010; Kutame, 2008). The living environments are described as hazardous; they may contain volumes of newspapers, used food containers, and human or animal excrement (Pavlou & Lachs, 2006). The poor environmental conditions can extend outdoors to yard or garden and affect other lives and areas the community. The terms *domestic squalor* (Snowdon et al., 2012) and *Diogenes syndrome* are often used to define and diagnose extreme self-neglect (Pavlou & Lachs, 2006). Diogenes syndrome has been defined as extreme self-neglect, domestic squalor, social disengagement, affinity for hoarding (syllogomania), apathy, and sometimes lack of awareness of home living circumstances (Pavlou & Lachs, 2006). These behaviors and attributes are at the extreme end of the trajectory of squalor, and this definition would not be representative of all self-neglect cases (Pavlou & Lachs, 2006). Available evidence that self-neglect is a syndrome is sparse and has been questioned (Braye, Orr, & Preston-Shoot, 2011b; Halliday, Banerjee, Philpot, & Macdonald, 2000; Lauder et al., 2009). In Australia, self-neglect is viewed as neglect of self; domestic squalor is used to contextualize and describe extreme neglect of the environment; *collecting* is the accumulation of certain objects, and *hoarding* is the inability to throw objects away (McDermott, 2008). In severe cases of self-neglect, living environments are often described as hazardous; they may contain large volumes of newspapers, used food containers, and human or animal excrement (Choi, Kim, & Asseff, 2009; Pavlou & Lachs, 2006). Severe environmental neglect was a key factor used by nurses in the classification and judgments of self-neglect (Day, 2014; Lauder et al., 2001).

Cumulative behaviors and deficits are the second defining attribute. These can include malnourishment, poor hygiene, poor grooming, failure to pay bills, noncompliance with medication, nonadherence to self-care regimes, poor health management, withdrawal/poor engagement, fear, aggressive behaviors, misplaced trust, and noncooperativeness or unwillingness to accept assistance (Dong et al., 2010; Dyer et al., 2006; Iris et al., 2010; Turner, Hochschild, Burnett, Zulfiqar, & Dyer, 2012). Dimensions used in judgment and classification of self-neglect by nurses were self-care status and poor personal hygiene (Lauder et al., 2001), which identified characteristics as "combination of lack of food in the home, low body weight, difficult with meal preparation and shopping, potential nutritional frailty with potential to exacerbate medical problems" (p. 300). Poor compliance and nonadherence to medication regimes are very prevalent among older adults who self-neglect (Leibbrandt, 2007; Turner et al., 2012), as is nonadherence to treatment regimens (Kutame, 2008). Malnutrition (Adams & Johnson, 1998; Ernst & Smith, 2011; Smith et al., 2006), obesity (Ernst & Smith, 2011), and incontinence (Alexa, Ilie, Morosanu, Emmanouil-Stamos, & Raiha, 2012; Lauder, 1999) are associated with self-neglect. Cumulative behaviors and deficits can be attributed to multiple losses, homelessness (Lauder et al., 2009), alcohol/substance abuse (Choi et al., 2009; Gibbons, 2009; Halliday et al., 2000; Lauder et al., 2009; Tierney et al., 2004), defiant behavior (Lauder, 1999), life history (Band-Winterstein et al., 2012), and discordant and fractured lifestyles (Day, Mulcahy, Leahy-Warren, & Downey, 2015; Day et al., 2013; Lauder et al., 2009).

DEFINITION

Elder self-neglect (ESN) encompasses environmental neglect and cumulative behaviors and deficits, with potential for serious adverse outcomes that impact on health, safety, and well-being of the person and may extend beyond to the community.

MODEL CASE

Mr. M is a 68-year-old single man, a diabetic, who has poor mobility, appears frail, and lives alone. The Public Health Nurses (PHNs) undertook a home visit and had difficulty in gaining access to the house. They observed severe environmental neglect. There was barely room to walk in; clutter, dirty beer bottles, and empty food cartons were everywhere, and it was extremely cold. An offensive odor of animal excrement pervaded the house. Assessment identified cumulative behaviors and deficits. Mr. M's face, hands, nails, and clothes were deeply ingrained with dirt and he was malnourished. Mr. M had not obtained medical treatment and had not kept hospital appointments; he had a leg ulcer that was very infected and toes that were gangrenous. Mr. M reported that he was fighting with his neighbors; he had no social supports, was socially isolated, and appeared to be indifferent to his situation; he was refusing services. Initial assessment suggested that Mr. M had capacity.

In this case, Mr. M's home environment was described as portraying severe environmental neglect and accumulation of animal excrement added a very offensive odor to the home environment. There were cumulative behaviors and deficits relating to personal care, nutrition, nonattendance at hospital appointments, and poor attention to health care regimens that posed serious threats to Mr. M's well-being and safety. Social isolation, absent social support, personality, behaviors, and indifference of Mr. M compounded his vulnerability. In essence, this case is complex and presents an array of health and safety challenges. In protecting and safeguarding Mr. M, the PHN and primary care team members need to work through a number of ethical issues: for example, self-determination, choice, capacity, and best interest.

RELATED CASE

Related cases have some of the defining attributes. An example is that of Mr. T, who lives in a very unclean home that has numerous health and safety hazards (environmental neglect). Mr. T agreed to host a charity golf classic as a fundraiser for cancer services. He was disorganized, not a team player, and disregarded the amount of detailed planning required. He was late advertising the event in local papers, so only a few tickets were sold. Tom's self-neglect of the details had far-reaching consequences that meant the event had to be cancelled, to his dismay and embarrassment.

This case reveals environmental neglect that is hidden from sight of Mr. T's friends and neighbors, as he does not invite people into his home. He is a very private man and presents well to others. However, Mr. T had no insight into the effort necessary to take on a project like hosting a golf classic. An accumulation of poor behavior by Mr. T, including neglect of and indifference to project planning and late advertising, led to huge disappointment and resulted in the cancellation of the golf event (failed cumulative behaviors and deficits).

BORDERLINE CASE

Mr. B is a diabetic, partially blind, and has been experiencing pain due to a chronic infected leg ulcer in recent weeks. He was prescribed antibiotics, but he has not been taking them. Mr. B's mobility has deteriorated; he is having physical difficulty caring for himself, his home, and his four cats. He appears to have lost weight recently. He has poor contact with neighbors, his family do not live close by, and he is refusing home help (cumulative behaviors and deficits). However, his home environment is clean.

In the case of Mr. B, there is one defining attribute: cumulative behaviors and deficits. For example, the infected leg ulcer, not taking prescribed antibiotics, refusing services, poor mobility, reduced self-care, weight loss, social isolation, and poor social support are creating vulnerabilities for his health, safety, and well-being. Mr. B needs support and he is not coping; however, he is not self-neglecting (failed environmental neglect). Self-neglect occurs on a continuum of severity, and he is vulnerable.

CONTRARY CASE

Mrs. H, a 75-year-old widow, is an insulin-dependent diabetic with coronary heart disease. She lives on her own and has good support from family and neighbors, and she is involved with community groups. She monitors and records her blood glucose levels daily, using a glucometer, and diet is taken as advised by nutritionist. Home environment is very welcoming. In this case, there is no vulnerability, and there is failed environmental neglect or cumulative behaviors and deficits. Mrs. H is engaged with her community and all critical attributes of self-neglect are absent.

ANTECEDENTS

The antecedents of self-neglect (SN) are multiple comorbidities, mental health issues, and absence of social networks. There is a close relationship between alcohol/substance abuse, mental health issues, and self-neglect (Halliday et al., 2000; Leibbrandt, 2007; Spensley, 2008). Dyer, Goodwin, Pickens-Pace, Burnett, and Kelly (2007) suggest that the presence of one or more comorbidities (depression, dementia, diabetes, psychiatric illness, cerebrovascular disease, functional decline, and nutritional deficiency) can lead to ED. ED can affect capacity and cause inability for self-care and protection (Dyer et al., 2007); it also can inhibit appropriate decision making and problem solving (Hildebrand, Taylor, & Bradway, 2013). Tierney et al. (2004) found that individuals with increased cognitive deficits and ED were more likely to self-neglect and experience harm. This signals that individuals who self-neglect may refuse services because they lack the necessary skills, capacity, and insight or problem-solving ability for safe independent living. ED was associated with greater risk and greater severity for reported and confirmed self-neglect (Dong et al., 2010), and is likely to be an important factor in older adults who self-neglect (Pickens et al., 2013).

Certain client characteristics may contribute to the risk of self-neglect; these antecedents include older age, living alone, marital status, absence of social networks, childhood abuse, drug/alcohol abuse, poor self-related health (Hurley et al., 2000), traumatic life history (Band-Winterstein et al., 2012; Lauder et al., 2009), poverty, and frugality (Day et al., 2013). Self-neglect is associated with absent and reduced social engagement and poorer social networks (Ernst & Smith, 2011), and these were associated with increased reporting of self-neglect (Dong, Simon, Beck, & Evans, 2010; Spensley, 2008) and greater self-neglect severity (Dong et al., 2010). Leibbrandt (2007) reported that self-neglect clients engaged in fewer activities, had a preference for staying at home, and often refused services (Hurley et al., 2000). Self-neglect can be intentional or nonintentional, and Gibbons (2009) concluded that personal beliefs and coping abilities were factors in intentional self-neglect. Therefore, self-neglecting behaviors should be seen in the context of people's life experiences and life stories (Band-Winterstein et al., 2012; Bozinovski, 2000; Day et al., 2013, Gibbons, 2009; Kutame, 2008). Resistance by individuals who self-neglect may be a way of coping, trying to take control over their death and destiny (Braye et al., 2011; Gibbons, 2009).

CONSEQUENCES

Consequences of Self-neglect are lower health status (Dong et al., 2010), increased mortality (Reyes-Ortiz et al., 2014), and increased use of health services (Dong & Simon, 2013; Dong, Simon, & Evans, 2012c). People who self-neglect are at increased risk for nursing home placement (Lachs, Williams, O'Brien, & Pillemer, 2002), hospitalization (Dong, Simon, Mosqueda, & Evans, 2012), and hospice admission (Dong & Simon, 2013); their rate of annual visits to the emergency department are three times higher than those who did not self-neglect. A CHAP cohort study found that the annual rate of hospitalization for reported self-neglect participants was significantly higher when compared to participants without self-neglect. Elder self-neglect was linked to increased risk for subsequent caregiver neglect, financial exploitation, and multiple forms of elder abuse (Dong, Simon, Evans, 2013; Mardan et al., 2014).

EMPIRICAL REFERENTS

Empirical referents demonstrate current perspective on measureable ways to demonstrate the occurrence and recognition of self-neglect. A small number of researchers have developed and operationalized measures for self-neglect (Day, 2014; Dyer et al., 2006; Iris, Conrad, & Ridings, 2014). These include the Self-Neglect Severity Scale (SNSS) (Kelly, Dyer, Pavlik, Doody, & Jogerst, 2008), Assessment of Self-Neglect Severity (Dong, de Leon, & Evans, 2009); Elder Self-Neglect Assessment (ESNA-25; Iris et al., 2013), and the Self-Neglect (SN-37) Measurement Instrument (Day, 2014). However, self-neglect assessment tools are not being used widely by health and social care professionals (Braye et al., 2011; Day et al., 2012). Globally, lack of clarity in relation to a standardized definition of self-neglect and the absence of an instrument for identifying self-neglect have led to conceptual, assessment, and intervention problems for health and social care professionals (Fulmer, 2008; Iris et al., 2010; Kelly et al., 2008; Lauder, Anderson, & Barclay, 2005; McDermott, 2008; Pavlou & Lachs, 2006; Skelton, Kunik, Regev, & Naik, 2010).

The SNSS (personal hygiene, impaired function, and status of environment) was developed by the Consortium for Research in Elder Self-Neglect (CREST) at Baylor College of Medicine, Texas (Dyer et al., 2006). Field-testing with older adults ($n = 23$) enabled identification of self-neglect, but acceptable validity was not attained (Kelly et al., 2008). The Assessment of Self-Neglect Severity (15 items; Dong et al., 2009; Dong et al., 2012a) relates to assessment of health and safety risks. A trial in Chicago yielded an interrater reliability coefficient greater than 0.70, and face and content validity and predictive validity were established (Illinois Department of Aging, 1989). Iris et al. (2013) developed the Elder Self-Neglect Assessment (ESNA-25) tool, which has two subscales: Environmental Conditions and Behavioral Characteristics. This tool, also tested in Chicago, had an explained variance of 39.1%, person reliability of 0.83, Cronbach's alpha of 0.87, and a residual variance of 15.3% (no substantial rival dimension).

Day (2014) developed the Self-Neglect (SN-37) Measurement Instrument, and exploratory factor analysis identified a five-factor solution that explained 55.6% of the cumulative variance. Factors were labelled "Environment," "Social Networks," "Emotional and Behavioral Liability," "Health Avoidance," and "Self-Determinism." Preliminary construct validity was supported by findings in relation to the content validity and factor analysis results.

Halliday et al. (2000) used the 13-item Living Conditions Rating Scale (Samios, 1996) to describe and rate 76 living environments. In Australia, Snowdon et al. (2013) used the Environmental Cleanliness and Clutter Scale (ECCS) to rate home environments of 203 people referred to the Domestic Squalor Project. Principal component analysis conducted on 186 cases identified two factors: Factor 1 (7 squalor items) explained 33.7% of the variance, and Factor 2 (3 items on reduced accessibility and accumulation of items) explained 17.6% of the variance. Findings reported that 105 cases (56%) scored high in both squalor and accumulation; 38% had high squalor and 15% were high for squalor and accumulation. Cronbach's alpha for scale was 0.72, demonstrating good internal consistency. Further research is necessary to establish the construct- and criterion-related validity of instruments across different populations (Figure 2.1).

SUMMARY

Globally, self-neglect is a public health issue that has very serious adverse outcomes yet is largely hidden. The concept of self-neglect remains elusive, and the absence of a common definition has hampered research. The goal of this concept analysis of self-neglect for theory development was to clearly establish the critical attributes that will enable self-neglect to be readily identified. This will make explicit the meaning of self-neglect and promote consistency in using the concept in nursing dialogue and research. This concept

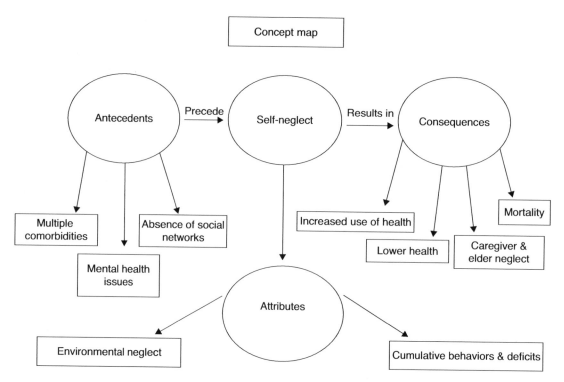

FIGURE 2.1 Elder self-neglect.

analysis has identified the antecedents, defining attributes, and consequences of self-neglect. A synthesis of the literature concluded that self-neglect can manifest both externally and internally (e.g., hoarding of rubbish, poor self-care, gross domestic squalor, refusal of medical treatment or lack of attention to medical regimens).

REFERENCES

Adams, J., & Johnson, J. (1998). Nurses' perceptions of gross self-neglect amongst older people living in the community. *Journal of Clinical Nursing, 7*(6), 547–552.

Alexa, I. D., Ilie, A. C., Morosanu, A., Emmanouil-Stamos, P., & Raiha, I. (2012). Self-neglect in elders: A worldwide issue ignored in Romania. *Romania Journal of Bioethics, 10*, 141–148.

Band-Winterstein, T., Doron, I., & Naim, S. (2012) Elder self neglect: A geriatric syndrome or a life course story? *Journal of Aging Studies, 26*(2), 109–118.

Bozinovski, S. D. (2000). Older self-neglecters: Interpersonal problems and the maintenance of self-continuity. *Journal of Elder Abuse & Neglect, 12*(1), 37–56. doi:10.1300/J084v12n01_06

Braye, S., Orr, D., & Preston-Shoot, M. (2011). *Self-neglect and adult safeguarding: Findings from research* (DOH trans.). London, UK: Social Care Institute for Excellence.

Braye, S., Orr, D., & Preston-Shoot, M. (2013). *A scoping study of workforce development for self-neglect work.* University of Sussex & University of Bedfordshire, UK. Retrieved from http://www.skillsforcare.org.uk/Document-library/NMDS-SC,-workforce-intelligence-and-innovation/Research/Self-Neglect-Final-Report-301013-FINAL.pdf

Choi, N. G., Kim, J., & Asseff, J. (2009). Self-neglect and neglect of vulnerable older adults: Re-examination of etiology. *Journal of Gerontological Social Work, 52*(2), 171–187. doi:10.1080/01634370802609239

Clark, A. N. G., Mankikar, G. D., & Gray, I. (1975). Diogenes syndrome clinical study of gross self-neglect in old age. *Lancet, 1*(7903), 366–368.

Day, M. R. (2014). *Self-neglect: Development and evaluation of a self-neglect (SN-37) measurement instrument* (Unpublished doctoral thesis). National University of Ireland, University College Cork, Cork, Ireland.

Day, M. R., Leahy-Warren, P., & McCarthy, G. (2013). Perceptions and views of self-neglect: A client-centred perspective. *Journal of Elder Abuse and Neglect, 25*(1), 76–94.

Day, M. R., & McCarthy, G. (2015). A national cross sectional study of community nurses' and social workers' knowledge of self-neglect. *Age and Ageing, 44*(4), 717–720. doi:10.1093/ageing/afv025

Day, M. R, McCarthy, G., & Leahy-Warren, P. (2012). Professional social workers' views on self-neglect: An exploratory study. *British Journal of Social Work, 42*(4), 725–743. doi:10.1093/bjsw/bcr082

Day, M. R., Mulcahy, H., Leahy-Warren, P., & Downey, J. (2015). Self-neglect: A case study and implications for clinical practice. *British Journal of Community Nursing, 20*(2), 585–590.

Dong, X., de Leon, C. F. M., & Evans, D. A. (2009). Is greater self-neglect severity associated with lower levels of physical function? *Journal of Ageing and Health, 21*(4), 596–610.

Dong, X., & Simon, M. A. (2013). Association between elder self-neglect and hospice utilization in a 207 community population. *Archives of Gerontology and Geriatrics, 56*(1), 192–198. doi:10.1016/j.archger.2012.06.008

Dong, X., & Simon, M. A. (2015). Prevalence of elder self-neglect in a Chicago Chinese population: The role of cognitive physical and mental health. *Geriatrics & Gerontology International.* doi: 10.1111/ggi.12598. Retrieved from http://onlinelibrary.wiley.com/doi/10.1111/ggi.12598/pdf

Dong, X., Simon, M., Beck, T., & Evans, D. (2010). A cross-sectional population based study of elder self-neglect and psychological, health, and social factors in a biracial community. *Aging and Mental Health, 14*(1), 74–84.

Dong, X., Simon, M. A., & Evans, D. (2010). Cross-sectional study of the characteristics of reported elder self-neglect in a community-dwelling population: Findings from a population-based cohort. *Gerontology, 56*, 325–334.

Dong, X., Simon, M. A., & Evans, D. (2012a). Prevalence of self-neglect across gender, race, and socioeconomic status: Findings from the Chicago Health and Aging Project. *Gerontology, 58*(3), 258–268.

Dong, X., Simon, M. A., & Evans, D. (2012b). Prospective study of the elder self-neglect and ED use in a 205 community population. *American Journal of Emergency Medicine, 30*(4), 553–561.

Dong, X., Simon, M. A., & Evans, D. (2012c). Elder self-neglect and hospitalization: Findings from the Chicago Health and Aging Project. *Journal of the American Geriatrics Society, 60*(2), 202–209. doi:10.1111/j.1532-5415.2011.03821.x

Dong, X., Simon, M. A., & Evans, D. (2013). Elder self-neglect is associated with increased risk for elder abuse in a community-dwelling population: Findings from the Chicago Health and Aging Project. *Journal of Aging and Health, 25*(1), 80–96. doi:10.1177/0898264312467373

Dong, X., Simon, M., Fulmer, T., de Leon, C. F. M., Rajan, B., & Evans, D. A. (2010). Physical function decline and the risk of elder self-neglect in a community-dwelling population. *Gerontologist, 50*, 316–326.

Dong, X., Simon, M. A., Mosqueda, L., & Evans, D. A. (2012). The prevalence of elder self-neglect in a community-dwelling population: Hoarding, hygiene, and environmental hazards. *Journal of Aging Health, 24*(3), 507–524. doi:10.1177/0898264311425597

Dong, X., Simon, M. A., Wilson, R. S., de Leon, C. F. M., Rajan, K. B., & Evans, D. A. (2010). Decline in cognitive function and risk of elder self-neglect: Finding from the Chicago Health Aging Project. *Journal of the American Geriatrics Society, 58*(12), 2292–2299.

Doron, I., Band-Winterstein, T., & Naim, S. (2013). The meaning of elder self-neglect: Social workers' perspective. *International Journal of Aging and Human Development, 77*(1), 12–36. Retrieved from http://www.ncbi.nlm.nih.gov/pubmed/23986978

Dulick, K. C. (2010) Self-neglect among the elderly: Knowledge and perceptions of MSW students. In *Department of Social Work, California State University, Long Beach,* Vol. Partial fulfillment of the requirements for the degree Master of Social Work, California State University, Long Beach, California.

Dyer, C. B., Goodwin, J. S., Pickens-Pace, S., Burnett, J., & Kelly, P. A. (2007). Self-neglect among the elderly: A model based on more than 500 patients seen by a geriatric medicine team. *American Journal of Public Health, 97*(9), 6.

Dyer, C. B., Kelly, P. A., Pavlik, V. N., Lee, J., Doody, R. S., Regev, T., … Smith, S. M. (2006). The making of the self-neglect severity scale. *Journal of Elder Abuse and Neglect, 18*(4), 13–24.

Ernst, J. S., & Smith, C. A. (2011). Adult protective services clients confirmed for self-neglect: Characteristics and service use. *Journal of Elder Abuse and Neglect, 23*(4), 289–303.

Fulmer, T. (2008). Barriers to neglect and self-neglect research. *Journal of the American Geriatrics Society, 56,* S241–S243. doi:10.1111/j.1532-5415.2008.01975.x

Gibbons, S. (2009). Theory synthesis for self-neglect: A health and social phenomenon. *Nursing Research, 58*(3), 194–200.

Gibbons, S., Lauder, W., & Ludwick, R. (2006). Self-neglect: A proposed new NANDA diagnosis. *International Journal of Nursing Terminologies and Classifications, 17*(1), 10–18. doi:10.1111/j.1744-618X.2006.00018.x

Gunstone, S. (2003). Risk assessment and management of patients who self-neglect: A "grey area" for mental health workers. *Journal of Psychiatric & Mental Health Nursing, 10*(3), 287–296. doi:10.1046/j.1365-2850.2003.00568.x

Halliday, G., Banerjee, S., Philpot, M., & Macdonald, A. (2000). Community study of people who live in squalor. *Lancet, 355*(9207), 882–886. doi:10.1016/s0140-6736(99)06250-9

Health Service Executive. (2013). *Open your eyes: There is no excuse for elder abuse.* Kildare, Ireland: Author.

Health Service Executive. (2014). *Open your eyes: There is no excuse for elder abuse.* Kildare, Ireland: Author.

Hildebrand, C., Taylor, M., & Bradway, C. (2013). Elder self-neglect: The failure of coping because of cognitive and functional impairments. *Journal of the American Association of Nurse Practitioners.* doi:10.1002/2327-6924.12045. Retrieved from http://onlinelibrary.wiley.com/doi/10.1002/2327-6924.12045/abstract

Hurley, M., Scallan, E., Johnson, H., & De La Harpe, D. (2000). Adult service refusers. *Irish Medical Journal, 93*(7), 208–211. Retrieved from http://www.ncbi.nlm.nih.gov/pubmed/11142956

Illinois Department on Aging. (1989) *Determination of need revision final report* (Vol. I). Chicago, IL: Illinois Department on Aging.

Iris, M., Conrad, K.J. & Ridings, J. (2014) Observational Measure of Elder Self-Neglect. *Journal of Elder Abuse and Neglect, 26*(4), 365–397.

Iris, M., Ridings, J. W., & Conrad, K. J. (2010). The development of a conceptual model for understanding elder self-neglect. *Gerontologist, 50*(3), 303–315. doi:10.1093/geront/gnp125

Kelly, P. A., Dyer, C. B., Pavlik, V., Doody, R., & Jogerst, G. (2008). Exploring self-neglect in older adults: Preliminary findings of the self-neglect severity scale and next steps. *Journal of the American Geriatrics Society, 56*, S253–S260. doi:10.1111/j.1532-5415.2008.01977.x

Kutame, M. M. (2008). *Understanding self-neglect from the older person's perspective* (doctoral dissertation). Retrieved from https://etd.ohiolink.edu/!etd.send_file?accession=osu1186597966&disposition=inline

Lachs, M. S., Williams, C. S., O'Brien, S., & Pillemer, K. A. (2002). Adult protective service use and nursing home placement. *Gerontologist, 42*(6), 734–739. doi:10.1093/geront/42.6.734

Lauder, W. (1999). Constructions of self-neglect: A multiple case study design. *Nursing Inquiry, 6*(1), 48–57.

Lauder, W., Anderson, I., & Barclay, A. (2005). Housing and self-neglect: The responses of health, social care and environmental health agencies. *Journal of Interprofessional Care, 19*(4), 317–325. Retrieved from http://informahealthcare.com/doi/abs/10.1080/1356182500223172

Lauder, W., Anne Scott, P., & Whyte, A. (2001). Nurses' judgements of self-neglect: A factorial survey. *International Journal of Nursing Studies, 38*(5), 601–608. doi:10.1016/S0020-7489(00)00108-5

Lauder, W., Roxburgh, M., Harris, J., & Law, J. (2009). Developing self-neglect theory: Analysis of related and atypical cases of people identified as self-neglecting. *Journal of Psychiatric & Mental Health Nursing, 16*(5), 447–454.

Leibbrandt, S. M. V. (2007). *Factors associated with self-neglect in community-dwelling older adults* (doctoral dissertation). Case Western Reserve University, Cleveland, OH.

Mardan, H., Jaehnichen, G., & Hamid, T. A. (2014). Is self neglect associated with the emotional and financial abuse in community-dueling? *International Journal of Nursing and Health Science, 3*(3), 51–56. Retrieved from http://www.iosrjournals.org/iosr-jnhs/papers/vol3-issue3/Version-4/F03345156.pdf

McDermott, S. (2008). The devil is in the details: Self-neglect in Australia. *Journal of Elder Abuse & Neglect, 20*(3), 231–250.

McDermott, S. (2010). Professional judgements of risk and capacity in situations of self-neglect among older people. *Ageing & Society, 30*(06), 1055–1072. doi:10.1017/S0144686X10000139

National Center on Elder Abuse. (2005). *Elder abuse prevalence and incidence.* Washington, DC: Author.

Pavlik, V. N., Hyman, D. J., Festa, N. A., & Bitondo Dyer, C. (2001). Quantifying the problem of abuse and neglect in adults—analysis of a state-wide database. *Journal American Geriatric Society, 49*(1), 45–48.

Pavlou, M. P., & Lachs, M. S. (2006). Could self-neglect in older adults be a geriatric syndrome? *Journal of the American Geriatrics Society, 54*(5), 831–842. doi:10.1111/j.1532-5415.2006.00661.x

Pickens, S., Ostwald, S. K., Pace, K., Murphy, D., Burnett, J., & Dyer, C. B. (2013). Assessing dimensions of executive function in community-dwelling older adults with self-neglect. *Clinical Nursing Studies, 2*(1), 17.

Reyes-Ortiz, C. A., Burnett, J., Flores, D. V., Halphen, J. M., & Dyer, C. B. (2014). Medical implications of elder abuse: Self-neglect. *Clinics in Geriatric Medicine, 30*(4), 807–823.

Skelton, F., Kunik, M. E., Regev, T., & Naik, A. D. (2010). Determining if an older adult can make and execute decisions to live safely at home: A capacity assessment and intervention model. *Archives of Gerontology and Geriatrics, 50*(3), 300–305. doi:10.1016/j.archger.2009.04.016

Smith, S. M., Mathews Oliver, S. A., Zwart, S. R., Kala, G., Kelly, P. A., Goodwin, J. S., & Dyer, C. B. (2006). Nutritional status is altered in the self-neglecting elderly. *Journal of Nutrition, 136*(10), 2534–2541.

Snowdon, J., Halliday, G., & Banerjee, S. (Eds.). (2012). *Severe domestic squalor.* Cambridge, UK: Cambridge University Press.

Snowdon, J., Halliday, G., & Hunt, G.E. (2013). Two types of squalor: Findings from a factor analysis of the Environmental Cleanliness and Clutter Scale (ECCS). *International Psychogeriatric, 25*(07), 1191–1198.

Spensley, C. (2008). The role of social isolation of elders in recidivism of self-neglect cases at San Francisco adult protective services. *Journal of Elder Abuse and Self-Neglect, 20*(1), 43–61.

Teaster, P. B., Dugar, T., Mendiondo, M., Abner, E. L., Cecil, K. A., & Otto, J. M. (2006). *The 2004 survey of adult protective services: Abuse of adults 60 years of age and older.* National Committee for the Prevention of Elder Abuse/National Adult Protective Services Association. The National Center on Elder Abuse, Washington, DC.

Tierney, M. C., Charles, J., Naglie, G., Jaglal, S., Kiss A., & Fisher, R. H. (2004). Risk factors for harm in cognitively impaired seniors who live alone: A prospective study. *Journal of the American Geriatric Society, 52*(9), 1435–1441.

Turner, A., Hochschild, A., Burnett, J., Zulfiqar, A., & Dyer, C. B. (2012). High prevalence of medication non-adherence in a sample of community-dwelling older adults with adult protective services-validated self-neglect. *Drugs & Aging, 29*(9), 741–749. doi:10.1007/s40266-012-0007-2

3

EXERCISE ADHERENCE

Health benefits related to exercise are well established, and those benefits increase with adherence to a program with regular duration and frequency (Powell, Paluch, & Blair, 2011; U.S. Department of Health and Human Services [USDHHS], 2008). Overall, exercise adherence has many desired benefits that include physical and mental health, longevity, and reduction in weight, cardiovascular disease risk, and cancer risk (Bertram et al., 2011; Blanchard, Courneya, & Stein, 2008; Irwin et al., 2009; McCullough et al., 2011; Shay, 2008). However, studies that have examined exercise adherence often use different terms, leading to confusion in the literature and in practice. Therefore, clarification of exercise adherence is necessary to help understand how best to promote exercise adherence in the clinical setting in order to improve health-related outcomes.

Research relating exercise adherence to health has blossomed over the past two decades, and shows consistent benefits to nearly all individuals (USDHHS, 1996, 2008). Exercise plays a critical role in preventing or reducing the sequelae of chronic illness (Nunan, Mahtami, Roberts, & Heneghan, 2013; USDHHS, 2008). The American College of Sports Medicine (ACSM) and American Heart Association (AHA) recommend at least 30 minutes of moderate- to vigorous-intensity exercise on most days of the week (McArdle, Katch, & Katch, 2014). Yet, despite these recommendations, the Centers for Disease Control and Prevention (CDC) determined that less than 50% of Americans are adhering to these recommendations (CDC, 2014). The ACSM additionally recommends flexibility and muscular strength training 2 to 3 days per week. Unfortunately, less than half of the individuals who initiate an exercise program are still exercising 6 months later, and almost one-quarter of our population reports no exercise within the last month (CDC, 2014). Exercise adherence throughout life is essential in health prediction. In fact, nonadherence predicts negative health consequences more than such risk factors as high blood pressure, high cholesterol, obesity, and family history (McArdle et al., 2014).

In literature, there is often overlapping of similar terms, which can make disease management confusing to individuals. The terms *adherence, compliance, concordance, maintenance,* and *sustenance* are often used interchangeably. However, there are significant differences between these words. *Adherence* is nonjudgmental and describes a mutual desire to achieve behaviors. Adherence to exercise is foundational in a healthy lifestyle.

In 2002, the Department of Health and Human Services described adherence as an antonym of noncompliance. Van Dulmen et al. (2007) describe adherence to be much more comprehensive in that it describes a shared nonjudgmental decision-making process to continue with a medical plan.

Exercise as a concept is generally clearer, but is still dynamic in nature and our understanding continues to improve. The terms *exercise* and *physical activity* are frequently used as overlapping terms. However, exercise is much clearer in its scope; being planned, structured, and purposeful.

Shepard and Balady (1999) defined *exercise* as being planned, structured, repetitive, and purposeful and paramount in cardiovascular therapy. Catenacci and Wyatt (2007) additionally looked at exercise and a similar term, *physical activity*. They noted that exercise was a type of physical activity and recommended that future research be done to determine the intensity, type, and frequency of activity required for health.

When paired, the terms *exercise* and *adherence* present a concept of a faithfully continued, structured physical activity for the benefit of health promotion and disease prevention and treatment. For the purposes of this chapter, the concept will be further refined to include exercise for disease prevention and treatment.

The Transtheoretical (stages of change) Theory has been used as a framework to study adherence in physical exercise (Prochaska & Velicer, 1997). This theory, developed in the 1990s, acknowledges that individuals go through five stages to change their behaviors: precontemplation, contemplation, preparation, action, and maintenance. Key concepts in this theory are based in other models of human behavior and how people change, with the main focus being on decision making. Hellman (1997) attempted to predict exercise adherence in the cardiac rehab patient, by studying perceived self-efficacy over the different stages of change. During the precontemplation stage, individuals are not exercising and they have no intention of initiating an exercise program. In the next stage, contemplation, although the person is still not exercising he or she is now thinking about starting a program. The preparation stage allows the individual to actually start a program, though the actual exercise is inconsistent and/or limited in nature. Action, the next stage on the continuum, is when exercise becomes regular (for instance, 3 times per week for 30 minutes per session). Still, in the action phase, the behavior is performed for less than a 6-month period. In the final phase, maintenance, the individual's behavior has continued for a period of more than 6 months' duration.

DEFINING ATTRIBUTES

The defining attributes of exercise adherence are *self-efficacy promotion, active voluntary involvement,* and *relapse prevention.*

Self-efficacy promotion is the first defining attribute of exercise adherence. By examining a variety of strategies to improve adherence in diabetes self-management, Schechter and Walker's (2002) meta-analysis concluded that even a combination of interventions yielded only small improvements. They did find that the most successful approaches included improving self-efficacy and coping skills. Young, Friedberg, Ulmer, Cho, and Natarajan (2009) also determined that improved self-efficacy along with social support were key in exercise adherence for diabetic patients. A 4-week study on a home exercise program for individuals with chronic low back pain yielded positive predictions for adherence with improved self-efficacy and social support, along with duration of the exercise session.

Positive strategies to address adherence included education, professional support, and improving self-efficacy. Self-efficacy interventions, such as mindfulness-based stress reduction to enhance mood, social support, and reinforcement, aided the seniors with adherence. Self-efficacy is a promoter of exercise and exercise adherence promotes self-efficacy (Schnoll & Zimmerman, 2001). Mastery of exercise is one of the strongest sources of self-efficacy and can be facilitated with identifying past successes both mentally and physically and using goal setting to continuously promote exercise (Jackson, 2010).

Active voluntary involvement is the second defining attribute for exercise adherence. Treatment adherence is challenging in chronic illness management, and health outcomes can be directly tied to patients taking a voluntary active role in their care. An active role versus a passive role in one's care in diabetes and in obesity have been correlated with better engagement in all aspects of self-care (Delamater, 2006). Patients with low back pain were shown to improve faster when they took an active role in physical therapy, both during their visits and at home (Fritz, Cleland, & Brennan, 2007).

Relapse prevention is the third attribute for exercise adherence. Choosing to exercise is a daily choice, and there are many reasons why people do not exercise: "I am too tired" and "I do not have enough time" are reasons commonly given not to exercise. Understanding this is critical in exercise adherence. Jones and Rose (2005) described relapse prevention as necessary for older patients to continue with their exercise plan, because lapses are certain to occur at some point. They identified cognitive and behavioral plans that could prevent individuals from succumbing to high-risk situations that would make a brief lapse in exercise into a permanent condition.

DEFINITION

Exercise adherence is defined as active voluntary involvement in exercise characterized by self-efficacy promotion and relapse prevention.

MODEL CASE

Mr. W, recently diagnosed with noninsulin-dependent diabetes, is 75 pounds overweight (BMI 30.9%) and leads a sedentary lifestyle. His physician encouraged Mr. W to start exercising and stressed the importance of adherence to the program. Mr. W received a packet of information from his doctor and joined a local fitness center. A personal trainer taught him how to use the equipment and provided instruction for the first 2 weeks. This initial support provided by his personal trainer, along with continuous encouragement by his wife, facilitated Mr. W's going to the gym for his workouts at least 4 days per week. Mr. W also developed logs of his workouts, monitoring his physical activity and incorporating what he learned from the trainer. After a month, he was sleeping better, he had lost 5 pounds, and his hemoglobin A1-C was in the normal range. To prevent relapsing, he found a workout buddy and also started to track his diet and exercise on his smartphone (active voluntary involvement and self-efficacy promotion). At his 6- and 12-month doctor's appointments, Mr. W reviewed his log during his doctor's appointment and discussed the improved lab values. His improved health keeps Mr. W motivated to exercise on a daily basis (relapse prevention).

RELATED CASE

Ms. V is 25 and she decided to run a half marathon with her best friend to raise money for breast cancer research. Ms. V is a couch potato and really prefers curling up with a good book and a bowl of popcorn. Although she felt better than she had in years after training for the marathon and completing the race (active voluntary involvement), she did not make any plans to prevent relapse (failed self-efficacy promotion and relapse prevention), and she returned to her previous lifestyle, spending most of her free time on the couch.

BORDERLINE CASE

Mrs. T is a 53-year-old, obese female who has a strong family history of hypertension and dyslipidemia. She lives a mostly sedentary lifestyle, eats a typical American diet high in simple carbohydrates, and is a nonsmoker. She started seeing a personal trainer after having two elevated readings on her home blood pressure monitor. She believed she could make some health lifestyle changes that could help prevent chronic health problems, but knew there was no one that would support her efforts. Mrs. T started going to the gym every other day and would ride the bike for 30 minutes (active voluntary involvement). She lost 45 pounds and her blood pressure returned to normal, but she is thinking of discontinuing her gym membership due to cost and has no plans for sustaining her current exercise routine (failed relapse prevention and failed self-efficacy promotion).

CONTRARY CASE

Mrs. A is a 57-year-old with heart disease and arthritis, who is moderately obese and enjoys a sedentary life. She was told by her physician that she needed to exercise 5 days a week for at least 60 minutes to manage her weight and blood pressure. Mrs. A's physician said that if she did not start and adhere to an exercise program, she would need to be on more medication. Mrs. A is scheduled for a follow-up visit in 6 weeks. Upon getting home, Mrs. A told her husband what the doctor said and his reply was, "You'll never do that. You have tried exercise a dozen times before and you just quit and I am not paying for another gym membership." A few minutes later, Mr. A went to go pick up Pizza Hut's Meat Lovers pizza for dinner. In this example, Mrs. A did not have any of the defining attributes reflecting the concept of adhering to exercise (failed active voluntary involvement, self-efficacy promotion, and relapse prevention).

ANTECEDENTS

The antecedents of exercise adherence are the biomedical status of the individual, the self-efficacy, and the motivation. Boyette et al.'s (2002) literature review identified barriers to exercise in older adults. They found that adherence was limited by biomedical status, education, socioeconomic status, and past participation in exercise. Furthermore, they identified factors that did not impact exercise adherence, which included age, ethnicity, gender, occupation, and smoking status (Figure 3.1).

Cuaderes, Parker, and Burgin (2004) addressed leisure time and exercise issues with Native Americans. They identified gender, self-motivation, physical self-efficacy, support, and addressing barriers as keys to adherence, whereas body mass index and age were not. Schutzer and Graves (2004) thought that adherence to exercise was best in those with high self-efficacy. They additionally thought that physical environment and physician influence played a role. Speck and Harrell (2003) found that history of relapse from exercise predicted long-term nonadherence and also that spousal support increased adherence.

Resnick (2002) reported on high self-efficacy expectations: Older adults would adhere to an exercise program if they had positive outcome expectations (if they believed that the exercise would improve their strength, function, or overall health). Resnick, Luisi, and Vogel (2008) again studied elderly adults and noted that negative outcome expectations, along with fear of falling, age, and pain, impacted adherence. A systematic review of exercise adherence in the elderly by Picorelli, Pereira, Pereira, Felicio, and Sherrington (2014) identified that low socioeconomic status and living alone negatively influenced exercise adherence.

McArthur, Dumas, Woodend, Beach, and Stacey (2014) identified factors influencing adherence to regular exercise in middle-aged women. They determined that routines, intrinsic motivation, biophysical issues, psychosocial commitments, environmental factors, and resources all contribute to a

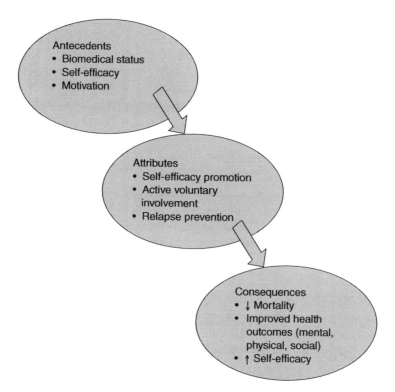

FIGURE 3.1 Exercise adherence.

woman's exercise adherence. They did not find that lack of time or menopause symptoms affected adherence.

CONSEQUENCES

The consequences that result from exercise adherence are decreased mortality; higher self-efficacy; and improved outcomes, including improved mental, physical, and social health. Improved health outcomes can be manifested mentally, physically, and socially. Miller et al. (2014) evaluated the health benefits of adhering to an exercise program in adults and found that exercise adherence health indicators were improvement in anthropometric measures and cardiovascular risk factors. Exercise improves sleep, provides more energy, and can make one more toned, which often allows clothes to fit better (Anshel, 2007). The endorphins that are released with regular aerobic exercise can improve mood and concentration, which allows individuals to focus on the exercise activity itself with an increased desire to adhere to doing the exercise. Higher self-efficacy can further support adherence to exercise and the positive effects of physical exercise.

EMPIRICAL REFERENTS

A multidimensional literature review identified instruments for the defining attributes; no single tool measures exercise adherence. Price et al. (2008) compared self-report tools of physical activity in adults to five direct report instruments. Existing self-report scales lacked quality measures. Tools like the Sports Injury Rehabilitation Scale (SIRAS), an observational scale measuring adherence to exercise for rehabilitation, was limited by the need for direct observation. Furthermore, none of the direct report instruments in Price and colleagues' (2008) study had content validity. The Self-Efficacy for Exercise Instrument, developed by Wilcox, Sharpe, Hutto, and Granner (2005) can be used to measure one's motivation (i.e., self-efficacy) with a higher scores of self-efficacy paralleling greater exercise. Motivation to exercise, an essential part of exercise adherence, can also be measured with the Behavioral Regulation in Exercise Questionnaire (BREQ), which was developed by Mullan, Markland, and Ingeldew (1997) and tested for validity by Wilson, Rodgers, and Fraser (2002), and is a widely used tool in exercise psychology. Refinements to this scale continue with attempts to fully capture the concept of motivation in exercise. The BREQ 2 was developed by Markland et al. (2004) to measure motivation in exercise, while the third version of the BREQ 3 (Wilson et al, 2006), is designed to capture an individual's initial motivation to engage in exercise.

SUMMARY

Exercise adherence is a phenomenon that is necessary to help nurses create a foundation for knowledge and develop interventions to improve health outcomes. Identification of antecedents, attributes, and consequences helps nurses understand how the concept is used within the discipline. Furthermore, identifying what is essential and providing cases to describe how different scenarios meet the whole or parts of the definition will help standardize the meaning. This will enhance the understanding among health care professionals in both practice and research. Clarity and consistency may be the first step in implementing interventions and therefore improving measurable health outcomes.

REFERENCES

Anshel, M. (2007). Conceptualizing applied exercise psychology. *Journal of American Board of Sports Psychology*, *1*(2). Retrieved from http://www.americanboardofsportpsychology.org/portals/24/absp-journalanshel1.pdf

Bertram, L., Stefanick, M., Saquib, N., Natarajan, L., Patterson, R., Bardwell, N., & Pierce, J. (2011). Physical activity, additional breast cancer events, and mortality among early stage breast cancer survivors: Findings from WHEL study. *Cancer, Causes & Control*, *22*(3), 427–435.

Blanchard, C., Courneya, K., & Stein, K. (2008). Cancer survivor's adherence to lifestyle behavior recommendations and associations with health-related quality of life. *Journal of Clinical Oncology*, *26*, 2198–2204.

Boyette, L., Lloyd, A., Boyette, J., Watkins, A., Furbush, L., Dunbar, L., & Brandon, L. (2002). Personal characteristics that influence exercise behavior of older adults. *Journal of Rehabilitation Research & Development*, *39*, 95–103.

Catenacci, V., & Wyatt, H. (2007). The role of physical activity in producing and maintaining weight loss. *Endocrinology and Metabolism*, *3*, 518–529.

Centers for Disease Control and Prevention. (2014). *How much physical activity do you need?* Retrieved from http://www.cdc.gov/physicalactivity/everyone/guidelines/index.html

Cuaderes, E., Parker, D., & Burgin, C. (2004). Leisure time activity in adult Native Americans. *Southern Online Journal of Nursing, 1,* 5.

Delamater, A. (2006). Improving patient adherence. *Clinical Diabetes, 24*(2), 71–77.

Fritz, J., Cleland, J., & Brennan, G. (2007). Does adherence to the guideline recommendation for active treatments improve the quality of care for patients with acute low back pain delivered by physical therapists? *Medical Care, 45*(10), 973–980.

Hellman, E. A. (1997). Use of the stages of change in exercise adherence model among older adults with a cardiac diagnosis. *Journal of Cardiopulmonary Rehabilitation, 17,* 145–155.

Irwin, M., Alvarez-Reeves, M., Cadmus, L., Mierzejewski, E., Mayne, S., Yu, H., & DiPietro, L. (2009). Exercise improves body fat, lean mass, and bone mass in breast cancer survivors. *Obesity, 17,* 1534–1541.

Jones, C. J., & Rose, D. J. (2005). *Strategies to increase exercise adherence in older adults.* Champaign, IL: Human Kinetics.

Markland, D., & Tobin, V. (2004). A modification of the Behavioral Regulation in Exercise Questionnaire to include an assessment of amotivation. *Journal of Sport and Exercise Psychology, 26*(2), 191–196.

McArdle, W., Katch, F., & Katch, V. (2014). *Exercise physiology: Nutrition, energy and human performance* (8th ed.). Amsterdam, The Netherlands: Wolters Kluwer.

McArthur, D., Dumas, A., Woodend, K., Beach, S., & Stacey, D. (2014). Factors influencing adherence to regular exercise in middle-aged women: A qualitative study to inform clinical practice. *Womens Health, 14,* 49. Retrieved from http://www.biomedcentral.com/1472-6874/14/49

McCullough, M., Patel, A., Kushi, L., Patel, R., Willet, W., Doyle, C., ... Gapstur, S. (2011). Following cancer prevention guidelines reduces risk of cancer, cardiovascular disease and all-cause mortality. *Cancer Epidemiology, Biomarkers and Prevention, 20,* 1089–1097.

Miller, F., O'Connor, D., Herring, M., Sailors, M., Jackson, A., Dishman, R., & Bray, M. (2014). Exercise dose, exercise adherence, and associated health outcomes in the TIGER study. *Medical Science in Sports and Exercise, 46*(1), 69–75.

Mullan, E., Markland, D., & Ingledew, D.K. (1997). A graded conceptualisation of self-determination in the regulation of exercise behaviour: Development of a measure using confirmatory factor analytic procedures. *Personality and Individual Differences, 23,* 745–752.

Nunan, D., Mahtami, K., Roberts, N., & Heneghan, C., (2013). Physical activity for the prevention and treatment of major chronic disease: An overview of systematic reviews. *Systematic Reviews, 2,* 56. doi:10.1186/2046-4053-2-56

Picorelli, A., Pereira, L., Pereira, D., Felicio, D., & Sherrington, C. (2014). Adherence to exercise programs for older people is influencing program characteristics and personal factors: A systematic review. *Journal of Physiotherapy, 60,* 151–156.

Powell, K., Paluch, A., & Blair, S. (2011). Physical activity for health: What kind? How much? How intense? On top of what? *Annual Review of Public Health, 32,* 349–365.

Prince, S., Adamo, K., Hamel, M., Hardt, J., Gorber, S., & Tremblay, M. (2008). A comparison of direct versus self-report measures for assessing physical activity in adults: A systematic review. *International Journal of Behavioral Nutrition and Physical Activity, 5,* 56.

Prochaska, J., & Velicer, W. (1997). The transtheoretical model of health behavior change. *American Journal of Health Promotion, 12*, 38–48.

Resnick, B. (2002). Testing the effect of the WALC intervention on exercise adherence in older adults. *Journal of Gerontological Nursing, 28*, 40–49.

Resnick, B., Luisi, D., & Vogel, A. (2008). Testing the Senior Exercise Self-Efficacy Project (SESEP) for use with urban dwelling minority older adults. *Public Health Nursing, 25*(3), 221–234.

Schechter, C., & Walker, E. (2002). Improving adherence to diabetes self-management recommendations. *Diabetes Spectrum, 15*, 170–175.

Schnoll, R., & Zimmerman, B. (2001). Self-regulation training enhances dietary self-efficacy and dietary fiber consumption. *Journal of the American Dietetic Association, 101*, 1006–1011.

Schutzer, K. A., & Graves, B. S. (2004). Barriers and motivations to exercise in older adults. *Preventive Medicine, 39*, 1056–1061.

Shay, L. (2008). A concept analysis: Adherence and weight loss. *Nursing Forum, 43*(1), 42–52.

Shepard, R., & Balady, G. (1999). Exercise as cardiovascular therapy. *Circulation, 99*, 963–972.

U.S. Department of Health and Human Services. (1996). *Physical activity and health: A report of the Surgeon General*. Atlanta, GA: U.S. Department of Health and Human Services Centers for Disease Control and Prevention, National Center for Chronic Disease Control and Prevention and Health Promotion.

U.S. Department of Health and Human Services. (2008). *2008 physical activity guidelines for Americans: Be active, healthy and happy*. Atlanta, GA: U.S. Department of Health and Human Services Centers for Disease Control and Prevention, National Center for Chronic Disease Control and Prevention and Health Promotion. Retrieved from www.health.gov/paguidelines

Van Dulmen, S., Sluijs, E., van Dijk, L., de Ridder, D., Heerdink, R., & Bensing, J. (2007). Patient adherence to medical treatment: A review of reviews. *BMC Health Services Research, 7*, 55.

Wilcox, S., Sharpe, P., Hutto, B., and Granner, M. (2005). Psychometric properties of the Self-Efficacy for Exercise Questionnaire in a diverse sample of men and women. *Journal of Physical Activity & Health, 2*, 3.

Wilson, P., Rodgers, W., & Fraser, S. (2002). Examining the psychometric properties of the Behavioral Regulation in Exercise Questionnaire. *Physical Education and Exercise Science, 6*, 1–21.

Wilson, P.M., Rodgers, W.M., Loitz, C.C., & Scime, G. (2006). "It's who I am…really!" The importance of integrated regulation in exercise contexts. *Journal of Biobehavioral Research, 11*, 79–104.

Young, N., Friedberg, J., Ulmer, M., Cho, H., & Natarajan, S. (2009, November). *Exercise adherence in diabetes: Evaluating the role of behavioral factor in managing diabetes*. Paper presented at American Public Health Association AOHA 137th Meeting and Expo, Philadelphia, PA.

4

HARDINESS IN STROKE

Hardiness improves health by buffering or moderating the effects of stress (Bartone, Roland, Picano, & Williams, 2008; Kobasa, Maddi, & Kahn, 1982). Hardiness is believed to develop early in life and remain stable over time, although changes in hardiness are also possible (Kobasa et al., 1982). Kobasa described hardiness in terms of three personality traits: commitment, control, and challenge. Nonetheless, the concept has not been examined in many chronic conditions such as stroke.

Hardiness enables individuals to deal with stressful events rather than deny or avoid them, and transform them from potential disasters into opportunities and accomplishments (Bartone et al., 2008; Maddi & Khoshaba, 2001; Maddi & Kobasa, 1984). Aspects of hardiness also influence the interpretation of an event (e.g., as stressful or nonstressful) and the imaginative ways the individual confronts or copes with events appraised as stressful (Kobasa, Maddi, Puccetti, & Zola, 1985). Bartone, Kelly, and Matthews (2013) demonstrated that the facets of commitment, control, and challenge can operate somewhat differently with respect to important performance outcomes; therefore, the concept should be examined within its separate dimensions as well as in total. Lang et al. (2001) conducted a concept analysis on hardiness in the context of perinatal bereavement using Wilson's concept analysis method. This analysis only provided a perspective for understanding hardiness with regard to perinatal loss.

The positive influence of hardiness has been reported in sports players and athletes (Sheard & Golby, 2007), military personnel (Bartone, 2006), and stressful work environments (Maddi, 2006; McCalister et al., 2006). In nursing, hardiness has been studied primarily when nurses confront death and dying in hospice settings (Hutchings, 1997), adaptation to chronic illness (Pollock, 1986, 1989), burnout with regard to management (Duquette, Kérouac, Sandhu, Ducharme, & Saulnier, 1995; McCranie, Lambert, & Lambert, 1987), and family adaptation to stressors (McCubbin, McCubbin, Thompson, & Thompson, 1998). Pollock (1986) demonstrated that health-related hardiness

(HRH) significantly relates to higher psychosocial adaptation in individuals with chronic illnesses such as diabetes mellitus, hypertension, and rheumatoid arthritis. HRH has been reported by other researchers to be an effective indicator of adaptation to numerous health problems, chronic obstructive pulmonary disease (Narsavage & Weaver, 1994), human immunodeficiency virus infection (Farber, Schwartz, Schaper, Moonen, & McDaniel, 2000), and multiple sclerosis (Pollock & Duffy, 1990). Hardiness has also been examined in aging studies and has been characterized as the ability to overcome or endure hardship (van Wormer et al., 2011). Thus, there has been successive strong support for measuring hardiness; however, there is a dearth of empirical research on hardiness after a stroke.

DEFINING ATTRIBUTES

The defining attributes of hardiness are *perception of the changed situation as stressful, finding of meaning and a sense of purpose,* and *ability to influence the situation.*

The first attribute, perception of the changed situation as stressful, is derived from the belief that change rather than stability is normal in life, and that it is an interesting incentive for growth (challenge) rather than a threat to security. A hardy person views change as a normal part of life and an opportunity for personal growth rather than a threat. Those who view change as a challenge remain healthier than those who view it as a threat (Kobasa, 1979). Challenge, as described by Kobasa (1979), involves an appreciation for change and a motivation to learn and grow by trying new things. Maddi (1967) used the term *ideal identity* to describe the person who lives a vigorous and proactive life, with an abiding sense of meaning and purpose, and a belief in his or her own ability to influence things. This is contrasted with the "existential neurotic" who shies away from change, seeking security, and sameness in the environment (Bartone et al., 2013). Bartone et al. (2013) highlight that challenge involves an abiding acceptance of change in life, and a proclivity for variety.

The second attribute identified was an individual's ability to find meaning and a sense of purpose. This relates to the sense of meaning and perseverance attributed to one's existence. This attribute is closely related to the component of commitment, as Bartone et al. (2013) highlighted that people high in commitment are more intimately engaged with the world, seeing their experience as generally meaningful and important. Hence, they are more interested in what is going on around them, more attentive, and thus more likely to perceive different aspects of situations, as well as to envision multiple possible response alternatives. This attribute reflects the persons' confidence in their ability to cope with different circumstances (Holahan & Moos, 1985) and increase the sense of independence (Howard et al., 1986).

The ability to influence the situation is the third attribute and demonstrates one's sense of autonomy and perceived ability to influence one's experiences. According to Bartone et al. (2013), the control component of hardiness is derived from the concept of locus of control (Lefcourt, 1973; Rotter, Seeman, & Liverant, 1962). Kobasa's emphasis on control was also influenced by extensive experimental research showing that when subjects have control over aversive stimuli, the stress effects are substantially reduced (Averill, 1973; Seligman, 1975).

DEFINITION

Hardiness is the individual's perception of a changing situation as stressful, finding of meaning and a sense of purpose, and ability to influence the situation.

MODEL CASE

Jane, an active 76-year-old woman, was diagnosed with a stroke (perception of a changing situation as stressful). Subsequently, she had motor impairments of the upper and lower limbs on the left side of her body. Despite her eagerness to return home, she agreed to admission to the rehabilitation unit. She knew her rehabilitation therapy would require effort and dedication if she was to regain use of her affected side (find meaning and a sense of purpose). Jane's attitude was one of determination and being active in helping herself. Jane met regularly with the physiotherapist and occupational therapist while in the unit, where she learned how to use aids and adopt new skills to manage independently. A home visit as part of the occupational therapist assessment improved Jane's knowledge and increased her confidence about managing her recovery. This motivated Jane to continue with the exercises, which helped overcome her impairments and develop new skills to adapt to her life poststroke (ability to influence the situation). Thus, all defining attributes are present in this case.

RELATED CASE

Jane, an active 76-year-old woman, was diagnosed with a stroke (perception of a changing situation as stressful). Subsequently, she had motor impairments of the upper and lower limbs on the left side of her body. Despite Jane's anxieties and helplessness with regard to her impairments, she wanted to return home rather than be admitted to a rehabilitation unit. After much encouragement by her family, Jane agreed to be admitted to the rehabilitation unit. She quickly perceived the effort and expectation that was required during her rehabilitation therapy and she also determined to overcome her impairments (finds meaning and a sense of purpose). Jane met regularly with the physiotherapist and occupational therapist while in the unit, where she learned how to use aids and adopt new skills to manage independently. Jane's family and friends who visited regularly were very supportive and took her out on the weekends. A home visit as part of the occupational therapist assessment was organized. Jane did not believe that she would persist with her rehabilitation (failed ability to influence the situation).

BORDERLINE CASE

Jane, an active 76-year-old woman, was diagnosed with a stroke (perception of a changing situation as stressful). Subsequently, she had motor impairments of the upper and lower limbs on the left side of her body. Despite her eagerness to return home, she agreed to admission to the rehabilitation unit. She knew her rehabilitation therapy would require effort and dedication if she was to regain use of her affected side. Jane's attitude was one of determination and being active in helping herself (find meaning and a sense of purpose). Jane met regularly with the physiotherapist and occupational therapist while in the unit to learn how to use aids and adopt new skills. However, she had difficulty in using the aids and lacked motivation, as the aids demonstrated to her that she would no longer be active as she had been prior to her stroke (failed ability to influence the situation). A home visit as part of the occupational therapist assessment reinforced the loss she felt in her ability to engage in activities in the home; consequently, this affected her engagement in her community activities.

CONTRARY CASE

Jane, an active 76-year-old woman, was diagnosed with a stroke. Subsequently, she had motor impairments of the upper and lower limbs on the left side of her body. Jane became very withdrawn and thought that she would have another stroke (failed perception of a changing situation as stressful). Jane's refused admission to the rehabilitation unit (failed to accept change); however, family insisted on it. Jane had no motivation to engage in her rehabilitation therapy (failed finds meaning and a sense of purpose) and chose to use the wheelchair rather than a walking aid. When the therapist came to do exercises and teach new skills to Jane, she was in bed and reluctant to get dressed for the therapy (failed ability to influence the situation). Jane refused to attend the home visit with the occupational therapist and said that there was no point, as her house was not designed for a wheelchair. As the days passed, she alienated herself from those around her and believed she could no longer be active. This example does not exemplify the concept, as it does not have any defining attributes.

ANTECEDENT

The antecedent to hardiness is a stressful life event such as the diagnosis of a chronic illness. Illness is the single most notorious stressful life event. Any type of major illness is a significant stressor for the entire family. One person being ill does not affect just that person, but everyone around him or her. Many people who experience a major illness usually experience a dramatic change in their lives. Stroke is considered a stressful life event and it is well documented in the literature that the physical and psychosocial consequences of stroke often arrest previously cherished activities (Brewer, Horgan, Hickey, & Williams, 2013; Mukherjee, Levin, & Heller, 2006; Thompson & Ryan, 2009).

CONSEQUENCES

The consequences of hardiness poststroke can be positive, as measured by positive adaptation or improved quality of life; or negative, such as depression or powerlessness (Lee, 1994). Pollock (1993) identified that hardiness was positively related to psychosocial adaptation in insulin-dependent diabetics, individuals diagnosed with hypertension, and individuals diagnosed with multiple sclerosis. Brooks (2008) demonstrated that individuals with higher HRH scores had better psychosocial adaptation to illness. Hamama-Raz and Solomon (2006) also demonstrated that adaptation is better predicted by personal traits (hardiness and attachment style) than by their sociodemographic features and features of the illness.

Hardiness has ranged from low to moderate in individuals with chronic illnesses. It is evident that people who are chronically low in hardiness also tend to rely on negative, avoidance coping strategies in responding to stress (Bartone, 2006). According to Kobasa et al. (1982), hardiness reflects to what extent the individual is psychologically "buffered" from stress and illness. The absence of hardiness suggests that the individual may be more vulnerable to the negative effects of stress (i.e., may become ill more frequently when subjected to stress-related conditions). Hardiness protects against stress by altering perceptions of stress and by mobilizing effective coping strategies (Kobasa, 1982). Hardy people who draw on this resource believe that they can control or influence events they experience, have the ability to feel deeply involved in or committed (self-concept) to the activities of their lives, and anticipate change as an exciting challenge to further development (Kobasa, 1979). Hence, hardiness contributes to their adaptation to chronic illness or improved quality of life (see Figure 4.1).

EMPIRICAL REFERENTS

The Personal Views Survey, developed by Maddi and Kobasa (1984), contains 50 items with scores ranging from 50 to 250; a higher score indicates greater hardiness. The HRH Scale developed by Pollock and Duffy (1990) was a frequently used measure of hardiness (Brooks, 2008; Cataldo, 1994; Martin, Engle, & Graney, 1999; Navuluri, 2001; Nicholas & Leuner, 1999; Pollock, 1993). This 34-item, domain-specific, hardiness scale combined the two factors of challenge/commitment in 20 items and control was measured in 14 items. Scores ranged from 34 to 204, with higher scores indicating greater hardiness. The Dispositional Resilience Scale developed by Bartone (1989) stemmed from the original Hardiness Scale used by Maddi and Kobasa (1984). New items were added and some items were eliminated, and additional psychometric refinement led to improved versions from the 45-item to

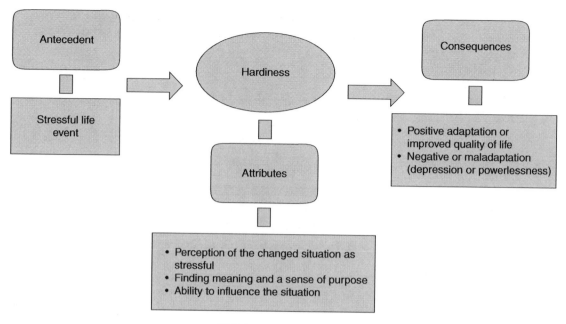

FIGURE 4.1 Hardiness.

the 15-item version. The Dispositional Resilience Scale displays good reliability and predictive validity in several samples, with respect to both health and performance under high-stress conditions (Bartone, 2007). Kobasa emphasizes that the three subcomponents of hardiness are not independent or mutually exclusive, but rather are inextricably intertwined aspects that bear a considerable resemblance to one another and, together, comprise the overall style of hardiness (Kobasa, 1979, p. 9).

SUMMARY

This concept analysis defined and identified defining attributes of hardiness. A definition of hardiness is proposed and the antecedent identified. The consequences of hardiness are significant in terms of positive or negative adaptation poststroke. The empirical referents, which ensure that the concept can be measured, were also identified. A schematic representation is provided to facilitate understanding of the concept (Figure 4.1).

REFERENCES

Averill, J. R. (1973). Personal control over aversive stimuli and its relationship to stress. *Psychological Bulletin, 80*, 286–303.

Bartone, P.T. (1989). Predictors of stress-related illness in city bus drivers. *Journal of Occupational Medicine, 3*, 657–663.

Bartone, P. T. (2006). Resilience under military operational stress: Can leaders influence hardiness? *Military Psychology, 18*(S), S131.

Bartone, P. T. (2007). Test-retest reliability of the Dispositional Resilience Scale-15, a brief hardiness scale. *Psychological Reports, 101*(3, pt. 1), 943–944.

Bartone, P. T., Kelly, D. R., & Matthews, M. D. (2013). Psychological hardiness predicts adaptability in military leaders: A prospective study. *International Journal of Selection and Assessment, 21*(2), 200–210.

Bartone, P. T., Roland, R. R., Picano, J. J., & Williams, T. J. (2008). Psychological hardiness predicts success in US Army Special Forces candidates. *International Journal of Selection and Assessment, 16*, 78–81.

Brewer, L., Horgan, F., Hickey, A., & Williams, D. (2013). Stroke rehabilitation: Recent advances and future therapies. *Quarterly Journal of Medicine, 106*(1), 11–25.

Brooks, M. V. (2008). Health-related hardiness in individuals with chronic illnesses. *Clinical Nursing Research, 17*(2), 98–117.

Cataldo, J. K. (1994). Hardiness and death attitudes: Predictors of depression in the institutionalized elderly. *Archives of Psychiatric Nursing, 8*(5), 326–332.

Duquette, A., Kérouac, S., Sandhu, B. K., Ducharme, F., & Saulnier, P. (1995). Psychosocial determinants of burnout in geriatric nursing. *International Journal of Nursing Studies, 32*(5), 443–456.

Farber, E. W., Schwartz, J. A., Schaper, P. E., Moonen, D. J., & McDaniel, J. S. (2000). Resilience factors associated with adaptation to HIV disease. *Psychosomatics, 41*(2), 140–146.

Hamama-Raz, Y., & Solomon, Z. (2006). Psychological adjustment of melanoma survivors: The contribution of hardiness, attachment, and cognitive appraisal. *Journal of Individual Differences, 27*(3), 172.

Holahan, C. J., & Moos, R. H. (1985). Stress and health: Personality, coping, and family support in stress resistance. *Journal of Personality and Social Psychology, 49*(3), 739–747.

Hull, J. G., Van Treuren, R. R., & Virnelli, S. (1987). Hardiness and health: A critique and alternative approach. *Journal of Personality and Social Psychology, 53*, 518–530.

Hutchings, D. (1997). The hardiness of hospice nurses. *American Journal of Hospice & Palliative Care, 14*(2), 110–113.

Kobasa, S. C. (1979). Stressful life events, personality and health: An inquiry into hardiness. *Journal of Personal and Social Psychology, 37*, 1–11.

Kobasa, S. C., Maddi, S. R., & Kahn, S. (1982). Hardiness and health: A prospective study. *Journal of Personality and Social Psychology, 42*(1), 168.

Kobasa, S. C., Maddi, S. R., Puccetti, M. C., & Zola, M. A. (1985). Effectiveness of hardiness, exercise and social support as resources against illness. *Journal of Psychosomatic Research, 29*(5), 525–533.

Lang, A., Goulet, C., Aita, M., Giguère, V., Lamarre, H., & Perreault, E. (2001). Weathering the storm of perinatal bereavement via hardiness. *Death Studies, 25*(6), 497–512.

Lee, Y. A. (1994). A concept analysis of hardiness. *Journal of Korean Academy of Nursing, 24*(4), 616–622.

Lefcourt, H. M. (1973). The function of the illusions of control and freedom. *American Psychologist, 28*, 417–425.

Maddi, S. R. (1967). The existential neurosis. *Journal of Abnormal Psychology, 72*(4), 311.

Maddi, S. R. (2006). Hardiness: The courage to grow from stresses. *Journal of Positive Psychology, 1*(3), 160–168.

Maddi, S. R., & Khoshaba, D. M. (2001). *Personal Views Survey III-R: Test development and Internet instruction manual*. Newport Beach, CA: Hardiness Institute.

Maddi, S. R., & Kobasa, S. C. (1984). *The hardy executive: Health under stress*. Homewood, IL: Dow Jones-Irwin.

Martin, J. C., Engle, V. F., & Graney, M. J. (1999). Determinants of health-related hardiness among urban older African-American women with chronic illness. *Holistic Nursing Practice, 13*(3), 62–70.

McCranie, E. W., Lambert, V. A., & Lambert, C. E., Jr. (1987). Work stress, hardiness, and burnout among hospital staff nurses. *Nursing Research, 36*(6), 374–378.

McCubbin, H. I., McCubbin, M. A., Thompson, A. I., & Thompson, E. A. (1998). Resiliency in ethnic families: A conceptual model for predicting family adjustment and adaptation. *Resiliency in Native American and Immigrant Families, 2*, 3–48.

Mukherjee, D., Levin, R. L., & Heller, W. (2006). The cognitive, emotional, and social sequelae of stroke: Psychological and ethical concerns in post-stroke adaptation. *Topics in Stroke Rehabilitation, 13*(4), 26–35.

Narsavage, G. L., & Weaver, T. E. (1994). Physiologic status, coping, and hardiness as predictors of outcomes in chronic obstructive pulmonary disease. *Nursing Research, 43*(2), 90–94.

Navuluri, R. B. (2001). Do hardiness and attitude promote self-care adherence to physical activity among adults with diabetes? *Internet Journal of Internal Medicine, 3*(1), 23–37.

Nicholas, P. K., & Leuner, J. D. M. (1999). Hardiness, social support, and health status: Are there differences in older African-American and Anglo-American adults? *Holistic Nursing Practice, 13*(3), 53–61.

Pollock, S. E. (1986). Human responses to chronic illness: Physiologic and psychosocial adaptation. *Nursing Research, 35*(2), 90–97.

Pollock, S. E. (1989). The hardiness characteristic: A motivating factor in adaptation. *Advances in Nursing Science, 11*(2), 53–62.

Pollock, S. E. (1993). Adaptation to chronic illness: A program of research for testing nursing theory. *Nursing Science Quarterly, 6*, 86–92.

Pollock, S. E., & Duffy, M. E. (1990). The health-related hardiness scale: Development and psychometric analysis. *Nursing Research, 39*(4), 218–222.

Rotter, J. B., Seeman, M., & Liverant, S. (1962). Internal vs. external locus of control of reinforcement: A major variable in behavior theory. In N. F. Washburne (Ed.), *Decisions, values and groups* (pp. 473–516). London, UK: Pergamon Press.

Seligman, M. E. P. (1975). *Helplessness*. San Francisco, CA: Freeman.

Sheard, M., & Golby, J. (2007). Hardiness and undergraduate academic study: The moderating role of commitment. *Personality and Individual Differences, 43*(3), 579–588.

Thompson, H. S., & Ryan, A. (2009). The impact of stroke consequences on spousal relationships from the perspective of the person with stroke. *Journal of Clinical Nursing, 18*(12), 1803–1811.

van Wormer, K., Sudduth, C., & Jackson, III, D. W. (2011). What we can learn of resilience from older African-American women: Interviews with women who worked as maids in the deep South. *Journal of Human Behavior in the Social Environment, 21*(4), 410–422.

5

HELP-SEEKING BEHAVIOR FOR BREAST CANCER SYMPTOMS

Help-seeking behavior (HSB) has been studied in the context of mental health, chronic pain, and a wide array of cancer symptoms. However, lack of clarity surrounds the concept. An overview of how the concept is described in the literature is presented here.

An earlier review of the literature on help seeking for cancer symptoms defined *help seeking* as a response to health changes and part of the broader process of health-seeking behavior (O'Mahony & Hegarty, 2009). A concept analysis on HSB for health problems generally (Cornally & McCarthy, 2011) described HSB as a problem-focused, planned behavior, involving interpersonal communication with a particular health care professional (HCP). In a study on the factors influencing women's HSB for breast cancer symptoms, the concept of HSB was operationalized as "the time from symptom discovery to presentation of the symptom to a general practitioner (GP)" (O'Mahony, McCarthy, Corcoran, & Hegarty, 2013). Within this study, help-seeking following symptom discovery was categorized as either "prompt" (i.e., presentation of symptoms to a HCP within 1 month [4 weeks] of symptom discovery) or "delayed" (i.e., presentation of symptoms to a HCP more than 1 month [more than 4 weeks] after symptom discovery). An earlier phase of this study sought to validate the appropriateness of its guiding framework through a qualitative exploration of women's HSB for a self-discovered breast symptom. Interviews focused on women's ($n = 10$) experience of finding a breast symptom and their associated HSB (O'Mahony, Hegarty, & McCarthy, 2011). Thus, help seeking and HSB are used synonymously in the literature. Additionally, since one of the outcomes associated with help seeking is "delay" or postponed help seeking, an earlier pilot study sought to identify the extent of delay and the factors influencing women in seeking help from a HCP on self-discovery of a breast symptom (O'Mahony & Hegarty, 2009). Therefore, any discussion on help seeking or HSB must consider prompt or delay as consequences of the process.

The referenced studies on HSB for breast cancer symptoms were guided in part by the Judgment to Delay (J-Delay) model (Facione, Miaskowski, Dodd, & Paul, 2002), which theoretically integrates factors associated with delay behavior (e.g., demographics, knowledge and beliefs, affective responses, relationship constraints, health service system variables, and health-seeking habits). The J-Delay model proposes that these factors, together with symptom appraisal, lead to a decision around problem resolution which is described as "seeking evaluation" (help seeking) versus "patient delay" (Facione et al., 2002). However, certain elements of the model required further clarification; hence the development of the "help-seeking behavior and influencing factors" framework (O'Mahony et al., 2011, 2013) to guide the studies on women's HSB for self-discovered breast symptoms.

Other studies on help seeking for cancer symptoms have identified many important aspects of HSB. Grant, Silver, Bauld, Day, and Warnakulasuriya (2010) reported an exploratory study on the experiences of younger patients with oral cancer in Scotland. The study focused in particular on patients' response to "emerging symptoms" and the time taken for specialist referral and diagnosis. A meta-ethnographic synthesis of qualitative studies ($n = 13$) identified the key concepts of symptom detection, initial symptom interpretation, symptom monitoring, social interaction, emotional reaction, priority of medical help, appraisal of health services, and personal-environmental factors, as the factors influencing HSB of women with self-discovered breast cancer symptoms (Khakbazan, Taghipour, Latifnejad Roudsari, & Mohammadi, 2014). Thus, HSB for breast cancer symptoms is a complex, multidimensional concept.

The complex nature of HSB was reiterated in a recent study of individuals with lung cancer symptoms and the relationship of perceived lung cancer stigma on the timing of medical HSB (Carter-Harris, 2015). The theoretical underpinnings for this study were provided by the "Model for Understanding Delayed Presentation with Breast Cancer" (Bish, Ramirez, Burgess, & Hunter, 2005). This model is based on the premise that delayed medical HSB is influenced by multiple complex interactions between sociodemographic, clinical, cognitive, and behavioral variables (Bish et al., 2005). Again, the need to include delay as a possible consequence of any help-seeking process is emphasized.

Help seeking for "cancer alarm" symptoms was the focus of a recent U.K. community-based qualitative study ($n = 48$; Whitaker, Macleod, & Wardle, 2015). Findings highlighted the complexity around decision making for cancer "alarm" symptoms. The decision to seek or not seek help was influenced by an array of emotional (fear), cognitive (symptom awareness), and attitudinal (not wanting to make a fuss; lack of confidence that the GP could help) variables. The need to address barriers to help seeking was also emphasized.

Lim (2011) reviewed models ($n = 6$) of patient delay and help seeking for breast cancer in studies ($n = 7$) over a period of 7 years (2003–2010). The review found that while some degree of consistency existed among the models' ability to explain HSB, overall there was a lack of consensus in the terminology used to define the key constructs and variables. The need for greater consensus and a shared "conceptual language" was highlighted. Thus, a concept analysis of HSB for breast cancer symptoms is timely.

DEFINING ATTRIBUTES

The attributes of HSB for breast cancer symptoms are *response to a self-discovered breast symptom, symptom appraisal, symptom interpretation,* and *decision making to consult with a HCP* (GP).

A response to self-discovered breast symptoms is something that a woman does when she detects a breast change. In order to respond, the woman needs to be breast aware, that is, have the confidence to "look at and feel" her breasts so that she knows what is normal for her own body and what changes to look and feel for (Irish Cancer Society, 2015; National Comprehensive Cancer Network [NCCN], 2014; NHS Breast Cancer Screening Programme, 2015). An understanding of the implications of these changes, and the need to consult promptly with a HCP, is also necessary (MacBride, Pruthi, & Bevers, 2012). The next phase of the response involves symptom appraisal.

According to Facione et al. (2002), symptom appraisal is understood to be a cognitive decision-making process dependent on the estimation of the potential risk posed by the symptom. This is part of the process of initial symptom interpretation as described earlier by Khakbazan et al. (2014). Hence, cognitive processes play an important role throughout the phase of symptom appraisal and initiate the process of symptom interpretation.

Symptom interpretation is highlighted as an important part of the process of HSB (Grant et al., 2010; Khakbazan et al., 2014). According to Grant et al. (2010), symptom interpretation is primarily based on comparing the nature of the symptom with pre-existing knowledge and experiences regarding disease symptoms. Knowledge and beliefs are key to appropriate interpretation of symptoms. Weller et al. (2012) provide an "Aarhus checklist" to promote greater transparency in early cancer diagnosis research. Within this framework, the appraisal interval is described as being the time taken to interpret bodily changes/symptoms. Therefore, symptom interpretation is part of symptom appraisal and an important part of the help-seeking process.

Decision making around HSB is also a complex process and is influenced by an array of factors (Facione et al., 2002; Lim, 2011). These factors range from socio demographic, cognitive, emotional, social, attitudinal, breast health-related habits, and access to health services (Facione et al., 2002; Lim, 2011; Meechan, Collins, & Petrie, 2002, 2003; O'Mahony & Hegarty, 2009; O'Mahony et al., 2011, 2013). In their model of pathways to treatment, Walter, Webster, Scott, and Emery (2012) outline the decision to consult with a HCP and arrange an appointment as part of the help-seeking process. In the context of help seeking for cancer symptoms, the decision can be to seek help promptly or to delay (postpone) help seeking.

DEFINITION

HSB for breast cancer symptoms is defined as: a response to a self-discovered breast symptom involving symptom appraisal, symptom interpretation, and decision making to consult with a HCP.

MODEL CASE

Mary is a 40-year-old woman who notices a swelling in her left breast while showering. She looks in the mirror to see if she can detect any changes (response to self-discovered breast symptom). She continues to feel her breast and, yes, is certain that this swelling resembles a lump that she never noticed before (symptom appraisal). She considers the date and how long it is since her last menstrual period—it is only 4 days. Therefore, this is a breast change that is not due to her menstrual cycle. It is a breast change/breast symptom that could be associated with breast cancer (symptom interpretation). Mary is worried and afraid that the lump could be breast cancer. She knows that the only way to relieve this worry is to go to her GP and have the symptom assessed. She makes a decision to consult with her GP and arrange an appointment as soon as possible (decision making). This case has all of the defining attributes of HSB for breast cancer symptoms.

RELATED CASE

Sarah is a 50-year-old woman who notices a pain in her left breast over the past few days. It is vague but she knows that she has not felt a pain like this before (symptom appraisal). She cannot remember if this is associated with her menstrual period or not, as her cycle has become quite irregular of late (failed symptom interpretation). She checks her diary to confirm when her next visit to her GP to renew her prescription for blood pressure medication is scheduled (response to a self-discovered breast symptom). She decides that she will mention this pain in her breast to the GP during her next visit in 2 weeks' time (decision making). This case has some of the attributes of HSB for breast cancer symptoms, but Sarah responds to the symptom in the context of general health-seeking behavior.

BORDERLINE CASE

Lydia is a 70-year-old woman who notices a crusted area on her left nipple as she showers. It is itchy, so she applies some moisturizer to it (response to a self-discovered breast symptom). She wonders what it could be (symptom appraisal). She thinks maybe it could be due to an allergy to washing powder or some clothing she is wearing (failed symptom interpretation). She wonders what is best to wear today and chooses cotton clothing that will not irritate her skin further. She thinks about the weekend and her planned trip to London with friends. She is really looking forward to it. Lydia decides to start packing her suitcase and to ensure that all her travel documents are in order (decision making). This case has only three of the four attributes of HSB for breast cancer symptoms, and is thus a borderline case.

CONTRARY CASE

Susan is 42 years of age. One night her husband notices a lump in her right breast. He mentions it to her immediately. She is not interested and does not respond (failed response to a self-discovered breast symptom). Her husband tries to persuade her to have it checked out, but Susan gets annoyed and tells him to "stop fussing" (failed symptom appraisal). Susan starts reading the novel that she just started last night, and she tells her husband to try and go to sleep and to stop worrying about silly things (failed symptom interpretation). Susan starts thinking about her plans for her husband's birthday party at the end of the month. She starts making out a "to do" list in her diary (failed decision making). This case contains none of the four attributes of HSB for breast cancer symptoms.

ANTECEDENTS

The antecedents to HSB for breast cancer symptoms are knowledge, beliefs, breast cancer awareness, and confidence to seek help. If a woman is to seek help for a self-discovered breast symptom, she requires knowledge of breast cancer and the associated breast cancer symptoms. In this regard, the concept of breast cancer awareness is relevant. To date, the concept of breast cancer awareness has been poorly understood. In the United Kingdom, the promoting early presentation (PEP) intervention has been developed to provide women with knowledge, skills, motivation, and confidence to present early with breast cancer symptoms (Burgess et al., 2009; Linsell et al., 2009; Forbes et al., 2011). To date, results demonstrate that the intervention has increased women's breast cancer awareness at 1 year (Linsell et al., 2009) and 2 years (Forbes et al., 2011) postdelivery. It is hypothesized that the intervention has potential to increase the likelihood of women seeking help promptly in the event of developing a breast cancer symptom (Forbes et al., 2011). Thus, increasing women's breast cancer awareness is likely to increase their confidence and motivation for prompt HSB (Figure 5.1).

CONSEQUENCES

The consequences of HSB for breast cancer symptoms depend on whether the help seeking is prompt or delayed. Early diagnosis and treatment of cancer are likely to achieve better outcomes (Jemal et al., 2011; Richards, 2009; Siegel, Naishadham, & Jemal, 2013). Early detection of breast cancer is promoted as being "the cornerstone of breast cancer control" (World Health Organization, 2015). Prompt HSB has potential to lead to early detection and diagnosis of breast cancer. This in turn has implications for early treatment and improved outcomes for women. In addition, prompt help seeking has potential to result

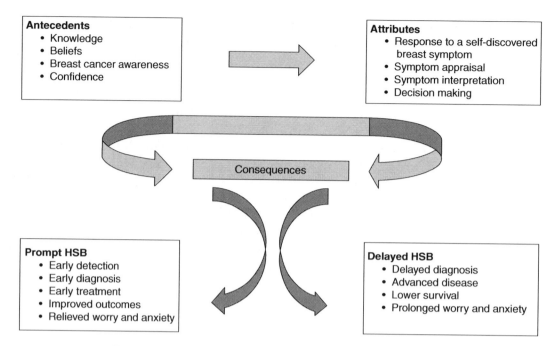

FIGURE 5.1 Help-seeking behavior for breast cancer symptoms.

in a benign diagnosis and relieved worry and anxiety for women following symptom discovery (Meechan et al., 2003; O'Mahony et al., 2013).

Conversely, delayed help seeking has the potential to result in more advanced disease at diagnosis. Prolonged delay (i.e., delay in excess of 3 months from onset of symptoms to diagnosis and treatment of breast cancer) is associated with a lower survival rate (Richards, 2009; Richards, Westcombe, Love, Littlejohns, & Ramirez, 1999). Delayed help seeking also has the potential to lead to prolonged worry and anxiety for women who fear a breast cancer diagnosis (O'Mahony et al., 2011).

EMPIRICAL REFERENTS

HSB for breast cancer symptoms has been measured in terms of the factors that influence HSB (O'Mahony & Hegarty, 2009; O'Mahony et al., 2011, 2013). In addition, it has been studied at various time points of the symptom trajectory: that is, prior to the occurrence of a symptom (Facione, Giancarlo, & Chan, 2000; Facione et al., 2002; Hunter, Grunfeld, & Ramirez, 2003); following symptom occurrence but prior to seeing the consultant in the breast clinic (de Nooijer, Lechner, & de Vries, 2002; Meechan et al., 2002, 2003; O'Mahony & Hegarty, 2009; O'Mahony et al., 2011, 2013); following symptom evaluation prior to diagnosis (Unger-Saldana & Infante-Castaneda, 2011); and following diagnosis of breast cancer or benign breast disease (Arndt et al., 2002; Burgess, Hunter, & Ramirez, 2001; O'Mahony, 2001).

The complex and multidimensional nature of HSB for breast cancer symptoms makes it an elusive concept to measure in its entirety. Therefore, tools have been developed to measure women's likelihood to delay by focusing on the factors proposed to influence delay behavior (Facione et al., 2002). Conversely, studies on HSB for actual breast symptoms have used a variety of researcher-developed tools, some of which are atheoretical (Meechan et al., 2003) and some of which are based on relevant theories and frameworks (O'Mahony et al., 2013). Inherent in these tools are measurements of the key attributes of HSB symptom appraisal, symptom interpretation, and a decision to consult a HCP. Symptom appraisal and interpretation have been measured by assessing women's knowledge and beliefs around breast symptoms (O'Mahony et al., 2013). Beliefs were measured using an adaptation of the Illness Perception Questionnaire (Weinman, Petrie, Moss-Morris, & Horne, 1996) which asked women their perceptions of the cause, duration, consequences, curability/controllability of their breast symptom. In addition, women's knowledge of their breast symptom was measured using an adaptation of the Breast Cancer Knowledge Scale (Facione et al., 2002). In the United Kingdom, the Breast Cancer Awareness Measure (BCAM) (Linsell et al., 2010) is a validated and reliable tool used to measure women's knowledge of breast cancer symptoms, age-related risk, and frequency of breast checking. Measurement of women's breast symptom knowledge and beliefs provides some insight into the process of women's symptom appraisal and interpretation and helps highlight any deficits in this regard.

The decision to seek help is influenced by women's knowledge and beliefs along with other social, psychological, and health service-related variables (O'Mahony et al., 2011, 2013). Measurement of the decision-making process to seek help is difficult; however, women can be asked to identify dates and time intervals as follows: (a) the date when the symptom/breast change is first noticed, (b) the time taken to interpret the symptom/breast changes (the appraisal interval), and (c) the time taken to act on the interpretations and seek help (the help-seeking interval; Weller et al., 2012). Therefore, empirical referents are available for the purpose of measuring and observing HSB for breast cancer symptoms. However, further research and review on this topic are necessary to identify optimum tools to fully ascertain the complex and multidimensional nature of HSB for breast cancer symptoms.

SUMMARY

Review of the literature and previous research highlighted that the terms *help seeking* and *HSB* are used synonymously. In addition, HSB has been studied in the context of its influencing factors and the time intervals from symptom discovery to consulting with a HCP. Key attributes of HSB for breast cancer symptoms were outlined as being: a response to a self-discovered breast symptom, symptom appraisal, symptom interpretation, and decision making to consult a HCP. Various tools have been used to measure HSB, some focusing on women's likelihood to delay and others on the factors influencing HSB. Globally, considerable efforts are being made to promote early presentation of cancer symptoms generally, and breast cancer symptoms specifically. Clarity around the concept of HSB for breast cancer symptoms is one step in the pathway toward achieving breast cancer control through the promotion of early detection, diagnosis, treatment, and improved outcomes for women who are diagnosed with breast cancer.

REFERENCES

Arndt, V., Sturmer, T., Stegmaier, C., Ziegler, H., Dhom, G., & Brenner, H. (2002). Patient delay and stage of diagnosis among breast cancer patients in Germany: A population based study. *British Journal of Cancer, 86,* 1034–1040.

Bish, A., Ramirez, A., Burgess, C., & Hunter, M. (2005). Understanding why women delay in seeking help for breast cancer symptoms. *Journal of Psychosomatic Research, 8,* 321–326.

Burgess, C. C., Hunter, M. S., & Ramirez, A. J. (2001). A qualitative study of delay among women reporting symptoms of breast cancer. *British Journal of General Practice, 51,* 967–971.

Burgess, C. C., Linsell, L., Kapari, M., Omar, L., Michell, M., Whelehan, P., ... Ramirez, A. J. (2009). Promoting early presentation of breast cancer by older women: A preliminary evaluation of a one-to-one health professional-delivered intervention. *Journal of Psychosomatic Research, 67,* 377–387.

Carter-Harris, L. (2015). Lung cancer stigma as a barrier to medical help-seeking behavior: Practice implications. *Journal of the American Association of Nurse Practitioners, 27*(5), 240–245.

Cornally, N., & McCarthy, G. (2011). Help-seeking behaviour: A concept analysis. *International Journal of Nursing Practice, 17*(3), 280–288.

de Nooijer, J., Lechne, L., & de Vries, H. (2002). Early detection of cancer: Knowledge and behavior among Dutch adults. *Cancer Detection and Prevention, 26,* 362–369.

Facione, N. C., Giancarlo, C. A., & Chan, L. (2000). Perceived risk and help-seeking behavior for breast cancer: A Chinese-American perspective. *Cancer Nursing, 23*(4), 258–267.

Facione, N. C., Miaskowski, C., Dodd, M. J., & Paul, S. M. (2002). The self-reported likelihood of patient delay in breast cancer: New thoughts for early detection. *Preventive Medicine, 34,* 397–407.

Forbes, L. J., Linsell, L., Atkins, L., Burgess, C., Tucker, L., Omar, L., & Ramirez, A. J. (2011). A promoting early presentation intervention increases breast cancer awareness in older women after 2 years: A randomised controlled trial. *British Journal of Cancer, 105*(1), 18–21.

Grant, E., Silver, K., Bauld, L., Day, R., & Warnakulasuriya, S. (2010). The experiences of young oral cancer patients in Scotland: Symptom recognition and delays in seeking professional help. *British Dental Journal, 208*(10), 465–471.

Hunter, M. S., Grunfeld, E. A., & Ramirez, A. J. (2003). Help-seeking intentions for breast cancer symptoms: A comparison of the self-regulation model and the theory of planned behaviour. *British Journal of Health Psychology, 8,* 319–333.

Irish Cancer Society. (2015). *Preventing breast cancer: Becoming breast aware.* Retrieved from http://www.cancer.ie/cancer-information/breast-cancer/prevention

Jemal, A., Bray, F., Center, M. M., Ferlay, J., Ward, E., & Forman, D. (2011). Global cancer statistics. *CA: Cancer Journal for Clinicians, 61,* 69–90.

Khakbazan, Z., Taghipour, A., Latifnejad Roudsari, R., & Mohammadi, E. (2014). Help seeking behavior of women with self-discovered breast cancer symptoms: A meta-ethnographic synthesis of patient delay. *PLoS ONE, 9*(12), e110262. doi:10.1371/journal.pone.0110262

Lim, J. N. (2011). Empirical comparisons of patient delay and help seeking models for breast cancer: Fitness of models for use and generalisation. *Asian Pacific Journal of Cancer Prevention, 12*(6), 1589–1595.

Linsell, L., Forbes, L. J., Burgess, C., Kapari, M., Thurnham, A., & Ramirez, A. J. (2010). Validation of a measurement tool to assess awareness of breast cancer. *European Journal of Cancer, 46*(8), 1374–1381.

Linsell, L., Forbes, L. J., Kapari, M., Burgess, C., Omar, L., Tucker, L., & Ramirez, A. J. (2009). A randomised controlled trial of an intervention to promote early presentation of breast cancer in older women: Effect on breast cancer awareness. *British Journal of Cancer, 101*(Suppl. 2), S40–S48.

MacBride, M. B., Pruthi, S., & Bevers, T. (2012). The evolution of breast self-examination to breast awareness. *Breast Journal, 18*(6), 641–643.

Meechan, G., Collins, J., & Petrie, K. J. (2002). Delay in seeking medical care for self-detected breast symptoms in New Zealand women. *New Zealand Medical Journal, 115*, U257.

Meechan, G., Collins, J., & Petrie, K. J. (2003). The relationship of symptoms and psychological factors to delay in seeking medical care for breast symptoms. *Preventive Medicine, 36*, 374–378.

Morse, K. (2010) What factors are associated with parental concern regarding their child's weight? Journal of Pediatric Health Care 24: e8–e9.

National Comprehensive Cancer Network. (2014). *Guidelines 2014.* Retrieved from www.nccn.org/professionals/physician_gls/pdf/breast-screening.pdf

NHS Breast Cancer Screening Programme. (2015). *National Office of NHS Cancer Screening Programmes, Public Health England: NHS Breast Cancer Screening Programme 2015.* Retrieved from www.cancerscreening.nhs.uk/breastscreen/breastawareness.html

O'Mahony, M. (2001). Women's lived experience of breast biopsy: A phenomenological study. *Journal of Clinical Nursing, 10*, 512–520.

O'Mahony, M., & Hegarty, J. (2009). Factors influencing women in seeking help from a health care professional on self discovery of a breast symptom, in an Irish context. *Journal of Clinical Nursing, 18*(14), 2020–2029.

O'Mahony, M., Hegarty, J., & McCarthy, G. (2011). Women's help seeking behaviour for self discovered breast cancer symptoms. *European Journal of Oncology Nursing, 15*, 410–418.

O'Mahony, M., McCarthy, G., Corcoran, P., & Hegarty, J. (2013). Shedding light on women's help seeking behaviour for self discovered breast symptoms. *European Journal of Oncology Nursing, 17*(5), 632–639.

Richards, M. A. (2009). The size of the prize for earlier diagnosis of cancer in England. *British Journal of Cancer, 101*, S125–S129.

Richards, M. A., Westcombe, A. M., Love, S. B., Littlejohns, P., & Ramirez, A. J. (1999). Influence of delay on survival in patients with breast cancer: A systematic review. *Lancet, 353*, 1119–1126.

Siegel, R., Naishadham, D., & Jemal, A. (2013). Cancer statistics, 2013. *CA: Cancer Journal for Clinicians, 63*(1), 11–30.

Unger-Saldana, K., & Infante-Castaneda, C. B. (2011). Breast cancer delay: A grounded model of help-seeking behaviour. *Social Science & Medicine, 72*(7), 1096–1104.

Walter, F., Webster, A., Scott, S., & Emery, J. (2012). The Andersen model of total patient delay: A systematic review of its application in cancer diagnosis. *Journal of Health Services Research & Policy, 17*(2), 110–118. doi:10.1258/jhsrp.2011.010113

Weinman, J., Petrie, K. J., Moss-Morris, R., & Horne, R. (1996). The illness perception questionnaire: A new method for assessing the cognitive representation of illness. *Journal of Psychology and Health, 11,* 431–445.

Weller, D., Vedsted, P., Rubin, G., Walter, F. M., Emery, J., Scott, S. E., ... Neak R. D. (2012). The Aarhus statement: Improving design and reporting of studies on early cancer diagnosis. *British Journal of Cancer, 106,* 1262–1267. doi:10.1038/bjc.2012.68

Whitaker, K. L., Macleod, U., & Wardle, J. (2015). Help seeking for cancer "alarm" symptoms: A qualitative interview study of primary care patients in the UK. *British Journal of General Practice, 65*(631), e96–e105. doi:10.3399/bjgp15X683533

World Health Organization. (2015). *Breast cancer: Prevention and control.* Retrieved from http://www.who.int/cancer/detection/breastcancer/en

JOAN MURPHY AND MOIRA O'DONOVAN

6

HOPE IN MENTAL HEALTH RECOVERY

Hope is a concept that has been applied and investigated by many disciplines, including philosophy, theology, anthropology, psychology, psychiatry, sociology, and nursing. Walker and Avant (2011) contend that the attributes of a concept may change in different contexts. Significantly, there is no concept analysis of hope in relation to mental health recovery where *recovery* is defined as the fulfilment of a meaningful life and a positive sense of identity founded on hope and self-determination (Andresen, Oades, & Caputi, 2003). In this context, hope has been identified as integral and fundamental to recovery (Andresen, Oades, & Caputi, 2011; Gerhart, 2012; Schrank, Bird, Rudnick, & Slade, 2012). This is reflected in strategic documents outlining how professionals should work in recovery-oriented ways (e.g., Australian Health Ministers Advisory Council, 2013). We are told that if mental health nurses need to think about recovery, they need to think about hope (Clarke, Oades, Crowe, Capuit, & Deane, 2009). Therefore, it is imperative to have a clear concept of what hope means from a mental health perspective.

Long before the advent of the recovery approach to care, Menninger (1959), a psychiatrist, emphasized the pragmatic relational capacity of the hope of health care professionals to increase the hope of others. However, it was not until the 1970s onward that the influence of nursing on the development of hope theory became significant. DuFault and Martocchio (1985) are credited with being the first to encapsulate the multidimensionality of hope in acknowledging its conceptual richness and complexity. Thereafter, hope has been investigated in diverse populations including patients with chronic illness (Cutcliffe & Grant, 2001), cancer (Herth, 1990), stroke (Tutton, Seers, Langstaff, & Westwood, 2011), HIV/AIDS (Zinck & Cutcliffe, 2013), the older person (Cutcliffe & Grant, 2001), palliative care (Duggleby et al., 2010), and to a lesser extent people experiencing mental health problems (Hobbs & Baker, 2012; McCann, 2002; Noh, Choe, & Yang, 2008) and bereavement (Cutcliffe, 2006). All authors depict hope as a positive attribute necessitating the involvement of others, as being future and goal oriented with positive health outcomes. However, a consistent observation in the mental health literature has been the significant absence of discourse and research on hope (Cutcliffe, 2009; Schrank, Stanghellini, Slade, 2008). Given the adoption of the recovery paradigm into mental health care, in which hope is a key component, this absence must be addressed. At the outset, hope has been presented as an abstract concept, leading to some complexity in determining its defining attributes (Nekolaichuk, 2005). Indeed, Kinghorn (2013) argues that hope defies absolute definition, citing the challenge of encapsulating its deepest meaning in human language. The unidimensionality of hope is captured in the seminal work of Stotland (1969) and Snyder et al. (1991). Theoretically, hope has evolved from being viewed as unidimensional to now being accepted as a multidimensional phenomenon (Nekolaichuk, 2005). The *Oxford English Dictionary* (Simpson & Weiner, 1989) has defined hope as both a noun and a verb. As a noun, hope is identified as a feeling of expectation and desire for a particular thing to happen. As a verb, it is described as the act of desiring, of having confidence, of believing, or trusting in something or someone. When used in this way, hope is seen as being intentional and active.

DEFINING ATTRIBUTES

The attributes are *cognitive goal-directed process, enabling the possible, interrelational process, personality trait*, and *attribution of meaning*.

The first defining attribute of hope derived from this work is that of a cognitive goal-directed process expressed in pathways and agency to achieve selected goals which are perceived as being achievable (Snyder et al., 1991). This agency involves the evolution of hope into motivation, energy, and activation (Farran, Herth, & Popovich, 1995; Ridgway, 2003). It is intrinsically dynamic because its intensity and nature change over time (Hobbs & Baker, 2012; Ridgway, 2003).

The second linked attribute of hope is enabling the possible, making it vital to life by providing psychological nourishment in challenging times and by increasing awareness of one's own inner resources (Hall, 1990). In this context, hope has been attributed many positive representations including a key change agent (Larsen & Stege, 2010), a key psychosocial resource, an inner strength or power (Cutcliffe & Grant, 2001; Duggleby et al., 2010), and a coping mechanism in the face of crisis (Soundy, Stubbs, Freeman, Coffee, & Roskell, 2014).

This process is underpinned by the third attribute of hope as a basic developmental personality trait with the existence of high- and low-hope individuals (Snyder et al., 1991). Snyder et al.'s (1991) conceptualization of hope is that people with high hope levels will report more goals, perceive that they will reach these goals, and will be more successful in actual goal attainment.

The fourth attribute of hope which is intrinsic to this cognitive process of hope is the attribution of meaning. This process has recently been extended to include a more existential transcendent perspective, with hope enabling the integration of past experiences to bring about new meaning

(Hobbs & Baker, 2012; Schrank et al., 2008) and the ability to transcend current difficulties (McCann, 2002).

This dynamism of hope encapsulates its fifth and final attribute: its interrelational process (Cutcliffe & Zinck, 2011; Herrestad & Biong, 2010). A sense of relatedness to others is consistently articulated in the literature (Duggleby & Wright, 2007; Farran et al., 1995; Morse & Doberneck, 1995). Thus, one is influenced by the others' hope presence, and this embodies the possibility of "holding hope" for others (Chandler & Hayward, 2009). This is particularly important when engaging with individuals experiencing mental distress, as professionals hold the potential to trigger and maintain hope in others, which is fundamental to the person's recovery journey (Andersen et al., 2011; Hobbs & Baker, 2012). Therein, Kinghorn (2013) argues that it is this sustaining context, whether it is relationships or one's higher power, that makes hope intelligible.

DEFINITION

Hope is a dynamic developmental personality trait which enables the possible through cognitive goal-directed processes of pathways and agency, where levels are influenced through attribution of meaning and interrelational processes.

MODEL CASE

A 52-year-old man, Tom, with a diagnosis of depression for 20 years, currently attends the local mental health day-care facility. Tom describes himself when well as an optimistic, hopeful character (personality trait). He loves his daily chats with other clients, the mental health nurse, and other members of the multidisciplinary team (interrelational processes). The center has recently rented a small allotment and Tom has accepted the task of planning the vegetables to be planted and feels energized about this venture (goal-directed process). He has secured some seeds from a local farmer and describes an inner strength to succeed (enabling the possible). Now, when Tom reviews his years of mental distress, he philosophically reflects that perhaps he needed to go through it to be able to appreciate where he is now (attribution of meaning). Thus, all defining attributes are present in this case.

RELATED CASE

John is a 21-year-old man who had a chaotic childhood; both of his parents had significant mental health problems, and John was placed in a number of foster homes (failed interrelational processes). Despite this, John gained a place in college (enabling the possible). He failed his first year and had to take a year out. Later John returned to college and secured a degree in nursing (goal-directed process). Subsequently, he was involved in a traffic accident, was hospitalized, and missed initial chances of employment. However, with careful planning and significant energy, he continued in his job search and achieved successful employment some 15 interviews later. This case is related in that it contains some of the elements necessary for hope, including the goal-directed process and enabling the possible.

BORDERLINE CASE

Rose has been a resident in a mental health unit for the past 10 years. She has articulated that she would like to live in the community with her brother, and plans are afoot to make this a reality (goal-directed process). She describes some members of staff as being like her family and says that they have sustained her through some very difficult circumstances (interrelational processes). She is, therefore, philosophical about the extended time she has spent as a resident of the mental health services (attribution of meaning). She describes herself when well as having an optimistic disposition (personality trait). However, Rose is susceptible to frequent periods of low mood and anxiety when she lacks the inner strength and confidence to pursue her plans with any sense of interest, belief, or vigor (failed enabling the possible). This is thus a borderline case, as it contains four of the five essential attributes of hope but one failed attribute (enabling the possible) is missing.

CONTRARY CASE

Mary is a 63-year-old woman who has a diagnosis of recurrent depression, has no hope for the future (failed personality trait), and describes herself as merely existing (failed enabling the possible and failed goal-directed process). She is presently homeless, refuses to engage with services, has no friends, and has very little access to other humans (failed interrelational process). She sees no meaning in life, has no plans for the future or energy to engage in making plans, and often thinks that she would be better off dead (failed attribution of meaning). This is a contrary case, as Mary lacks all five of the essential attributes of hope as it relates to recovery.

ANTECEDENTS

The antecedents are challenging life event(s), uncertainty, belief that recovery is possible, meaningful information, fighting to get better, and nurturing environment. Antecedents are underpinned by the experience of a challenging life event that provokes mental distress, the experience of infirmity, suffering, loss, and uncertainty (Cutcliffe, 2006; Miller, 2007). In particular, encountering uncertainty is a key antecedent to hope. Logically, if certainty exists, then hope is unnecessary; thus, based on degree of uncertainty, levels of hope fluctuate (Duggleby et al., 2010). A belief that recovery is possible is a required antecedent for the engagement and maintenance of hope (Andresen et al., 2011). Families identified meaningful information as being key to this belief (Jönsson, Skärsäter, Wijk, & Danielson, 2011; Tranvag & Kristoffersen, 2008).

Andresen et al. (2011) found that being angry was a pivotal experience for some individuals to trigger hope and move forward in their mental health recovery. In addition, an associated antecedent—fighting to get better—was identified as critical in triggering hope in individuals experiencing mental distress (O'Doherty & Doherty, 2010). Fighting was associated with a revolt against being labelled with an illness, along with discovery of one's intrinsic motivation for recovery. Finally, the presence of a nurturing environment with hopeful individuals makes the emergence of hope more likely (Farran et al., 1995).

CONSEQUENCES

Consequences are new perspectives/meaning in life, having the energy and ability to engage in the process of recovery, life satisfaction, making sense of one's experience, increased trust in others, being free and in control, and improved physical and psychological health. O'Doherty and Doherty (2010) describe the role of hope in strengthening the belief that recovery from mental distress is possible. This may include the development of a new perspective and meaning in life and a sense of mastery, as evidenced by having the energy and ability to engage in the process of recovery (Hobbs & Baker, 2012). Hope may also serve as a protection against experiencing failure and disappointment during this process (Herrestad & Biong, 2010).

In the context of recovery, Chan, Chan, Ditchman, Phillips, and Chou (2013) consider life satisfaction as key hope outcomes. This aligns with the ability to construct and respond to the future positively, which is variously recorded in the literature as the capacity to make sense of one's experience and to have increased trust in others (Nunn, 1996), happiness in life, to be free and in control (Hobbs & Baker, 2012; Noh et al., 2008), and to have improved physical and psychological health (Werner, 2012). For Snyder et al. (1991), the consequences of hope are congruent with its conceptualization as a goal-directed motivational force: successful (a) agency (goal-directed energy) and (b) pathways (planning to meet goals). This emerges as a strong theme throughout the literature in the context of increased pathways to wellness as experienced by service users (McCann, 2002).

EMPIRICAL REFERENTS

Empirical referents are measurable ways to demonstrate the occurrence of a concept. Logically, these are usually found in instruments to measure the concept. Significantly, a number of individuals have developed hope measures based on different conceptual frameworks (Nekolaichuk, 2005). Thus, one needs to be cognizant that one is not comparing like with like. Likewise, scales have been developed and validated for their use in nuanced areas and thus are neither valid nor reliable for generic use. Realistically, given the complexity of hope, with its tangible and intangible elements, it will always be challenging—if nigh on impossible—to obtain an absolute measurement of hope. However, this has not curtailed the growth of such instruments.

Presently, there are 32 scales for assessing hope (Shrank et al., 2008). Snyder et al.'s (1991) Hope Scales are quite distinctive, with their aforementioned narrow emphasis on goals and perceived agency and pathways to achieve goals. These have been tested more often than other scales in mental health care (Schrank et al., 2012). Recently, hope subscales as part of a larger Recovery Assessment Scale (Corrigan, Salzer, Ralph, Sangster, & Keck, 2004) have become popular. These explore goal orientation but also personal characteristics and future orientation (Schrank et al., 2012). Apart from the subscale, none of the other 32 scales was developed or validated for use in mental health care. However, some progress has occurred in this area recently, with three scales having been validated specifically for mental health use.

Van Gestel-Timmermans, Van den Bogaard, Brouwers, Herth, and Van Nieuwenhuizen (2010) validated the Herth Hope Index for use with Dutch mental health service users. This instrument has three main factors: temporality and the future, positive readiness and expectancy, and interconnectedness with self and others. In the same year, Schrank, Woppmann, Sibitz, and Lauber (2010) developed an Integrative Hope Scale for use with people experiencing severe mental distress. It covers four factors: trust and confidence, positive future orientation, social relations, and personal perspective. Finally, and most recently, Choe (2013) developed a Schizophrenia Hope Scale. Three core elements of hope are represented: positive expectations for the future, confidence in life and the future, and meaning in life. Congruence between all three sets of factors includes positivity, meaning in life, and to a lesser degree social interconnectedness.

Referents from qualitative studies also correlate well with these hope elements and include sense of meaning in life (McCann, 2002), spiritual relationship with God (Noh et al., 2008), supportive and reciprocal relationships (Houghton, 2007), and feeling understood by mental health service staff (Houghton, 2007). Finally, a recent review by Schrank et al. (2012) revealed some of the frequently occurring referents of hope in the quantitative literature as perceived recovery, self-efficacy, self-esteem, empowerment, spirituality, and social support.

SUMMARY

As seen in this chapter, hope in the context of mental health recovery is an emerging concept. It is a multidimensional dynamic process involving internal and external resources, and it is firmly rooted in the interpersonal process. The literature reviewed for this analysis was primarily situated within a positivist paradigm. Furthermore, there is a noticeable absence of first-person accounts of hope in the current empirical literature. Based on the concept analyses, defining attributes, antecedents, consequences, and empirical referents of hope have been identified. A schematic representation is provided in Figure 6.1.

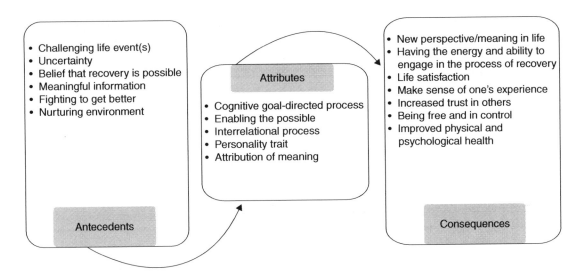

FIGURE 6.1 Hope in mental health recovery.

REFERENCES

Andresen, R., Oades, L., & Caputi, P. (2003). The experience of recovery from schizophrenia: Towards an empirically validated stage model. *Australian and New Zealand Journal of Psychiatry, 37*(5), 586–594.

Andresen, R., Oades, L., & Caputi, P. (2011). *Psychological recovery: Beyond mental illness.* Oxford, UK: Wiley-Blackwell.

Australian Health Ministers Advisory Council. (2013). *A national framework for recovery oriented mental health services: Guide for practitioners and providers.* Canberra, Australia: Author.

Chan, J., Chan, F., Ditchman, N., Phillips, B., & Chou, C. (2013). Evaluating Snyder's hope theory as a motivational model of participation and life satisfaction for individuals with spinal cord injury. *Rehabilitation Research, Policy, and Education, 27*(3), 171–185.

Chandler, R., & Hayward, M. (Eds.). (2009). *Voicing psychotic experiences: A reconsideration of recovery and diversity.* Brighton, UK: OLM-Pavilion.

Choe, K. (2013). Development and preliminary testing of the Schizophrenia Hope Scale, a brief scale to measure hope in people with schizophrenia. *International Journal of Nursing Studies, 2309,* 1–7.

Clarke, S., Oades, L., Crowe, T., Capuit, P., & Deane, F. (2009). The role of symptom distress and goal attainment in promoting aspects of psychological recovery for consumers with enduring mental illness. *Journal of Mental Health, 18*(5), 389–397.

Corrigan, P., Salzer, M., Ralph, R., Sangster, Y., & Keck, L. (2004). Examining the factor structure of the recovery assessment scale. *Schizophrenia Bulletin, 30,* 1035–1041.

Cutcliffe, J. (2006). The principles and processes of inspiring hope in bereavement counselling: A modified grounded theory study. *Journal of Psychiatric and Mental Health Nursing, 13,* 604–610.

Cutcliffe, J. (2009). Hope: The eternal paradigm for psychiatric/mental health nursing. *Journal of Psychiatric and Mental Health Nursing, 16,* 843–847.

Cutcliffe, J., & Grant, G. (2001). What are the principles and processes of inspiring hope in cognitively impaired older adults within a continuing care environment? *Journal of Psychiatric and Mental Health Nursing, 8*(5), 427–436.

Cutcliffe, J., & Zinck, K. (2011). Hope maintenance in people living long-term with HIV/AIDS. *Qualitative Research Journal, 11,* 34–49.

DuFault, K., & Martocchio, B. (1985). Hope: Its spheres and dimensions. *Nursing Clinics of North America, 20,* 371–379.

Duggleby, W., Holtslander, L., Kylma, J., Duncan, V., Hammond, C., & Williams, A. (2010). Metasynthesis of the hope experience of family caregivers of persons with chronic illness. *Qualitative Health Research, 20*(2), 148–158.

Duggleby, W., & Wright, K. (2007). The hope of professional caregivers caring for persons at the end of life. *Journal of Hospice and Palliative Nursing, 9*(1), 42–49.

Farran, C., Herth, K., & Popovich, J. (1995). *Hope and hopelessness: Critical clinical constructs.* Thousand Oaks, CA: Sage.

Gerhart, D. (2012). The mental health recovery movement and family therapy, part I: Consumer-led reform of services to persons diagnosed with severe mental illness. *Journal of Marital and Family Therapy, 38*(3), 429–442.

Hall, B. (1990). The struggle of the diagnosed terminally ill person to maintain hope. *Nursing Science Quarterly, 4*(3), 177–184.

Herrestad, H., & Biong, S. (2010). Relational hopes: A study of the lived experience of hope in some patients hospitalized for intentional self-harm. *International Journal of Qualitative Studies on Health and Well-Being, 5*(1), 4651–4659. doi:10.3402/qhw.v5i1.4651

Herth, K. (1990). Fostering hope in terminally ill people. *Journal of Advanced Nursing, 15,* 1250–1259.

Hobbs, M., & Baker, M. (2012). Hope for recovery—How clinicians may facilitate this in their work. *Journal of Mental Health, 21*(2), 144–153.

Houghton, S. (2007). Exploring hope: Its meaning for adults living with depression and for social work practice. *Advances in Mental Health, 6*(3), 186–193.

Jönsson, P. D., Skärsäter, I., Wijk, H., & Danielson, E. (2011). Experience of living with a family member with bipolar disorder. *International Journal of Mental Health Nursing, 20*(1), 29–37.

Kinghorn, W. (2013). "Hope that is seen is no hope at all": Theological constructions of hope in psychotherapy. *The Menninger Foundation, 77*(4), 369–394.

Larsen, D., & Stege, R. (2010). Hope focused practices during early psychotherapy sessions, part 1: Implicit approaches. *Journal of Psychotherapy Integration, 20,* 271–292.

McCann, T. (2002). Uncovering hope with clients who have psychotic illness. *Journal of Holistic Nursing, 20*(1), 81–99.

Menninger, K. (1959). The academic lecture: Hope. *American Journal of Psychiatry, 116,* 481–491.

Miller, J. (2007). Hope: A construct central to nursing. *Nursing Forum, 42*(1), 12–19.

Morse, J. M., & Doberneck, B. (1995). Delineating the concept of hope. *Image Journal of Nursing Scholarship, 27*(4), 277–285.

Nekolaichuk, C. (2005). Diversity or divisiveness? A critical analysis of hope. In J. Cutcliffe & H. McKenna (Eds.), *Essential concepts of nursing* (pp. 179–212). London, UK: Elsevier.

Noh, C., Choe, K., & Yang, B. (2008). Hope from the perspective of people with schizophrenia (Korea). *Archives of Psychiatric Nursing, 22*(2), 69–77.

Nunn, K. (1996). Personal hopefulness: A conceptual review of the relevance of the perceived future to psychiatry. *British Journal of Medical Psychology, 69,* 227–245.

O'Doherty, Y., & Doherty, D. (2010). Recovering from mental health problems: Giving up and fighting to get better. *International Journal of Mental Health Nursing, 19*, 3–15.

Ridgway, P. A. (2003). *Hope and mental health recovery: Co-constructing new paradigm knowledge* (unpublished dissertation proposal). University of Kansas School of Social Welfare, Lawrence, KS.

Schrank, B., Bird, V., Rudnick, A., & Slade, M. (2012). Determinants, self-management strategies and interventions for hope in people with mental disorders: Systematic search and narrative review. *Social Science and Medicine, 74*, 554–564.

Schrank, B., Stanghellini, G., & Slade, M. (2008). Hope in psychiatry. *Acta Psychiatrica Scandinavica, 118*, 421–433.

Schrank, B., Woppmann, M., Sibitz, I., & Lauber, C. (2010). Development and validation of an integrative scale to assess hope. *Health Expectations, 14*, 417–428.

Simpson, J., & Weiner, E. (1989). *The Oxford English dictionary* (2nd ed.). Oxford, UK: Clarendon Press.

Snyder, C., Harris, C., Anderson, J., Holleran, S., Irving, L., & Sigmon, S. (1991). The will and the ways: Development and validation of an individual-differences measure of hope. *Journal of Personality and Social Psychology, 60*, 570–585.

Soundy, A., Stubbs, B., Freeman, P., Coffee, P., & Roskell, C. (2014). Factors influencing patients' hope in stroke and spinal cord injury: A narrative review. *International Journal of Therapy and Rehabilitation, 21*(5), 210–218.

Stotland, E. (1969). *The psychology of hope*. San Francisco, CA: Jossey-Bass.

Tranvag, O., & Kristoffersen, K. (2008). Experience of being the spouse/cohabitant of a person with bipolar affective disorder: A cumulative process over time. *Scandinavian Journal of Caring Science, 22*, 5–18.

Tutton, E., Seers, K., Langstaff, D., & Westwood, M. (2011). Staff and patient views of the concept of hope on a stroke unit: A qualitative study. *Journal of Advanced Nursing, 68*(9), 2061–2069.

Van Gestel-Timmermans, H., Van den Bogaard, J., Brouwers, E., Herth, K., & Van Nieuwenhuizen, C. (2010). Hope as a determinant of mental health recovery: A psychometric evaluation of the Herth Hope Index-Dutch version. *Knowledge Centre for Self-Help and Consumer Expertise, 24*, 67–74.

Walker, L. O., & Avant, K. C. (2011). *Strategies for theory construction in nursing* (5th ed.). Upper Saddle River, NJ: Pearson Prentice Hall.

Werner, S. (2012). Subjective well-being, hope and needs of individuals with serious mental illness. *Psychiatry Research, 196*, 214–219.

Zinck, K., & Cutliffe, J. (2013). Hope inspiration among people living with HIV/AIDS: Theory and implications for counselors. *Journal of Mental Health Counseling, 35*(1), 60.

7

MEANING IN LIFE

There is a need for clarification of the *meaning in life* concept, which is closely related to other concepts such as spirituality and transcendence (Heintzelman & King, 2013; Parsian, 2009; Sessanna et al., 2007; Visser et al., 2009). For example, as part of the author's PhD research, a concept analysis of spirituality was conducted using Rodger's evolutionary framework (2000) that conceptualized spirituality as three dimensions: connectedness, transcendence, and meaning in life (Weathers et al., 2015). An instrument was then developed to operationalize this definition. The instrument was tested using factor analysis, and it emerged that meaning in life appeared to be similar to transcendence, with many of the items overlapping. Thus, the author thought it imperative to analyze the concept of meaning in life in order to achieve conceptual clarity. Furthermore, it is important for nurses and other health care professionals to have a clear understanding of the concept of meaning in life, especially in light of its importance during traumatic life events such as illness (Baldacchino, 2011; Molzahn et al., 2012).

Meaning in life has been conceptualized in several ways throughout the literature. For example, one definition proposed by Reker (2000) describes it as the cognizance of order, coherence, and purpose in one's existence, the pursuit and attainment of worthwhile goals and a sense of fulfilment. Other authors define it as pursuing personally valued goals or possessing a clear system of values that guide one's behavior (Crumbaugh & Maholick, 1964; Hicks et al., 2012; Krause, 2007). Indeed, a fundamental dilemma in the study of this concept is the nagging definitional ambiguity (Heintzelman & King, 2013). Yet, Heintzelman and King (2013) proposed that across the many diverse definitions, there are some commonalities: First, meaning in life is a subjective experience; second, it involves a sense of coherence; and finally, it comprises connections or relationships. For some theorists studying the concept of meaning, a meaningful life is one that "makes sense" (Baumeister, 1991; Baumeister & Vohs, 2002) or that possesses an overarching sense of coherence (Antonovsky, 1993; Antonovsky & Sourani, 1988). Baird (1985) differentiates between creating and searching for meaning in life: An individual may search for a personal meaning that had already existed in one's life; however, an individual might also need to create a new meaning in response to a current life event. Similarly, Clarke (2006) states that a person might have had a personal meaning in life in the past which needs to be revisited and redefined while searching for meaning in the current life situation.

One cannot discuss the concept of meaning in life without paying tribute to Dr. Viktor Frankl, a pioneer in the field. Viktor Frankl was a professor of neurology and psychiatry as well as a philosopher and a psychologist. Frankl (1988) proposed that the spiritual task of finding meaning in life through self-transcendence constitutes the core of existence. Frankl formulated the theory of meaning in life when he was a young boy, and was writing a book on the theory when he was captured by Nazis and imprisoned (Starck, 2008). His theory of meaning developed further as a result of his experiences in Nazi concentration camps where he observed the other prisoners. These experiences in the concentration camp served to validate his theory of meaning in life, which Frankl called Logotheory.

In Logotheory, the concept of person is based upon three core tenets: the freedom of will, the will to meaning, and meaning in life. The first of these is the freedom of human will, that is, the freedom to choose our attitude in response to any given situation (Frankl, 1988). According to Frankl (1988), a human's freedom is not freedom from conditions, but rather freedom to take a stand on whatever conditions might confront him. Logotheory purports that every person is responsible for what they become and for any choices they make; that is, a sense of responsibility to self, to life, and to others (Frankl, 1988). The second core principle of Logotheory is the will to meaning. Frankl (1988) states that every person must choose to find meaning. In other words, human beings have an inner motivation to find meaning in their lives, and they can choose to live a purposeful life (Schulenberg et al., 2008; Wong, 2011). The final core tenet of Logotheory is the meaning of life. Frankl (1985, 1988, 2011) holds that every person can find the unique meaning of each individual life situation. For Frankl (1988), there is both a meaning of life for which humanity has been searching and the freedom to embark on the fulfilment of this meaning. Frankl's theory has been expanded and several nursing research studies have used Frankl's Logotheory to frame research (Baldacchino, 2011; Coward, 2003, Coward & Kahn, 2004, 2005).

A sample of 35 empirical and theoretical papers was sourced. The author analyzed these papers to identify the defining attributes, conceptual definition, antecedents, consequences, and empirical referents of the concept. Cases were also presented that exemplified the concept of meaning in life. This concept analysis was rooted in Frankl's Logotheory and supported with conceptual and empirical evidence. It was thought that the use of a well-established theory would allow the clear delineation of the concept of meaning in life (Brandstatter et al., 2012).

DEFINING ATTRIBUTES

The defining attributes of meaning in life are *creative values, experiential values,* and *attitudinal values.*

Creative values are the first defining attribute of meaning in life. This is defined by Frankl (1988) as what we give to the world in terms of our talents and activities. For example, there is literature describing engagement in meaningful activity (Eakman, 2013; Krause, 2007). This can be anything that is meaningful to an individual, for example, gardening, playing music, painting, collecting flower petals, and so on.

Experiential values are the second defining attribute. This pertains to what we experience in the world (Frankl, 1988): for example, the relationships in our lives and our connections with self, others, a higher power, or nature. One of the eight major sources of meaning identified in the literature is interpersonal relationships (DeVogler & Ebersole, 1981). Experiential values could also include our religious practices or beliefs (Krause, 2008).

Attitudinal values are the third defining attribute. This relates to a person's attitude toward life in general and particularly toward suffering. Suffering can be physical or mental in nature and can be caused by experiencing a difficult or traumatic life event. Attitudinal values may consist of a deepened connection with a higher power, or the belief that there is an overarching pattern in life and everything happens for a reason (Molzahn et al., 2012). Changing one's attitude toward life and suffering may encourage and improve adaptation during recovery from illness (Baldacchino et al., 2011; Frankl, 1988; Walton, 2002). This may be because meaning enables the patient not only to endure illness, but also to use illness as a strengthening life experience (Baldacchino, 2003; Walton, 2002). Similarly, the ability to forgive another human being exemplifies attitudinal change (Hantman & Cohen, 2010).

DEFINITION

Meaning in life is defined as a subjective experience that provides a sense of coherence and is achieved through creative values, experiential values, and attitudinal values.

MODEL CASE

John is a 55-year-old taxi driver who smokes. He was admitted to the emergency department last week with severe chest pain and shortness of breath. John was quickly diagnosed with a myocardial infarction and underwent a percutaneous coronary intervention (PCI) to dilate the arteries of the heart. He was told by the medical team that he was lucky to be alive. On speaking to John about his experience, he says: "I was so afraid I was going to die. The fear was ever-present during my heart attack. Now, I have realized how precious my health and family are (experiential values). I now appreciate the small things that I used to take for granted. I used to be an avid cyclist but I haven't cycled over the past few years. It was not a priority in my life, even though I absolutely loved it and I know it is good for my health. So I have decided to pull the bike out of the garage and start training for the annual local charity cycle (creative values). And I'm determined to stop smoking (attitudinal values). I'm hoping that I won't have another heart attack and I'll do my best to return to normal life."

RELATED CASE

Consider the case of Jane, a 65-year-old recently retired nurse who lives alone. Jane joined a senior citizens group recently and attends a meeting once a week in the local community center. At the meeting, Jane enjoys chatting with the other retirees (experiential values). However, Jane never wishes to participate in the activities organized by the group, even though one of the events was an art class and Jane used to love painting in her younger years (failed creative values). Jane does not have much motivation to take up any of her prior hobbies or to try anything new. She is sometimes quite down on herself and questions her life (failed attitudinal values).

BORDERLINE CASE

Take, for example, the same case of John the taxi driver, who is now 1 year post-PCI; his heart attack experience is beginning to become a distant memory. On speaking to John now about his life, he says: "Oh, yes . . . that was a frightening experience I had last year. But the docs have told me the stent should keep things at bay. Sure, at least it's over now and I'm back to normal. I suppose I do spend a lot more time with my wife and children now though— I would be lost without them (experiential values). At the weekend, my family and I usually go cycling together and we did a local charity cycle last year together (creative values)." After the conversation, John enquires about where the smoking room is (failed attitudinal values).

CONTRARY CASE

Consider the case of George, who is 35 years old and homeless. He has no contact with his family and has no friends he can depend on (failed experiential values). George is also addicted to heroin and spends his days trying to get his hands on some money to buy more heroin (failed creative values). He has never engaged with the support services that sometimes approach him offering help. George has no wish to fight his heroin addiction and has never made an attempt to seek help (failed attitudinal values).

ANTECEDENTS

Firstly, the person must have experienced suffering such as a traumatic life event or a spiritual crisis (Agrimson & Taft, 2009). For example, the experience of a life-threatening illness can force a reconstruction of meaning to

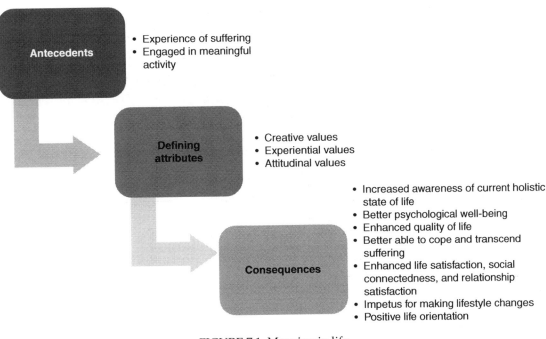

FIGURE 7.1 Meaning in life.

survive the most unfavorable conditions in life (Baldacchino, 2003; Barnard, 1984; Frankl, 1988; Taylor et al., 2000). Secondly, in order to achieve each of the defining attributes, a person must be engaged in meaningful activity (Eakman, 2013; Krause, 2007). This is particularly applicable for the creative values attribute (Figure 7.1).

CONSEQUENCES

A range of consequences occur when a person expresses meaning in life. These consequences include: increased awareness of current holistic state of life (Baldacchino et al., 2011); better psychological well-being (Eakman, 2013; Jaarsma et al., 2007; Steger et al., 2010); enhanced quality of life (Jafary et al., 2011; Krause, 2007; Krause & Shaw, 2003); better able to cope with and transcend suffering (Krause, 2007; Wong, 2013); enhanced life satisfaction, social connectedness, and relationship satisfaction (Bohlmeijer et al., 2008; Steger et al., 2010); impetus for making lifestyle changes (Baldacchino et al., 2011); and positive life orientation (Fagerstrom, 2010).

EMPIRICAL REFERENTS

In terms of operationalizing the concept of meaning in life, a range of instruments has been developed. Brandstatter et al. (2012) conducted a review of 59 meaning-in-life instruments. Results showed that 48 of the instruments apply nomothetic measurement, whereas 11 instruments use an idiographic approach. Of the nomothetic instruments, half are unidimensional ($n = 25$).

Brandstatter et al. (2012) concluded that there is a need for more integrative theorizing and research on meaning in life.

Each defining attribute of meaning in life requires an empirical referent. Yet, several authors have warned of the need to carefully choose measures that have demonstrated validity and ensure that the measures adequately tap the concept of meaning (Leontiev, 2013; Park & George, 2013). With regard to quantitatively measuring the concept, Leontiev (2013) refers to the Purpose in Life (PIL) test developed by Crumbaugh and Maholick (1964) or the Meaning in Life Questionnaire (MLQ) developed by Steger et al. (2006). In terms of the defining attributes outlined in this analysis (creative, experiential, and attitudinal values), either of these instruments would be appropriate. For example, the PIL test is a 20-item instrument designed to operationalize Frankl's concepts and to measure an individual's experience of meaning in life. It has been shown to have good reliability (Chamberlain & Zika, 1988; Seeman, 1991; Zika & Chamberlain, 1992) and some evidence of convergent and discriminant validity (Seeman, 1991). Each item is rated on a 7-point scale and total scores therefore range from 20 (low purpose) to 140 (high purpose). Examples of the 20 items include: "I am usually: completely bored (1)—exuberant, enthusiastic (7)"; "If I could choose, I would: prefer never to have been born (1)—like nine more lives just like this one (7)"; "As I view the world in relation to my life, the world: completely confuses me (1)—fits meaningfully with my life (7)," and "With regard to suicide, I have: thought of it seriously as a way out (1)—never given it a second thought (7)."

Similarly, the MLQ was developed by Steger et al. (2006) to measure the search for meaning in life and the presence of meaning in life. It consists of 10 items ranging on a scale of 1 (absolutely untrue) to 7 (absolutely true). Examples of items include: "I understand my life's meaning" and "I have discovered a satisfying life purpose." The MLQ is said to offer several improvements over other meaning-in-life measures, including no item overlap with distress measures, a stable factor structure, better discriminant validity, a briefer format, and the ability to measure the search for meaning (Steger et al., 2006). Furthermore, research has consistently supported the two-factor structure, the internal consistency of scale scores, and convergent validity of the scale (Steger & Yeon Shin, 2010). Both the MLQ and the PIL are suitable to operationalize meaning in life. However, some authors have recommended that other nonverbal methods of data collection (e.g., photography) be considered in future empirical research on meaning in life (Heintzelman & King, 2013; Steger et al., 2013).

SUMMARY

The concept of meaning in life is crucial to health care. It is central to experiences of illness and other traumatic life events. Hence, it is necessary that nurses, midwives, and other health care professionals have a good understanding of the concept. This concept analysis aimed to clarify the concept of meaning in life by identifying its antecedents, defining attributes, conceptual definition, consequences, and empirical referents. It is clear that a lot of progress has been made in research concerning the meaning in life, particularly from a theoretical or conceptual perspective. However, further empirical work is needed, including better understanding of appropriate variables of selected subgroups of instruments (Brandstatter et al., 2012) and further psychometric testing of instruments to help researchers choose the most appropriate for their research questions. This would further enhance the synthesis of the diverse empirical research findings on meaning in life and other variables. Leontiev (2013) identifies four key challenges in terms of advancing meaning research: the linguistic challenge (*meaning* is a word with multiple meanings); the dimensional challenge (meaning is multifaceted); the dynamic challenge (meaning as a living process); and the methodological challenge (how to catch meaning). Researchers interested in the concept of meaning in life would do well to heed the recommendations of Leontiev (2013) in terms of the complexity of the concept and its varied facets. Yet, it is hoped that this concept analysis provides some clarity and future direction regarding the concept of meaning in life.

REFERENCES

Agrimson, L. B., & Taft, L. B. (2009). Spiritual crisis: A concept analysis. *Journal of Advanced Nursing, 6*(2): 454–461.

Antonovsky, A. (1993). The structure and properties of the sense of coherence scale. *Social Science & Medicine, 36*(6): 725–733.

Antonovsky, A., & Sourani, T. (1988). Family sense of coherence and family adaptation. *Journal of Marriage and the Family, 50*, 79–92.

Baird, R. M. (1985). Meaning in life: Discovered or created? *Journal of Religion and Health, 24*(2), 117–124.

Baldacchino, D. (2003). *Spirituality in illness and care: Spiritual care: The views of patients, nurses, students and chaplains of Malta and Gozo.* Lancaster, UK: Veritas Press.

Baldacchino, D. (2011). Myocardial infarction: A turning point in meaning in life over time. *British Journal of Nursing, 2*(2): 107–114.

Barnard, D. (1984). Illness as a crisis of meaning: Psycho-spiritual agendas in health care. *Pastoral Psychology, 33*(2): 74–82.

Baumeister, R. F. (1991). *Meanings of life.* New York, NY: Guilford Press.

Baumeister, R. F., & Vohs, K. D. (2002). The pursuit of meaningfulness in life. In C. R. Snyder & S. J. Lopez (Eds.), *Handbook of Positive Psychology* (pp. 608–618), New York, NY: Oxford University Press.

Bohlmeijer, E. T., Westerhof, G. J., & Emmerik-de Jong, M. (2008). The effects of integrative reminiscence on meaning in life: Results of a quasi-experimental study. *Aging and Mental Health, 12*(5), 639–646.

Brandstätter, M., Baumann, U., Borasio, G. D., & Fegg, M. J. (2012). Systematic review of meaning in life assessment instruments. *Psycho-Oncology, 2*(10), 1034–1052.

Chamberlain, K., & Zika, S. (1988). Measuring meaning in life: An examination of three scales. *Personality and Individual Differences, 9*(3), 589–596.

Clarke, J. (2006). A discussion paper about "meaning" in the nursing literature on spirituality: An interpretation of meaning as "ultimate concern" using the work of Paul Tillich. *International Journal of Nursing Studies, 43*(7), 915–921.

Coward, D. D. (2003). Facilitation of self-transcendence in a breast cancer support group: II. *Oncology Nursing Forum, 30*(2), 291–300.

Coward, D. D., & Kahn, D. L. (2004). Resolution of spiritual disequilibrium by women newly diagnosed with breast cancer. *Oncology Nursing Forum, 31*(2), E24–31. doi:10.1188/04.onf.e24-e31

Coward, D. D., & Kahn, D. L. (2005). Transcending breast cancer: Making meaning from diagnosis and treatment. *Journal of Holistic Nursing, 23*(3), 264–283.

Crumbaugh, J. C., & Maholick, L. T. (1964). An experimental study in existentialism: The psychometric approach to Frankl's concept of noogenic neurosis. *Journal of Clinical Psychology, 20*(2), 200–207.

DeVogler, K. L., & Ebersole, P. (1981). Adults' meaning in life. *Psychological Reports, 49*(1), 87–90.

Eakman, A. M. (2013). Relationships between meaningful activity, basic psychological needs, and meaning in life: Test of the Meaningful Activity and Life Meaning model. *OTJR: Occupation, Participation and Health, 33*(2), 100–109.

Fagerström, L. (2010). Positive life orientation–an inner health resource among older people. *Scandinavian Journal of Caring Sciences, 24*(2), 349-356.

Frankl, V. E. (1985). *Man's search for meaning.* New York, NY: Simon & Schuster.

Frankl, V. E. (1988). *The will to meaning: Foundations and applications of logotherapy.* New York, NY: New American Library.

Frankl, V. E. (2011). *Man's search for ultimate meaning.* Chatham, UK: Random House Group Limited.

Hantman, S., & Cohen, O. (2010). *Forgiveness in late life. Journal of Gerontological Social Work, 53*(7), 613–630.

Heintzelman, S. J., & King, L. A. (2013). On knowing more than we can tell: Intuitive processes and the experience of meaning. *Journal of Positive Psychology, 8*(6), 471–482.

Hicks, J. A., Trent, J., Davis, W. E., & King, L. A. (2012). Positive affect, meaning in life, and future time perspective: An application of socioemotional selectivity theory. *Psychology and Aging, 27*(1), 181.

Jaarsma, T. A., Pool, G., Ranchor, A. V., & Sanderman, R. (2007). The concept and measurement of meaning in life in Dutch cancer patients. *Psycho-Oncology, 16*(3), 241–248.

Jafary, F., Farahbakhsh, K., Shafiabadi, A., & Delavar, A. (2011). Quality of life and menopause: Developing a theoretical model based on meaning in life, self-efficacy beliefs, and body image. *Aging & Mental Health, 15*(5), 630–637.

Krause, N. (2007). Longitudinal study of social support and meaning in life. *Psychology and Aging, 22*(3), 456.

Krause, N. (2008). The social foundation of religious meaning in life. *Research on Aging, 30*(4), 395–427.

Krause, N., & Shaw, B. A. (2003). Role-specific control, personal meaning, and health in late life. *Research on Aging, 25*(6), 559–586.

Leontiev, D.A. (2013) Personal meaning: A challenge for psychology. *Journal of Positive Psychology, 8*(6), 459–470.

Molzahn, A., Sheilds, L., Bruce, A., Stajduhar, K., Makaroff, K. S., Beuthin, R., & Shermak, S. (2012). People living with serious illness: Stories of spirituality. *Journal of Clinical Nursing, 21*(15–16), 2347–2356.

Park, C. L., & George, L. S. (2013). Assessing meaning and meaning making in the context of stressful life events: Measurement tools and approaches. *The Journal of Positive Psychology, 8*(6), 483–504.

Parsian, N. (2009). Developing and validating a questionnaire to measure spirituality: A psychometric process. *Global Journal of Health Science, 1*(1), 2.

Reker, G. T. (2000). Theoretical perspective, dimensions, and measurement of existential meaning. In G. T. Reker & K. Chamberlain (Eds.), *Exploring existential meaning: Optimizing human development across the life span* (pp. 39–55). Thousand Oaks, CA: Sage.

Rodgers, B. L. (2000). Concept analysis: An evolutionary view. In B. L. Rodgers & K. A. Knafl (Eds.), *Concept Development in Nursing: Foundations, Techniques, and Applications* (pp. 77–102). Philadelphia, PA: Saunders.

Schulenberg, S. E., Hutzell, R. R., Nassif, C., & Rogina, J. M. (2008). Logotherapy for clinical practice. *Psychotherapy: Theory, Research, Practice, Training, 45*(4), 447.

Seeman, M. (1991). Alienation and anomie. *Measures of personality and social psychological attitudes, 1*, 291–371.

Sessanna, L., Finnell, D., & Jezewski, M. A. (2007). Spirituality in nursing and health-related literature: A concept analysis. *Journal of Holistic Nursing, 25*(4), 252–262.

Starck, P. (2008). Theory of Meaning. In M. J. Smith & P. Liehr (Eds.), *Middle range theory for nursing*. New York, NY: Springer Publishing Company.

Steger, M. F., & Yeon Shin, J. (2010). The relevance of the Meaning in Life Questionnaire to therapeutic practice: A look at the initial evidence. *International Forum for Logotherapy, 33*(2), 95.

Steger, M. F., Frazier, P., Oishi, S., & Kaler, M. (2006). The Meaning in Life Questionnaire: Assessing the presence of and search for meaning in life. *Journal of Counseling Psychology, 53*(1), 80.

Steger, M. F., Littman-Ovadia, H., Miller, M., Menger, L., & Rothmann, S. (2013). Engaging in work even when it is meaningless: Positive affective disposition and meaningful work interact in relation to work engagement. *Journal of Career Assessment, 21*(2), 348–361.

Steger, M. F., Pickering, N. K., Adams, E., Burnett, J., Shin, J. Y., Dik, B. J., & Stauner, N. (2010). The quest for meaning: Religious affiliation differences in the correlates of religious quest and search for meaning in life. *Psychology of Religion and Spirituality, 2*(4), 206.

Taylor, S. E., Kemeny, M. E., Reed, G. M., Bower, J. E., & Gruenewald, T. L. (2000). Psychological resources, positive illusions, and health. *American Psychologist, 55*(1), 99.

Visser, A., Garssen, B., & Vingerhoets, A. (2009). Spirituality and well-being in cancer patients: A review. *Psycho-Oncology, 19*, 565–572.

Walton, J. (2002). Finding a balance: A grounded theory study of spirituality in hemodialysis patients. *Nephrology Nursing Journal: Journal of the American Nephrology Nurses' Association, 29*(5), 447–456.

Weathers, E., McCarthy, G., & Coffey, A. (2015). Concept analysis of spirituality: An evolutionary approach. *Nursing Forum*, early online publication. Retrieved from http://www.ncbi.nlm.nih.gov/pubmed/25644366

Wong, P. T. (2011). Positive psychology 2.0: Towards a balanced interactive model of the good life. *Canadian Psychology, 52*(2), 69.

Wong, P. T. (Ed.). (2013). *The Human Quest for Meaning: Theories, Research, and Applications*. London, UK: Routledge.

Zika, S., & Chamberlain, K. (1992). On the relation between meaning in life and psychological well-being. *British Journal of Psychology, 83*(1), 133–145.

SERENA M. FITZGERALD and ELAINE LEHANE

8

MEDICATION HABITS

Habit is an undervalued construct in health and adherence research. The importance of habits in facilitating medication-adherent behavior specifically, is documented within empirical adherence literature particularly from the patients' perspective (Lehane & McCarthy, 2007).

Habits encompass automatic links between cues in the environment and behaviors that are associated with these cues. The automatic qualities and reliance on stimulus control for habits are deemed powerful strategies that influence regulatory success of a specific behavior through the ease with that responses are executed (Neal et al., 2006; Wood et al., 2005). Reach (2005) suggests that habit formation is advantageous for the individual trying to maintain therapeutic adherence in three main ways. Firstly, habit forming helps individuals to avoid all unpleasant (if any) thoughts related to the disease each time they take their medication, unconsciously helping them to cope with a chronic condition. A second advantage relates to the calming effect of forming a habit. It is proposed that it is easier to complete a task that one is used to performing, thereby making it easier to perform the task than to submit to the temptation not to act, or to have to decide to act (for example, brushing your teeth). Finally, habit represents an effective alternative to memory, as memory relies on intent and conscious decision making. Habit enables individuals to recall events related to the time of the day.

To date, no concept analysis has been conducted to explain the various dimensions of medication habits and the complexities related to this concept with regard to how medications are managed.

DEFINING ATTRIBUTES

The defining attributes are *habitual automaticity, cues in the environment, behavior routinization,* and *volitional control.*

The first attribute, habitual automaticity, derives from the concept of habit strength. Phillips, Leventhal, and Leventhal (2013) describe habit strength as one of three theorized constructs for successful long-term treatment adherence. Phillips et al. (2013) describe *habit* as long-term behavior maintenance, specifically making it a daily occurrence without thought. Issues in relation to taking medication can become a normal part of a patient's life, becoming a habitual process (Moen et al., 2009). Elderly patients often view medication taking as a consequence of age, which in turn requires medication taking to become a habit; it is during this process that changes in daily routine begin (Henriques et al., 2012). Engaging in habit-forming behavior can be triggered automatically by environmental cues in a person's daily routine (Wood & Neal 2007).

The second attribute identified was cues in the environment, such as mealtime, wake-up, and sleep routines. Certain individuals within a person's life (e.g., a supportive family) can help in this cueing development process (Wu et al., 2008). Wu et al. (2008) state that developing a habit of taking medication daily is an essential facilitator of adherence. Ruppar's and Russell's (2009) study described how several participants developed habits to ensure that they took medications with food as necessary.

Behavior routinization, the third attribute, is described mainly through automaticity, expression of identity, and history of repetition (Boleman et al., 2011). Using structured care plans to establish routines may help older adults adhere to medication (O'Carroll, Chambers, Dennis, Sudlow, & Johnston, 2013). In a study conducted with kidney transplant recipients, many participants described taking medication as just being a part of their daily routine. However, having a "routine" was identified as an essential component of successful medication adherence for participants. When such routines were compromised, it created major difficulties in establishing medication-taking habits (Ruppar & Russell, 2009). Developing a habit is essential for long-term treatment adherence; it constitutes the functional characteristics of habit, that is, an individual performs behavior automatically as part of his or her daily routine (Phillips et al., 2013, p. 1137). Therefore, interventions should enhance the strength of a habit by encouraging repetition and identifying the significance of a daily routine. Notably, repetitive behavior can often become habitual and is therefore no longer under volitional control.

The fourth attribute identified was volitional control. Habit development may consist of an individual not having to utilize their cognitive resources in remembering and performing certain behaviors (Phillips et al., 2014). Habits can be automatically triggered and can often occur in the absence of awareness and conscious control (Bargh, 1994). Radomski and Davis (2002) identify that semiautomatic habits assist in the proficiency of consistent performance due to a minimal demand on both an individual's memory and decision making processes. Although education is vital in providing key information for adherence to medication regimens, it is long-term adherence through volitional control that ultimately guides an individual's medication-taking habits (Ruppar, 2010).

DEFINITION

Medication habit is defined as habitual automaticity derived from behavioral routinization, triggered by cues in the environment, and influenced by a person's volitional control. Therefore, habit moderates or mediates the relationship between cognitions and behavior.

MODEL CASE

Mary was diagnosed with hypertension 10 years ago. Subsequently, she has been in and out of the hospital quite regularly with numerous medical conditions. On admission, the medical team ask Mrs. Murphy the same question: "Have you been compliant with your medication this month?" to which Mrs. Murphy responds, "I find it hard these days." She lives alone, which she finds difficult, and her daily routine (behavioral routinization) changes every day. Some days she would take her medication without thinking (volitional control), but this was very rare. When her husband was alive, he would always remind Mary to take her medication in the morning and evening, and this led to her having a better quality of life (cues in the environment). The medical team decided that Mary needed to develop her own new habits which would help remind her to take her medication automatically (habitual automaticity) as part of her daily routine.

RELATED CASE

The S.I.M.P.L.E intervention is a tool used to increase medication adherence (American College of Preventive Medicine, 2001). It assists in simplifying regimens, imparting knowledge, modifying patient beliefs and behavior, providing communication and trust, omitting bias, and evaluating adherence. This may include breaking behavior routines (behavior routinization), and/ or adjusting timing, frequency, amount, and dosage for each patient. Unfortunately, in Mary's case this could lead to Mary having to create a new medication-taking routine, and remove one that she already has in place (failed habitual automaticity). Furthermore, S.I.M.P.L.E involves patient's families if appropriate, ensures that patients understand their risks if they do not take their medications, incorporates patient input in treatment decisions (volitional control), and develops patient-centered communication. In Mary's case, health professionals should also identify what new environmental triggers are helping Mary take her medication (cues in the environment).

BORDERLINE CASE

Mary dislikes living alone; she finds it difficult to cope since her husband passed away. The recurrent inpatient stays in the hospital made life easier. When Mary was in the hospital, she felt like she could relax, as she did not have to think about taking her medication (volitional control). Mary did worry, however, that her family and general practitioner (GP) believed she did not take her medication on purpose, even though at times this was true (failed habitual automaticity). On one occasion in hospital, Mary spoke with the lady next to her: "I was fine at home when my husband was alive. I would take my medication in the morning and in the evening. We had a good system; I would always take them with my morning and evening cup of tea" (cues in the environment). "It's nice being in here sometimes, the nurses have the same routine," she laughs (behavior routinization).

CONTRARY CASE

Mary is newly diagnosed with hypertension. She is having difficulty understanding the need to take her newly prescribed medication. "I feel fine," she stated. She never had problems with her health before, and would only take medication if absolutely necessary (failed habitual automaticity). Mary spoke to other patients in the hospital and wondered how they remembered to take their medication every day, as some patients were on more than 10 tablets at a time (failed cues in the environment). The patients advised her that medication taking became part of their daily routine, and certain things throughout the day reminded them to take their medication. However, Mary voiced her concerns to the medical staff: "My routine changes every day, I am always out with friends and family, and I really don't think I would remember to take these tablets every day" (failed behavior routinization). Mary would prefer to deal with this matter without having to take medication. She made the decision to change her diet and increase her exercise (failed volitional control). In this case, none of the attributes of medication habit are presented.

ANTECEDENTS

The antecedents to medication habit are habit formation and previous behavior. Habit formation refers to the development of a habit when a specific behavior is performed frequently in an unvarying context (Lally et al., 2010; Wood & Neal, 2007). Habits have further been described as goal-directed acts (Verplanken et al., 2005). Habits do not develop randomly; they are, however, formed because they serve an individual. Habit can often develop in stable situations when a particular sequence of acts is functional and efficient for that specific individual (Verplanken et al., 2005). Habit behaviors are developed through a process of repetition, frequency, and measures of past behavior (Triandis, 1977). Investigating habit formation has the potential to assist in designing health behavior change interventions (Lally & Gardner, 2013).

Most of our everyday behaviors are recurrences or variants of behaviors that we have previously performed many times (Verplanken et al., 2005). Previous behavior was described in the context of long-term behavior maintenance (Philps et al., 2013). Additionally, van Es et al. (2002) reported on the significance of previous behavior as a predictor of adherence. Ruppar and Russell (2009) described taking medication as being a part of a patient's daily routine. Interestingly, participants in this study stated that they could not remember a time when they did not regularly take medication, drawing on the integral nature of past behaviors. Adams and Carter (2010) acknowledge the link between past behavior and habit, reporting patients being incapable of reversing years of bad habits. Measures of past behavioral frequency have shown predictability in the occurrence of future behavior beyond certain antecedents of behavior, for example, attitudes and intentions (Sutton, 1994; Verplanken & Wood, 2006).

CONSEQUENCES

Consequences of medication habit include habit strength and adherence behavior. Habit strength is a function of the frequency with which an action has been repeated in a stable context and the acquisition of a high degree of habitual automaticity (Orbell, 2013). Habit strength only increases as a result of frequent recurrences of positive reinforcements. Moreover, habit strength affects the decision individuals make, and decreases the amount of information acquired and applied before that decision is made (Aarts, Verplanken, & Knippenberg, 1998). Furthermore, habit strength reflects automatic processes that are not deliberate (Phillips et al., 2013). However, intentional nonadherence is also related, as individuals who skip or adjust doses of medication often do so because of treatment-related beliefs or bad experiences. Therefore, these individuals are less likely to develop strong medication taking habits (Phillips et al., 2013).

The next consequence is adherence behavior. *Adherence* to a medication regimen is commonly defined as the degree to which patients take medications as prescribed by their health care providers (Osterberg & Blaschke, 2005). It could be assumed that the stronger the habit behavior, the better the adherence level. As a result, the stronger the patient's adherence level, the stronger the habit. Consequently, this would improve the therapeutic efficacy of a drug regimen within a patient's clinical health outcomes. Teaching patients how to form habits integrated within their cognitive procedures could be used as a therapeutic educational technique aimed at improving their adherence to treatment (Reach, 2005). Lehane and McCarthy (2007) acknowledge that factors related to unintentional nonadherence, such as habits or formation of routines, must be addressed if an individual is to maintain long-term medication adherence.

EMPIRICAL REFERENTS

The Self-Report Habit Index (SRHI; Verplanken & Orbell, 2003) assesses habitual action: repetition, automaticity, and relevance to self-identity. The SRHI supports theoretical predictions in behavior and the moderating of intention/behavior relationships in stable decisional contexts (Lehane, McCarthy, Collender, Deasy, & O'Sullivan, 2010). However, to gain an in-depth understanding of medication habits in our patients, utilizing the Reasoning and Regulating Medication Adherence Instrument affords clinicians and researchers the opportunity to appreciate the nature of patients' adherent behavior through the examination of issues that may impede adherence (Lehane et al., 2013). Furthermore, the Medication Taking Questionnaire—Patterned Behavior (MTQ-PB; Johnson, 2002) focuses on nonadherence in relation to patterned behavior, which is embedded in the concepts of "regularity of lifestyle, access, and remembering" (Lehane et al. 2013, p. 66; Figure 8.1).

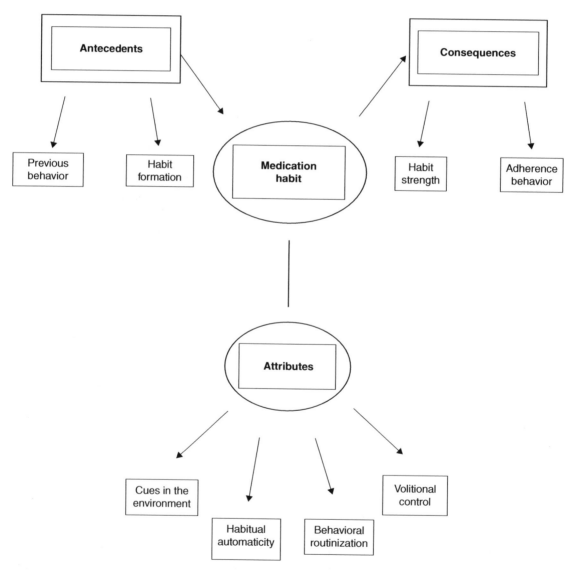

FIGURE 8.1 Medication habit.

SUMMARY

This concept analysis has identified key attributes within the concept of medication habit. These attributes have assisted in defining medication habit as habitual automaticity derived from behavioral routinization, triggered by cues in the environment, and influenced by a person's volitional control. Establishing antecedents and consequences further clarified the concept of medication habit by highlighting the significant influence of habit formation, previous behaviors, habit strength, and adherence behavior. The model case presents all defining attributes in the context of medication habit, whereas related, borderline, and contrary cases provide different perspectives to strengthen the understanding of the concept of medication habit.

REFERENCES

Aarts, H., Verplanken, B., & Knippenberg, A. (1998). Predicting behavior from actions in the past: Repeated decision making or a matter of habit? *Journal of Applied Social Psychology, 28*(15), 1355–1374.

Adams, O. P., & Carter, A. O. (2010). Diabetes and hypertension guidelines and the primary health care practitioner in Barbados: Knowledge, attitudes, practices and barriers—A focus group study. *BMC Family Practice, 11*, 96.

American College of Preventive Medicine. (2011). Medication adherence: Improving Health Outcomes Time Tool: A resource from the American College of Preventive Medicine. Retrieved from http://www.acpm.org/?MedAdhereTTProviders.

Bargh, J. A. (1994). The four horsemen of automaticity: Awareness, efficiency, intention, and control in social cognition. In R. S. Wyer, Jr., & T. K. Srull (Eds.), *Handbook of social cognition* (2nd ed., pp. 1–40). Hillsdale, NJ: Erlbaum.

Bolman, C., Arwert, T. G., & Völlink, T. (2011). Adherence to prophylactic asthma medication: Habit strength and cognitions. *Heart & Lung, 40*(1), 63–75.

Henriques, M. A., Costa, M. A., & Cabrita, J. (2012). Adherence and medication management by the elderly. *Journal of Clinical Nursing, 21*(21/22), 3096–3105.

Johnson, M. J. (2002). The medication-taking questionnaire for measuring patterned behaviour adherence. *Communicating Nursing Research, 35*, 65–70.

Lally, P., & Gardner, B. (2013). Promoting habit formation. *Health Psychology Review, 7*(Suppl. 1), S137–S158.

Lally, P., van Jaarsveld, C.H.M., Potts, H.W.W., & Wardle, J. (2010). How are habits formed: Modelling habit formation in the real world. *European Journal of Social Psychology, 40*, 998–1009.

Lehane, E., & McCarthy, G. (2007). Intentional and unintentional medication non-adherence: A comprehensive framework for clinical research and practice? A discussion paper. *International Journal of Nursing Studies, 44*(8), 1468–1477.

Lehane, E., McCarthy, G., Collender, V., Deasy, A., & O'Sullivan, K. (2013). The reasoning and regulating medication adherence instrument for patients with coronary artery disease: Development and psychometric evaluation. *Journal of Nursing Measurement, 21*(1), 64–79.

Moen, J., Bohm, A., Tillenius, T., Antonov, K., Nilsson, J.L., & Ring, L. (2009) "I don't know how many of these [medicines] are necessary…"—a focus group study among elderly users of multiple medicines. *Patient Education and Counselling, 74*, 135–141.

Neal, D. T., Wood, W., & Quinn, J. M. (2006). Habits: A repeat performance. *Current Directions in Psychological Science, 15*, 198–202.

O'Carroll, R. E., Chambers, J. A., Dennis, M., Sudlow, C., & Johnston, M. (2013). Improving adherence to medication in stroke survivors: A pilot randomised controlled trial. *Annals of Behavioral Medicine, 46*(3), 358–368.

Orbell, S. (2013). Habit strength. In M. Gellman & J. R. Turner (Eds.), *Encyclopedia of behavioral medicine* (pp. 885–886). New York, NY: Springer.

Osterberg, L., & Blaschke, T. (2005). Adherence to medication. *New England Journal of Medicine, 353*(5), 487–497.

Phillips, L. A., Leventhal, H., & Leventhal, E. A. (2013). Assessing theoretical predictors of long-term medication adherence: Patients' treatment-related beliefs, experiential feedback and habit development. *Psychology & Health, 28*(10), 1135–1151.

Radomski, M. V., & Davis, E. S. (2002). Optimizing cognitive abilities. In C. Trombly & M. Radomski (Eds.), *Occupational therapy for physical dysfunction* (5th ed., pp. 609–627). New York, NY: Lippincott Williams & Wilkins.

Reach, G. (2005). Role of habit in adherence to medical treatment. *Diabetic Medicine, 22*(4), 415–420.

Ruppar, T. M. (2010). Randomized pilot study of a behavioral feedback intervention to improve medication adherence in older adults with hypertension. *Journal of Cardiovascular Nursing, 25*(6), 470–479. doi:10.1097/JCN.0b013e3181d5f9c5

Ruppar, T. M., & Russell, C. L. (2009). Medication adherence in successful kidney transplant recipients. *Progress in Transplantation, 19*(2), 167–172.

Sutton, S. (1994). The past predicts the future: Interpreting behaviour–behaviour relationships in social psychological models of health behaviour. In D. R. Rutter & L. Quine (Eds.), *Social psychology and health: European perspectives* (pp. 71–88). Aldershot, UK: Avebury.

Triandis, H. C. (1977). *Interpersonal behavior*. Monterey, CA: Brooks/Cole.

Verplanken, B., Myrbakk, V., & Rudi, E. (2005). The measurement of habit. In T. Betsch & S. Haberstroh (Eds.), *The routines of decision making* (pp. 231–247). Mahwah NJ: Lawrence Erlbaum.

Verplanken, B., & Wood, W. (2006). Breaking and creating habits: Consequences for public policy interventions. *Journal of Public Policy & Marketing, 25*, 90–103.

Wood, W., Tam, L., & Guerrero Witt, M. (2005). Changing circumstances, disrupting habits. *Journal of Personality and Social Psychology, 88*, 918–933.

Wood, W., & Neal, D. T. (2007). A new look at habits and the habit–goal interface. *Psychological Review, 114*, 843–863.

Wu, J. R., Moser, D. K., Lennie, T. A., Peden, A. R., Chen, Y. C., & Heo, S. (2008). Factors influencing medication adherence in patients with heart failure. *Heart & Lung, 37*(1), 8.

9

MOTIVATION

Motivation is a complex, multifaceted term with many meanings that is used frequently in different contexts and environments (Dornyei & Ushioda, 2013). Although motivation is just one factor that influences performance, it is a vital determinant of achievement and critical element in success. Motivation is a theoretical construct used to explain the reasons underlying behavior relating to initiation, direction, and intensity of goal-directed behavior (Whelan & Barnes-Homes, 2013). It is an internal state that directs and maintains behavior. The origin of the concept of motivation stems from the early psychology literature (Gollwitzer & Oettingen, 2002). In nursing, motivation is not a new concept, appearing first in the literature in the 1980s (Toode, Routasalo, & Suominen, 2011). It is a central phenomenon in nursing and is critical to effective nursing leadership and management in health care organizations (Bishop, 2009). More specifically, motivation has been proposed as a key predictor in the practice of health promotion. Health behavior change can be difficult to predict or control, but motivation has been shown to be a powerful and consistent predictor of outcome. It is widely recognized as a key element influencing behavior change (Teixeria, Silva, Mata, Palmeria, & Markland, 2012).

Motivation is complex and understanding motivation has proven to be difficult. Several motivational theories have been developed to explain the concept. However, no single dominant theory fully explains motivation, though several have made a significant contribution to its understanding (Graham & Weiner, 1996). Because motivation is poorly defined in the literature, many researchers find it difficult to measure, due to its multiple interpretations. In light of this, undertaking a concept analysis is necessary to obtain greater clarity and gain an in-depth understanding about its meaning.

DEFINING ATTRIBUTES

The defining attributes of the concept are *self-determination*, *self-efficacy*, and *readiness to change*.

The first attribute, self-determination, concerns all aspects of intention and activation relating to the degree to which an individual's behavior is self-determined (Deci & Ryan, 1985). It relates to individuals who think about their actions reflectively and subsequently engage in those actions (Deci & Ryan, 2008). Individuals who are self-determined have the ability to make choices and exercise a high degree of control to initiate specific behavior (Pearson, 2011).

Self-efficacy, the second attribute, refers to individuals' beliefs about their capabilities to initiate and perform a certain activity regardless of obstacles (Bandura, 1977). According to Bandura (1991), individuals' self-efficacy beliefs determine their level of motivation. Zulkosky (2009) suggests that the higher the level of self-efficacy, the higher the levels of goals and the greater the result. Self-efficacy is frequently used across disciplines to assess an individual's beliefs about likelihood of engagement in certain behaviors.

The third attribute, readiness to change, involves a willingness to want to change behavior that will evolve into action. Kruglanski, Chernikova, Schori-eyal, and Kopetz (2014) describe readiness to change as a desire to satisfy a want, whether implicit or explicit. Once individuals are ready to change, achievement of certain goals is possible. This is important and significant, as this will fundamentally lead to better performance and ultimately behavior change (Marcus & Owen, 1992).

DEFINITION

Based on the preceding analysis, *motivation* is the driving force within individuals which causes a specific action or certain behavior that is underpinned by self-determination, self-efficacy, and readiness to change.

MODEL CASE

John, 78 years of age, is obese and was recently diagnosed with type 2 diabetes. He states that his weight has continued to increase over the past 5 years, and he is presently at the highest weight he has ever been. He has been repeatedly advised by his general practitioner to lose weight and exercise to improve his health status. He has decided to take part in a healthy aging initiative program that is being run in the day-care center where he attends 3 times weekly. The nurse has identified management goals and determined a plan of care with a focus on weight loss and improved diabetes control. John has tried on numerous occasions to lose weight and increase his exercise, but without success. He now feels more determined (self-determination) to change his behavior and believes (self-efficacy) he can lose weight this time. He admits to being ready to change (readiness to change) his unhealthy lifestyle and work toward achieving his realistic goals identified by him and the nurse.

In this case, all three attributes (self-determination, self-efficacy, and readiness to change) are present.

RELATED CASE

As part of a back-to-work initiative, John has been advised (self-efficacy) by his supervisor to set up a soccer team in his local area to create community engagement. John reluctantly begins to engage (failed self-determination) with the project and slowly organizes the event (readiness to change). Motivated by the thought of making money out of organizing the event, he charges 10 euro per person per night to participate. An average amount of people supported the event on the first night. However, every week thereafter the numbers dropped significantly due to the high participation fees.

This case shows some critical attributes of the concept of motivation (self-efficacy, readiness to change), but there is failed self-determination.

BORDERLINE CASE

Mark is 30 years old, married, with two young children. He weighs 280 pounds and has recently been complaining of breathlessness. He admits to being in denial about his weight, but his breathlessness has now inhibited him from playing with his children. His doctor has advised him to lose weight immediately for health reasons. Mark has struggled to lose weight in the past. Every time he loses weight, he regains it within a short time. Mark wants to take control over his situation and has made an appointment now to meet a dietician and join a gym. He is determined (self-determination) to lose weight and is ready to change (readiness to change) his behavior, as he wants to live a full and active life with his family. Despite his best intentions to change his situation, Mark is very apprehensive (failed self-efficacy) about his ability to lose weight, due to his past endeavors with successes and failures with diets and weight loss.

Mark's case has two defining attributes (self-determination and readiness to change). Self-efficacy is missing from this case study.

CONTRARY CASE

Paul is overweight and has been gaining weight steadily over the past 5 years (failed self-determination). He loves eating all kinds of food and does not believe in eating healthy, exercising, or dieting (failed self-efficacy, failed readiness to change).

In this case, there is no evidence of self-determination, self-efficacy, or readiness to change. No defining attributes of motivation are described here.

ANTECEDENTS

The antecedents of motivation are needs and goals. Motivation has been shown to be an internal state that activates behavior, driven by internal needs within individuals (Moody & Pesut, 2006). Ochsner, Scholz, and Hornung (2013) state that motivation occurs as a response to needs requiring fulfillment, as unsatisfied needs create an imbalance that activates behavior. According to Maslow (1954), needs are classified into five categories ranging from physiological needs, need for security, social needs, need for self-esteem, and need for self-realization. Collectively, these needs capture broad-ranging motivations and can be described as *intrinsic motivations*. These needs differ among individuals and evidence suggests that they form the basis of motivation (Maskin & Hopkins, 2014). Furthermore, motivation is described as the activation of *goal-oriented behavior*, which is defined as an internal drive that activates behavior that gives it direction (Singh, 2011). Goals play an imperative role as determinants of behavior and indicators of motivation, as they define an individual's primary reason for engagement (Ojun & Karoly, 2007; Schuz, Wurm, Warner, Wolff, & Schwarzer, 2014). Together, needs and goals are antecedents necessary for motivation to occur.

CONSEQUENCES

It is important to note that the consequences of motivation can only occur if the antecedents of motivation are in place. The consequences of motivation are success, sense of achievement, and change of behavior. Motivation is a complex issue determined by external and internal factors and is strongly associated with achievement, success, and change of behavior. Singh (2011) describes motivated individuals' performance as a subjective, internal, and psychological drive. One of the most important beliefs underpinning motivation is that it activates and guides behavior leading to accomplishment of goals (Schwarzer & Luszczynska, 2008). Regardless of this, it is important to note that motivated individuals do not always achieve success in attaining the desired changes. Moreover, an individual's motivational levels can fluctuate, and maintenance of motivation over time is of even greater complexity.

EMPIRICAL REFERENTS

Empirical referents, according to Walker and Avant (2005), are the ways in which a concept could be measured. Given that motivation sometimes, but not always, culminates in action, challenges exist in measuring motivation. Additionally, assessing cognitive aspects of motivation such as goals can be difficult, as they are not directly observable. Many measures of motivation use either self-reporting measures or rating scales.

Measurements of the attributes of motivation have been developed through the Weight Efficacy Life-Style Questionnaire (WEL; Clarke, Abrams, & Niaura, 1991), Self-Determination Scale (Sheldon, Ryan, & Reis, 1996), and Decision Balance Weight Management Scale (DBWM; Marcus, Selby, Niaura, & Rossi, 1992; Prochaska et al., 1994; Turner, Thomas, Wagner, & Moseley, 2008).

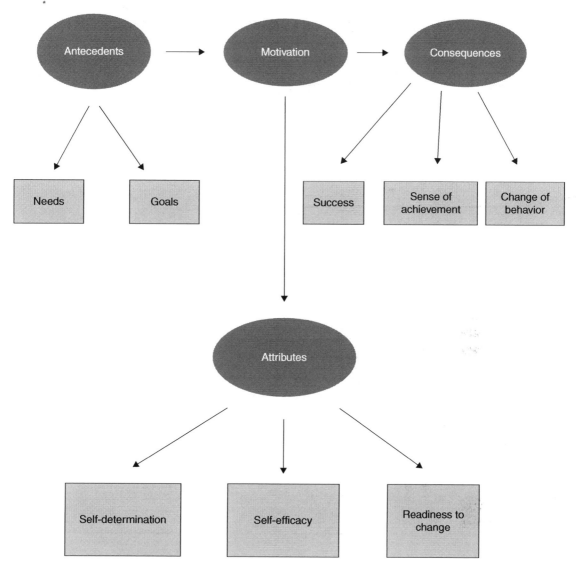

FIGURE 9.1 Motivation.

The relationships between the antecedents, attributes, and consequences are shown in Figure 9.1.

SUMMARY

Motivation is widely recognized as a key predictor of change. Examining the concept of motivation is important, as the concept has important implications and outcomes. The definition offers an understanding of what motivation represents and will potentially improve clarity relating to the concept. Having a clear and consistent understanding of the meaning of this concept and its empirical measurement is imperative.

REFERENCES

Bandura, A. (1977). Self-efficacy: Toward a unifying theory of behavioural change. *Psychological Review, 84*(2), 191–215.

Bandura, A. (1991). Self-efficacy mechanism in physiological activation and health promoting behaviour. In J. Maddem (Ed.), *Neuro-biology of learning, emotion and affect* (pp. 229–270). New York, NY: Raven Press.

Bishop, V. (2009). *Leadership for nursing & allied health care professions*. Berkshire, UK: Open University Press.

Clarke, M. M., Abrams, D. B., & Niaura, R. S. (1991). Self-efficacy in weight management. *Journal of Consulting and Clinical Psychology, 59*(5), 739–744.

Deci, E. L., & Ryan, R. M. (1985). *Intrinsic motivation and self-determination in human behaviour*. New York, NY: Plenum.

Deci, E. L., & Ryan, R. M. (2008). Self-determination theory: A macro-theory of human motivation, development, and health. *Canadian Psychology, 49*, 182–185.

Dornyei, Z., & Ushioda, E. (2013). *Teaching and researching motivation*. Abingdon, UK: Routledge.

Gollwitzer, P. M., & Oettingen, G. (2002). History of the concept motivation. In N. J. Smelser & P. B. Baltes (Eds.), *International encyclopaedia of the social & behavioural sciences* (pp. 10109–10112). New York, NY: Elsevier.

Graham, G., & Weiner, B. (1996). Theories and principles of motivation. In D. C. Berliner & R. C. Calfee (Eds.), *Handbook of educational psychology* (pp. 63–84). New York, NY: Macmillan.

Kruglanski, A. W., Chernikova, M., Schori-Eyal, N., & Kopetz, C. (2014). From readiness to action: How motivation works. *Psychological Bulletin, 45*(3), 259–267.

Marcus, B. H., & Owen, N. (1992). Motivational readiness, self-efficacy and decision-making for exercise. *Journal of Applied Social Psychology, 22*(1), 3–16.

Marcus, B. H., Selby, V. C., Niaura, R. S., & Rossi, J. S. (1992). Self-efficacy and the stage of behavioural change. *Research Quarterly for Exercise and Sport, 63*, 60–66.

Maskin, S., & Hopkins, A. (2014). Do incentives work? A qualitative study of managers' motivations in hazardous industries. *Safety Science, 70*, 419–428.

Maslow, A. H. (1954). *Motivation and personality*. New York, NY: Harper & Row.

Moody, R. C., & Pesut, D. J. (2006). The motivation to care: Application and extension of motivation theory to professional nursing work. *Journal of Health Organisation and Management, 20*(1), 15–48.

Ochsner, S., Scholz, U., & Hornung, R. (2013). Testing phase-specific self-efficacy beliefs in the context of dietary behaviour change. *Applied Psychology: Health and Well Being, 5*(1), 99–117.

Ojun, M. A., & Karoly, P. (2007). Perceived goal ownership, regulatory goal cognition, and health behavior change. *American Journal of Health Behaviour, 31*(1), 98–109.

Pearson, E. S. (2011). The "how-to" of health behaviour change brought to life; a theoretical analysis of the co-active coaching model and its underpinnings in self-determination theory coaching. *International Journal of Theory, Research and Practice, 4*(2), 89–103.

Prochaska, J. O., Velicer, W. F., Rossi, J. S., Goldstein, M. G., Marcus, B. H., Rakowski, W., … & Rossi, S. R. (1994). Stages of change and decisional balance for 12 problem behaviors. *Health Psychology, 13*, 39–46.

Schuz, B., Wurm, S., Warner, L. M., Wolff, J. K., & Schwarzer, R. (2014). Health motives and health behaviour self-regulation in older adults. *Journal of Behavioural Medicine, 37*, 491–500.

Schwarzer, R., & Luszczynska, A. (2008). How to overcome health-compromising behaviours: The health action process approach. *European Psychologist, 13*(2), 141–151.

Sheldon, K. M., Ryan, R., & Reis, H. (1996). What makes for a good day? Competence and autonomy in the day and in the person. *Personality and Social Psychology Bulletin, 22*(12), 1270–1279.

Singh, K. (2011). Study of achievement motivation relation to academic achievement of students. *International Journal of Educational Planning & Administration, 1*(2), 161–171.

Teixeria, P. J., Silva, M. N., Mata, J., Palmeria, A. L., & Markland, D. (2012). Motivation, self-determination, and long-term weight control. *International Journal of Behavioural Nutrition and Physical Activity, 9*(22), 1–13.

Toode, K., Routasalo, P., & Suominen T. (2011). Work motivation of nurses: A literature review. *International Journal of Nursing Studies, 48*, 246–257.

Turner, S. L., Thomas, A. M., Wagner, P. J., & Moseley, G. C. (2008). A collaborative approach to wellness: Diet, exercise, and education to impact behaviour change. *Journal of the American Academy of Nurse Practitioners, 29*(6), 339–344.

Walker, L. O., & Avant, K. C. (2005). *Strategies for theory construction in nursing.* Upper Saddle River, NJ: Pearson/Prentice Hall.

Whelan, R., & Barnes-Homes, D. (2013). Coming to terms with motivation in the behaviour-analytic literature. *Psychological Record, 63*, 655–660.

Zulkosky, K. (2009). Self-efficacy: A concept analysis. *Nursing Forum, 44*(2), 93–102.

10

PARENTAL CONCERN

The term *parental concern* is used liberally in the context of child health surveillance (Health Service Executive [HSE], 2005; Morse, 2010) as well as in primary care (Elshout et al., 2014), but without definition. Public health nurses (PHNs) and other health care professionals (HCPs) have key roles to play with parents in these areas of practice, in relation to identifying and acting on parental concern. Therefore, the concept has clinical significance.

Parents are naturally concerned about signs of acute illness, but it is also widely acknowledged that concern occurs even when children are growing and developing normally. High prevalence rates of parental concern have been identified. Coghlan et al. (2003) found that rate to be 30%, and in a Dutch representative sample of parents ($N = 4107$) of 14-month to 12-year-old children, 49.3% reported some concerns with their child, and 8.7% reported frequent concerns (Reijneveld, de Meer, Wiefferink, & Crone, 2008).

In the United States, Garbutt et al. (2012) found that the type of parental concerns about child health varied over time and by the child's age. Specifically, parents ($n = 1119$) identified allergies (26%), asthma (19%), acute infectious diseases (13%), and child development (10.2%) as concerns in their own preschool children; in contrast, these parents rated allergies (69%) as the greatest child health problem in their communities, followed by safety or disease-related issues. Findings from medical records of children under the age of 7 ($N = 273$) in Taiwan revealed six categories of parental concern: cognition, speech/language, motor, behavioral, psychosocial, global delay, and a nonspecific category (Chung et al., 2011). These sources of parental concern are well supported and most concerns identified are about boys (Kozlowski, Matson, Horovitz, Worley, & Neal, 2011; Mulcahy, 2014a; Porter & Ispa, 2012; Reijneveld et al., 2008). In the United States, Porter and Ispa (2012) analyzed parents' childrearing concerns ($N = 120$) and found that the most common were nutrition, sleep, discipline, and child development. A quarter of parents posted concerns, wondering if their child's behavior or development was "normal" or "off track," indicating a certain subtlety in presenting features.

Unlike child growth and development problems, signs of acute illness can naturally present at any age, and the degree to which they are noticed and concerning for parents depends on acuity. In contrast, developmental concerns are typically noticed when children are between 1 and 2 years old. Variations depend on gender and developmental domain, with motor delays being noticed earlier and neurodevelopmental problems later. Delay in the time from parents' first suspicion of a problem to expression of a concern to an HCP has been found to vary from 1 year for speech and mild cognitive delays (Watson, Kieckhefer, & Olshansky, 2006) to 2 to 4 years for autism (Noterdaeme & Hutzelmeyer-Nickels, 2010). In Mulcahy's (2014a) qualitative study, where parents delayed expressing concerns from 2 weeks to a year, there was a sense that parents delayed seeking help until the concern could be clarified and expressed. This strategy is supported in previous research in relation to overweight children (Edmunds, 2005) and for pervasive developmental delay (PDD), where the mean age of first symptom was 18.6 months but age at referral was 14 months later (Chakrabarti & Fombonne, 2005).

DEFINING ATTRIBUTES

The defining attributes of parental concern are: *parental/HCP interaction, parental uncertainty, child well-being,* and *verbal expression.*

Parental/HCP interaction is the first defining attribute because concern cannot be expressed in a vacuum. Parents may be reluctant, in denial (Glascoe, 2002), or unable for some other reason to express concern, but if the HCP is not interacting with the parent, the parental concern is not heard anyway.

Parental uncertainty is the second defining attribute. The author, in a recent study (Mulcahy, 2014b), identified *uncertainty* as a theme to describe parental sense-making of concerns about child growth or development in preschool children. Parents described themselves as uncertain, as well as using the word *concern* (Mulcahy, 2014b). The term *uncertainty* is different from parental concern, and there is some evidence from the literature of a lack of a common understanding of the term, perhaps related to language and culture (Kiing, Low, Chan, & Neihart, 2012). In purely semantic terms, *concern* implies that one has arrived at an appraisal, whereas being uncertain indicates a preceding or antecedent phase. *Uncertainty* is an attractive term, as often the issue of concern in child development is subtle.

Child well-being is also a defining attribute, as literature relating to parental concern relates primarily, but not exclusively, to developmental delay rather than illness (King et al., 2012). *Well-being* as a broader term could conceivably encapsulate concern about acute illness as well as growth or development problems.

Verbal expression is the usual way in which concern is expressed to an HCP. Although parental uncertainty could potentially be determined nonverbally, literature implies verbal expression (Hacker et al., 2006). Ellingson, Briggs-Gowan, Carter, and Horwitz (2004) found that few parents spoke to an HCP about their child's health concerns and concluded that HCPs needed to inquire systematically about parental concern. Perhaps parents' nonverbal cues in a well-child assessment context suggest that they are concerned, but parental concern is nevertheless an assumption until it is verbally expressed. In contrast, it is perhaps assumed in an illness context that parents bring their child for medical attention to a general practitioner (GP) or emergency department because they are concerned, but this may not be stated explicitly.

DEFINITION

Parental concern is defined as parental uncertainty about a child's current health or growth/development/behavioral stage (child well-being) verbally expressed during parental/HCP interaction.

MODEL CASE

A PHN does a home visit to carry out a developmental assessment of a 3-month-old girl. At the primary visit, the PHN had raised awareness of the developmental nature of developmental dysplasia of the hip (DDH), in line with best practice. In the course of the 3-month developmental assessment (parental/HCP interaction), the girl's mother says (verbal expression) that she is uncertain (parental uncertainty) about the range of movement of the child's left hip (child well-being). Thus, all defining attributes are present.

RELATED CASE

Related cases have some of the defining attributes. For example, a mother who brings her 3-year-old daughter to the child health clinic for a routine developmental assessment with the PHN (child well-being). She expresses no concerns (failed verbal expression and failed parental uncertainty) about her daughter's growth, despite her height measurements being consistently below the 0.3 percentile for age, because there is a family history of short stature. This case has a parental/HCP interaction in the context of child well-being in a routine developmental assessment, but there is failed parental uncertainty about growth or development (failed child well-being and verbal expression).

BORDERLINE CASE

Borderline cases contain most of the attributes. For example, a PHN carries out a home visit to a first-time mother to assess progress by a week-old infant boy. The PHN notices that the baby's muscle tone is a little lax. On assessment, the mother expresses generalized uncertainty and anxiety about caring for and handling her new baby, but nothing specific relating to muscle tone (failed parental uncertainty). This case has a parental/HCP interaction in the context of child well-being in a routine developmental assessment. Although there is verbal expression, there is failed parental uncertainty about development in the context of muscle tone and gross motor development.

CONTRARY CASE

A PHN does a home visit to a mother of a 12-month-old child who has failed to attend the developmental clinic on three occasions. There is no answer at the door (failed parental/HCP interaction and failed verbal expression). The PHN has never met the parents, but previously met the child's grandmother, who reported that the mother did not have any concerns (failed parental uncertainty) about her child (failed child well-being). She is concerned because the family has moved to a new address five times in the past year. This example does not exemplify the concept, as it does not have any defining attributes.

ANTECEDENTS

The antecedents of parental concern are knowledge, experience, personal control, personal threat, and accessibility and availability of health care providers.

Parents need to have knowledge and experience (Mulcahy, 2014a; Williams & Holmes, 2004) of a healthy child or normal child development in order to be uncertain or worried that there may be a deviation from this. From a theoretical perspective, uncertainty in the context of illness is first neutrally perceived until assessed as either an opportunity or a threat (Mishel & Clayton, 2003). Kai (1996) found that the two key motivators for expression of parental concerns in an illness context were perceived threat and personal control. This is supported by Garbutt et al. (2012).

Perceived threat and personal control could apply to acute illness or developmental delay. Parents are known to assess and compare their child's development and growth (Lucas et al., 2007; Mulcahy, 2014a). Similarly, parents watch and worry about severity in acute illness (Elshout et al., 2014). The obvious difference between child development and illness is the immediacy of the perceived threat with an acute illness.

In the author's own study, parents rarely described just one trigger that prompted them to take action in addressing their children's concern formally with a doctor or PHN. More often than not, there was a combination of a parent's "usual disposition"; the influence of family and friends; the impact on the child; and time passing (Mulcahy, 2014b). The impact of the child health concern on the child and family were previously identified by Ellingson et al. (2004). In Reijneveld et al.'s (2008) study, one of the reasons cited for not seeking help was confidence that the problem would resolve.

Once parents have decided to seek help (Cornally & McCarthy, 2011) or "to get the child's problem checked out" (Mulcahy, 2014a), there are decisions to be made in terms of what HCP to access. Participatory nurse/client relationships are known to be valued by parents in particular where there are previously satisfying experiences, positive peer influences, and trusting relationships (Mulcahy & McCarthy, 2008). In Reijneveld et al.'s (2008) study, lack of knowledge of an appropriate HCP and difficulties accessing help were cited by parents as reasons for not seeking help. However, those who had not sought help were from much-marginalized segments of the population, including the unemployed, immigrants, those on low income, one-parent family, young parent, or parents with low education level. Therefore, accessibility and availability are conducive to parents expressing concerns and consequently can be defined as antecedents.

CONSEQUENCES

The consequences of parental concern are increasing or decreasing anxiety, HCPs interventions, and positive or negative impact on child well-being.

The consequences of parental concern being expressed or elicited are that HCPs can intervene and concern can be explored and assessed. Parental concern was found to have a positive predictive value for confirmed disorders of language and motor domains (Glascoe, 2002). Predictive value was much less for cognitive disorders, global delay, or related behavior difficulties. Chung et al. (2011) suggest that a possible reason for the accuracy of parental concerns relating to motor and language may be the overtly visible nature of these domains. The variable nature of parental concern supports the need for HCPs to ask open questions for all health and developmental domains at each assessment (Garbutt et al., 2012).

Depending on the cause of the concern, the HCP may provide treatment, counseling, reassurance, or referral. A potential outcome is early identification of emerging behavioral, health problems, or subtle developmental problems (Williams, 2007). Early identification and treatment of acute illnesses have an obvious impact on child mortality and morbidity. A child's physical, psychological, educational, social, and other prospects can be seriously compromised by undetected or untreated growth or developmental problems (Williams & Holmes, 2004). There is widespread support for the commencement of early intervention services before school entry (Sices et al., 2007). Negative consequences may also emerge if parental concern is not addressed, such as increased parental anxiety or stress (Ellingson et al., 2004).

EMPIRICAL REFERENTS

Each defining attribute must have an empirical referent. Each element of parental/HCP interaction is separated as follows. Based on the literature included here, a *parent* is defined as mother, father, or guardian, although in reality the former is most likely (Morse, 2010). HCPs may be pediatricians, health visitors, GPs, PHNs, or public health doctors. Interaction between a parent and HCP can be defined as a communication exchange between parties as described earlier, occurring in an office, home setting, or potentially by telecommunication or electronic means.

The very nature of parental uncertainty means that this is a nebulous term. If one is uncertain, one is unsure or has doubts whether or not there is something wrong. In terms of child development, deviations from normal development can be very subtle. Normal growth may be statistically defined by HCPs. The authors' own qualitative study (Mulcahy, 2014a) found that parents experienced concern as uncertainty but they also, like others (Ellingson et al., 2004), used a variety of words interchangeably, such as *concern, doubt, unsure,* and *worry* when describing their experiences. The author believes that this is because one is unsure before one is certain of concern. Therefore, a dichotomized item of "concern/no concern" (Morse, 2010) or the Parents Evaluation of Developmental Status (PEDS) Scale (Glascoe, 2002) is likely to be insufficient to capture parental uncertainty. As a consequence, terms such as *concern, doubt, unsure, uncertainty,* and *worry* should be used in structured questionnaires to measure parental uncertainty regarding their children's well-being.

Most of the preceding studies related to growth or development, pointing to child well-being as opposed to childhood illness being the best attribute. This echoes the challenge of measuring health according to broad WHO definitions. Child well-being is considered a multidimensional concept that is challenging to define operationally (OECD, 2009). Therefore, it is proposed in this concept analysis that a potential empirical referent is the absence of any signs or symptoms of acute illness or deviations from normal growth or development.

Although parental concern was described in terms of verbal expression, data were often collected by written self-report instruments (Sices, 2007). Therefore, while verbal expression may be more usual in clinical practice, there is a general increase in telematic or electronic expressions. Thus, evidence of parental concern is possibly more likely to be collected in a written format for research purposes.

SUMMARY

Prevalence figures indicate that many parents are concerned about their children and that this can be related to any aspect of growth, development, or illness. As a result of this concept analysis, *parental concern* was defined and identified as containing four defining attributes. The consequences of parental concern are significant in terms of adverse effects on child and family health and well-being, thus emphasizing the clinical significance of the concept for HCPs. Each of the concept's attributes has potential empirical referents which ensure that the concept can be measured. A schematic representation is provided to facilitate an understanding of the concept (see Figure 10.1).

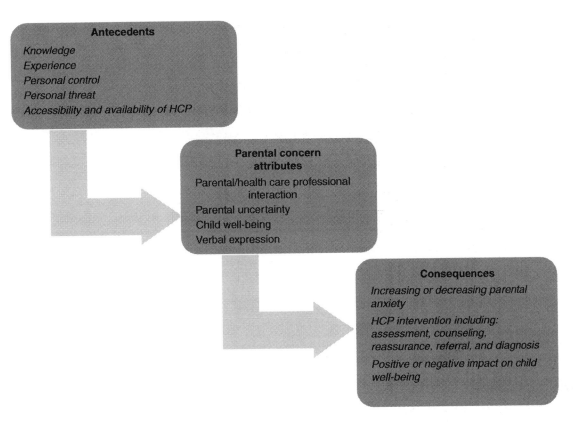

FIGURE 10.1 Parental concern.

REFERENCES

Chakrabarti, S., & Fombonne, E. (2005). Pervasive developmental disorders in preschool children: Confirmation of high prevalence. *American Journal of Psychiatry, 162*(6), 1133–1141. doi:10.1176/appi.ajp.162.6.1133

Chung, C.-Y., Liu, W.-Y., Chang, C.-J., Chen, C.-L., Tang, S. F.-T., & Wong, A. M.-K. (2011). The relationship between parental concerns and final diagnosis in children with developmental delay. *Journal of Child Neurology, 26*(4), 413–419. doi:10.1177/0883073810381922

Coghlan, D., Kiing, J. S. H., & Wake, M. (2003). Parents' evaluation of developmental status in the Australian day-care setting: Developmental concerns of parents and carers. *Journal of Paediatrics & Child Health, 39*(1), 49–54. doi:10.1046/j.1440-1754.2003.00084.x

Cornally, N., & McCarthy, G. (2011). Help-seeking behaviour: A concept analysis. *International Journal of Nursing Practice, 17*(3), 280–288. doi:10.1111/j.1440-172X.2011.01936.x

Edmunds, L. (2005). Parents' perceptions of health professionals' responses when seeking help for their overweight children. *Family Practice, 22*(3), 287–292. doi:10.1093/fampra/cmh729

Ellingson, K., Briggs-Gowan, M., Carter, A., & Horwitz, S. (2004). Parent identification of early emerging child behavior problems. *Archives of Pediatric Adolescent Medicine, 158*, 766–772.

Elshout, G., van Ierland, Y., Bohnen, A. M., de Wilde, M., Moll, H. A., Oostenbrink, R., & Berger, M. Y. (2014). Alarming signs and symptoms in febrile children in primary care: An observational cohort study in the Netherlands. *PLoS ONE, 9*(2), 1–6. doi:10.1371/journal.pone.0088114

Garbutt, J. M., Leege, E., Sterkel, R., Gentry, S., Wallendorf, M., & Strunk, R. C. (2012). What are parents worried about? Health problems and health concerns for children. *Clinical Pediatrics, 20*(10), 1–8.

Glascoe, F. P. (2002). *Collaborating with parents: Using Parents Evaluation of Developmental Status (PEDS) to detect and address developmental and behavioral problems.* Nashville, TN: Ellsworth and Vandermeer Press.

Hacker, K., Myagmarjav, E., Harris, V., Suglia, S., Weidner, D., & Link, D. (2006). Mental health screening in pediatric practice: Factors related to positive screens and the contribution of parental/personal concern. *Pediatrics, 118*(5), 1896–1906.

Health Service Executive. (2005). *Best health for children revisited—Report from the National Core Child Health Program Review Group.* Dublin, OH: HSE.

Kai, J. (1996). What worries parents when their pre-school children are acutely ill and why: A qualitative study. *British Medical Journal, 313*(7063), 983–986.

Kiing, J. S. H., Low, P. S., Chan, Y. H., & Neihart, M. (2012). Interpreting parents' concerns about their children's development with the parents' evaluation of developmental status: Culture matters. *Journal of Developmental and Behavioral Pediatrics, 33*(2), 179–183.

Kozlowski, A. M., Matson, J., Horovitz, M., Worley, J. A., & Neal, D. (2011). Parents' first concerns of their child's development in toddlers with autism spectrum disorders. *Developmental Neurohabilitation, 14*(2), 72–78.

Lucas, P., Arai, L., Baird, J., Kleijnen, J., Law, C., & Roberts, H. (2007). A systematic review of lay views about infant size and growth. *Archives of Disease in Childhood, 92*(2), 120–127. doi:10.1136/adc.2005.087288

Mishel, M., & Clayton, M. (2003). Theories of uncertainty in illness. In M. J. Smith & R. Liehr (Eds.), *Middle range theory for nursing* (pp. 25–48). New York, NY: Springer Publishing Company.

Morse, K. (2010). What factors are associated with parental concern regarding their child's weight? *Journal of Pediatric Health Care, 24*, e8–e9.

Mulcahy, H. (2014a). *Parents' experiences of child growth and development concerns: An interpretative phenomenological analysis* (Doctor of Nursing thesis). University College Cork, Cork, Ireland.

Mulcahy, H. (2014b). Triggers to action on child developmental concerns. *Boolean, 2014*, 93–97.

Mulcahy, H., & McCarthy, G. (2008). Participatory nurse/client relationships: Perceptions of public health nurses and mothers of vulnerable families. *Applied Nursing Research, 21*(3), 169–172. doi:10.1016/j.apnr.2006.06.004

Noterdaeme, M., & Hutzelmeyer-Nickels, A. (2010). Early symptoms and recognition of pervasive developmental disorders in Germany. *Autism, 14*(6), 575–588.

OECD. (2009). *Doing better for children. Chapter 2. Comparative child well-being across the OECD.* Paris, France: Author.

Porter, N., & Ispa, J. (2012). Mothers' online message board questions about parenting infants and toddlers. *Journal of Advanced Nursing, 69*(3), 559–568.

Reijneveld, S., de Meer, G., Wiefferink, C. H., & Crone, M. (2008). Parents' concerns about children are highly prevalent but often not confirmed by child doctors and nurses. *BMC Public Health, 8*(124), 1–10.

Sices, L. (2007). *Developmental screening in primary care: The effectiveness of current practice and recommendations for improvement.* Retrieved from http://www.commonwealthfund.org/Publications/Fund-Reports/2007/Dec/Developmental-Screening-in-Primary-Care-The-Effectiveness-of-Current-Practice-and-Recommendations-f.aspx

Watson, K. C., Kieckhefer, G. M., & Olshansky, E. (2006). Striving for therapeutic relationships: Parent-provider communication in the developmental treatment setting. *Qualitative Health Research, 16,* 647–662.

Williams, J. (2007). Learning from mothers: How myths, policies and practices affect the detection of subtle developmental problems in children. *Child: Care, Health and Development, 33*(3), 282–290. doi:10.1111/j.1365-2214.2006.00690.x

Williams, J., & Holmes, C. (2004). Improving the early detection of children with subtle developmental problems. *Journal of Child Health Care, 8*(1), 34–46.

11

PATIENT ENGAGEMENT

The movement toward patient-centered care (PCC), also referred to as *patient engagement* (PE; Pelletier & Stichler, 2014), has been driven by research supporting the importance of patients' involvement in their own health care (Luxford, Safran, & Delblanco, 2001). This momentum, increased in part by federal legislation, namely the American Recovery and Reinvestment Act (ARRA) in 2009 (*Health IT-Legislation and Regulations,* 2014), created the need to integrate the concept into the acute care setting by using technology.

Uses of PE and various definitions can be found when searching the literature. Barello et al. (2012) analyzed the academic literature from 2002 to 2012 for the concept of PE. These authors provided a summary of the top 10 cited publications where various definitions were found. Two medical perspectives defined PE as follows: Lehman et al. (2002) defined PE as individuals' actions performed to enhance adherence, thus leading to high-quality health care. Casale et al. (2007) defined PE as a behavioral activation that contributes to reduced resource abuse and improved health outcomes. From a nursing perspective, Hibbard, Stockard, Mahoney, and Tusler (2004) defined the term as a behavioral activation related to healthy behaviors and positive health outcomes.

In its report *Fostering Successful Patient and Family Engagement: Nursing's Critical Role*, the National Alliance for Quality Care cites the definition of PE from the Center for Advancing Health (CFAH), which defines engagement as "actions people take for their health and to benefit from health care" (Sofaer & Schumann, 2013, p. 9).

The term PE, as related to health information technology (HIT) and meaningful use (MU), has driven the concept from the regulatory and information technology (IT) side. Although it is cited as a requirement to meet the MU regulations, the term is not clearly defined. It is proposed via *meaningful use*, which includes the manner in which health care providers, patients, and families gain access to their records to more fully engage in their care (Ralston, Coleman, Reid, Handley, & Larson, 2010).

DEFINING ATTRIBUTES

The defining attributes of PE are *empowerment, collaboration, health information,* and *patient activation.*

The use of empowerment as a defining attribute is well supported in the literature. It is defined as a set of behaviors by the patient, family members, and health professionals and a set of organizational policies and procedures that foster inclusion of the patient and family as members of the health care team and partners (Pelletier & Stichler, 2013). Due to the encompassing nature of the term as so defined, it provides a sound foundation and cohesiveness for the concept of PE.

Collaboration is working with another person or group in order to achieve or do something. PE is driven by decisions and planning made by the health care team and patient. It cannot happen without all parties mutually agreeing upon a course of action or plan of care.

The selection of health information as a defining attribute was, at first, complex and delicate. However, as the process of the concept analysis progressed, it made greater sense to include this as an attribute. It places emphasis and importance on exchanges of information about the patient's health, such as teaching and planning care, versus everyday exchanges or polite conversation where information such as the weather is discussed.

Patient activation is the managing one's own health using knowledge, skills, and confidence (Hibbard et al., 2004). This attribute was selected as the final attribute because at the core of the concept is the patient and his or her participation and interest in his or her health care. If patient activation is not present, all other interventions, plans, or strategies for the concept would be irrelevant.

DEFINITION OF PE

PE is the empowerment of patients through collaboration with nurses and other HCPs to provide health information and promote patient activation.

MODEL CASE

The following model case demonstrates the presence of all the defining attributes. A patient is admitted to an acute care setting for a surgical repair of a leg fracture. During the admission process, the nurse introduces the patient to a tablet device which he can use to access his electronic medical records (EMRs) (empowerment). The patient accesses his health information and documents his level of pain (patient activation). The patient and nurse discuss pain management options and agree upon a regimen (collaboration). This example contains all defining attributes and exemplifies the meaning of the concept.

RELATED CASE

In this scenario, the patient is being discharged from the hospital following an exacerbation of her congestive heart failure (CHF). The nurse reviews all patient discharge instructions (health information) with the patient and her daughter, who will be caring for the patient (collaboration). The nurse reminds the patient that her discharge instructions and medical record are available anytime in her electronic patient portal (empowerment). The patient states that she relies on her daughter to help her manage her CHF (failed patient activation) and would prefer that her daughter have access to her portal account. However, they complete the discharge process without granting the patient's daughter access to the patient's portal account.

BORDERLINE CASE

During the review of his EMR, a patient notes a new and unfamiliar medication order (empowerment). That morning, when the nurse comes to the room to administer the morning medications, the patient asks the nurse about the new medication order (patient activation). The nurse reviews the EMR and responds by saying that she is unfamiliar with that particular medication and it is not due until bedtime (failed health information). However, she promises to return with more information about the medication (collaboration).

CONTRARY CASE

A patient is being treated at the hospital with a lengthy course of chemotherapy prior to bone marrow transplant. The patient has visitors who have finally been able to come from out of town. The nurse rushes into the room and states that the patient has been ordered for a stat CT scan. She insists that they must quickly prepare for transport, as this is the only time radiology can fit him in (failed empowerment). The patient asks why the CT scan was ordered, to which the nurse replies she does not know and has not had a chance to call the doctor (failed health information and failed collaboration). The patient accepts her explanation and reluctantly gets into the wheelchair (failed patient activation). In this example of a contrary case, the defining attributes are absent, as is the intent of the concept of PE.

ANTECEDENTS

In order for PE to exist, the following antecedents must be present: competency, knowledge, communication skills, and environment.

Multiple studies find that nurses require specific competencies in order for PE to be present. Pelletier and Stichler (2014) state that knowledge and competency on the part of the nurse are recommended in the areas of eliciting patient values, beliefs, and preferences, which are communicated to the care team and accounted for in the patient's plan of care. In addition, nurses are encouraged to understand the disease and the patient when developing the plan of care and caring for their patients (Abdelhadi & Drach-Zahavy, 2011). Finally, there must be knowledge to recognize the extent to which a patient or family is able to engage or choose to engage in care (Sofaer & Schumann, 2013), as this knowledge will determine actions or adjustments to the strategy for PE and, ultimately, the desired patient health outcomes.

In order for there to be patient activation and empowerment, patients must have knowledge and competency. Organizations must provide the tools for patients to be educated and informed in order to actively participate in their care (Pelletier & Stichler, 2014). This supports and drives empowerment and activation.

In order for there to be PE, nurses must have appropriate communication skills. Scholars agree that health care providers need to develop excellent communication skills, self-awareness, reflective listening, and adequate use of empathy. Improved communication skills have demonstrated better consultation style, use of empathy, and resolution of emotional problems that arise during the encounter (Abdelhadi & Drach-Zahavy, 2011).

Organizations that have been successful in building models for PE have considered the environment as an integral component. Environment is related to the organization's comprehensive approach to support PE (Luxford et al., 2001). It must be conducive to promoting and supporting all efforts of PE, from the perspective of the patient, staff, and family.

CONSEQUENCES

The consequences of PE are improved health outcomes and improved patient satisfaction.

Engagement, or how involved patients are in the management of their care, has shown a direct contribution to improved patient outcomes and decreased health care costs (Abdelhadi & Drach-Zahavy, 2011). In 2011, the National Strategy for Quality Improvement in Health Care also published reports highlighting the criticality of patients' being involved in their health care, because that engagement demonstrated improved clinical outcomes.

Improved patient satisfaction is also a consequence of PE, as demonstrated in improved Hospital Consumer Assessment of Healthcare Providers and Systems (HCAHPS) scores. In a pilot study of 254 hospitals that adopted a PE methodology, HCAHPS scores have consistently outperformed national benchmarks (Charmell & Frampton, 2008).

EMPIRICAL REFERENTS

The Patient Activation and Empowerment-Patient Activation Measure tool (PAM; Hibbard et al., 2004) may be used to measure the defining attributes of patient activation, empowerment, collaboration, and health information. This scale captures level of activation as well as beliefs the patient has about self-management, collaboration with providers, and maintainance of health. Additional scales are available to measure empowerment; however, they are disease specific.

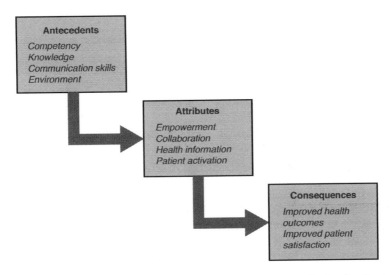

FIGURE 11.1 Schematic representation of concept analysis of patient engagement.

The Collaboration and Satisfaction About Care Decisions (CSACD) tool may also be used to measure collaboration (Gedney Baggs, 1994). The author acknowledges that although this scale is traditionally used to measure collaboration between nurses and physicians, it can be modified to include the patient.

Health information may appear broad and difficult to measure, but the literature references PE documentation on the plan of care. The author suggests that this be considered as a possible measurement point within the medical record. It has the potential to reflect collaboration, patient input, and exchange of health information that supports the concept. Another aspect to consider is direct documentation by the patient into the plan of care. Additional benefits of this method are capturing the patient's understanding of health information, driving greater activation, and empowerment (see Figure 11.1).

SUMMARY

The importance of PE in health care was demonstrated and a definition of PE was provided. The defining attributes of empowerment, collaboration, health information, and patient activation were identified, along with empirical referents for measurement. The antecedents and consequences were also provided, as well as a schematic representation thereof.

REFERENCES

Abdelhadi, N., & Drach-Zahavy, A. (2011). Promoting patient care: Work engagement as a mediator between ward service climate and patient centered care. *Journal of Advanced Nursing, 68*(6), 1276–1287.

Barello, S., Graffigna, G., & Vegni, E. (2012). Patient engagement as an emerging challenge for healthcare services: Mapping the literature. *Nursing Research and Practice, 2012*. doi:10.1155/2012/905934

Casale, A. S., Paulus, R. A., & Selna, M. J. (2007). "ProvenCareSM": A provider-driven pay-for-performance program for acute episodic cardiac surgical care. *Annals of Surgery, 246*(4), 613–621.

Charmell, P. A., & Frampton, S. B. (2008). Building the business case for patient-centered care. *Healthcare Financial Management, 62*(3), 80–85.

Gedney Baggs, J. (1994). Development of an instrument to measure collaboration and satisfaction about care decisions. *Journal of Advanced Nursing, 20,* 176–182.

Health IT-Legislation and Regulations. (2014, September 11). Retrieved from http://www .healthit.gov/policy-researchers-implementers/health-it-legislation

Hibbard, J. H., Stockard, J., Mahoney, E. R., & Tusler, M. (2004). Development of the patient activation measure (PAM): Conceptualizing and measuring activation in patients and consumers. *Health Services Research, 39*(4), 1005–1026.

Lehman, W. E. K., Greener, J. M., & Simpson, D. D. (2002). Assessing organizational readiness for change, *Journal of Substance Abuse Treatment, 22*(4), 197–209.

Luxford, K., Safran, D. G., & Delblanco, T. (2001). Promoting patient-centered care: A quality study of facilitators and barriers in healthcare organizations with a reputation for improving the patient experience. *International Journal for Quality in Health Care, 23*(5), 510–515.

Pelletier, L. R., & Stichler, J. F. (2013). Action brief: Patient engagement and activation: A health reform imperative and improvement opportunity for nursing. *Nursing Outlook, 61*(1), 51–54.

Pelletier, L. R., & Stichler, J. F. (2014). Patient-centered care and engagement: Nurse leaders' imperative for health reform. *Journal of Nursing Administration, 44*(9), 473–480.

Ralston, J. D., Coleman, K., Reid, R. J., Handley, M. R., & Larson, E. B. (2010). Patient experience should be part of meaningful-use criteria. *Health Affairs, 29*(4), 607–613.

Sofaer, S., & Schumann, M. J. (2013). *Fostering successful patient and family engagement: Nursing's critical role.* Washington, DC: Nursing Alliance for Quality Care.

CORAZON B. CAJULIS, LINDA AHN,
COLLEEN DeBOER, and DENISE O'DEA

12

QUALITY OF LIFE

The concept of quality of life (QoL) has been described in many ways, often in relevance to a situation or to an individual. As a concept, it follows that of a complex mental formulation of experience (Chinn & Kramer, 1995). It encompasses both objective and subjective indicators. Objective indicators include income, housing, and physical/functional capacity. Subjective indicators include attitudes, feelings, perception, or sense of well-being and value (Sarvimaki, 2000). Its analysis can provide better understanding of the concept and to some extent maximize its use. In health care, for example, it can be used for health needs assessment, resource allocation, planning of clinical patient care, and as an outcome measure for clinical research. It is also integral to patients as they decide own medical treatment plan together with the health care team.

QoL has been examined and used in health care, politics and economics, physical/mental health, education, recreation/leisure time, social belonging, and environment. Initially used to reference material goods after World War II (WWII), QoL has gradually expanded to personal, social, leisure, and enjoyment. It is a multidimensional concept that encompasses the objective environment, perceived QoL, behavioral competence, psychological well-being, social and emotional functioning, life satisfaction, standard of living, and social support (Mendlowicz & Stein, 2000). QoL is an interplay of an individual's expectation and values, adaptation, and overall well-being. It is the integration of both the subjective and objective indicators in a broad range of life domains together with an individual's values (Edgerton, Roberts, & von Below, 2012; Frisch, 2012). Sarvimaki (2000) stated that a person who has a reasonable degree of well-being sees some meaning and value in his or her life.

QoL has a wide contextual range and its definition is based on its use. There are many definitions of QoL, as differences exist for what individuals find valuable or important in their lives. These diverse QoL definitions and perspectives—such as quality of one's condition, one's satisfaction with life conditions, combination of life conditions and satisfaction, and combination of life conditions and satisfaction with emphasis on personal values, aspirations, and expectations—seek to explain issues of significance in one's life. Diverse as it may be in its definition and perspectives, contextually, similarities exist. It includes all areas of life and experience. Life experience with health, disease, treatment of disease, accompanying symptoms, and so on is all included as an individual goes through life.

QoL is often referred to as a degree of excellence in life based on an implied standard. This may pertain to health, economic condition, success in work, and relationships, to name a few (Frisch, 2013). Implied standard on QoL issues with a specific population such as the elderly, individuals with chronic diseases, and/or individuals with serious health condition can produce variable definitions of degrees of excellence in their life.

What determination can an individual consider as having QoL? What degree of symptom control, for example, does an individual with cancer consider as constituting QoL? As we know, cancer can occur anytime during life; however, when it does afflict the elderly population, it is even more challenging. Cancer and its treatment affect multiple aspects of a patient's life (Hacker, 2009), and short- and/or long-term effects on physical, functional, psychological, social, and/or financial aspects of a patient's life are often unavoidable. The patient's ability to perform the activities of living, control of symptoms, psychological and financial well-being all affect the patient's QoL.

DEFINING ATTRIBUTES

The defining attributes of QoL are *satisfaction with one's life, general perception of well-being*, and *autonomy/independence*.

Satisfaction with one's life is a subjective indicator; satisfaction can vary between individuals. An individual's judgment of conditions and their importance to life affect that individual's life satisfaction. Personal relationships influence general satisfaction with life (Plummer & Molzahn, 2009; Sanda et al., 2008). A patient with cancer, for example, determines what is important to him or her that makes her or him happy. For some, prolonging life with treatment despite accompanying side effects generally satisfies them, whereas others may feel satisfied with no treatment and/or symptom control. Some others note that changes in their functioning, such as sexual function, greatly affect their personal satisfaction and well-being (Sanda et al., 2008). Outcomes of cancer treatment affect general satisfaction in life and feeling of well-being.

General perception of well-being is another defining attribute of QoL. The total dimensions of well-being include the physical, functional, emotional, and social. Education and finances may also play a role in personal or social well-being (Mandzuk & McMillan, 2005). The level of education can directly or indirectly affect QoL. It is known that education is an important aspect of better life chances pertaining to health, social, and economic factors. However, individuals may have different views and allocation of different degrees of well-being pertaining to those previously mentioned. Individuals who are mentally (psychologically), physically, and physiologically healthy, and are surrounded by social support such as family and friends may, however, define QoL more favorably. For cancer patients, for example, well-controlled symptoms of the disease and/or treatment, improved functional capacity and activities, or meeting simple basic needs like a good night's sleep and absence of taste changes make up a feeling of well-being, an important attribute of QoL.

The autonomy to maintain or change life condition is relevant in the pursuit of happiness and satisfaction (Mandzuk & McMillan, 2005; Schalock, 2004). Several studies identified independence as a key indicator in QoL (Estebsari, Taghdisi, Mostafael, Jamshidi, & Latifi, 2013; Osborne, Bindemann, Noble, & Reed, 2014). Results of these studies on QoL at the last stage of life noted that independence (self-reliance, having control of one's life, environment, and events) is one of the key concepts, together with physical functioning and relationships, identified as most important to QoL. The level of independence in activities such as mobility, work capacity, and activities of daily living affect QoL.

DEFINITION OF QoL

QoL is a conscious general perception of well-being, satisfaction with one's life, happiness, and having the autonomy to grow and experience what is important to one as one defines life and well-being.

MODEL CASE

Mandy is a recently retired professional registered nurse in oncology. She was diagnosed with inoperable Stage IV metastatic lung cancer to bones and liver shortly after her retirement. She has lived a full, meaningful, and interesting life (satisfaction with one's life). She is well aware of her prognosis and well versed about her treatment plan. She receives chemotherapy for a chance to prolong her life. Her symptoms, such as pain and nausea, are well controlled, making her comfortable and able to improve her functional capacity (perception of well-being). Because her symptoms are well controlled, she is able to engage in conversation and spend valuable time with her family and friends. Her independence in performing basic activities of living such as eating, basic personal care, and ambulation (autonomy), and her spending time with family, make her happy (happiness). All the attributes are present in this case.

RELATED CASE

Edith is undergoing chemotherapy for metastatic angiosarcoma. She has failed four other lines of therapy. However, her current chemotherapy regimen greatly improved her disease condition, including her primary complaints of pain in her back and legs. Still, complaints of headache, decreased appetite, and inability to perform daily activities have gotten progressively worse with her current treatment; thus, she spends most of her day in bed (failed perception of well-being). Because of these reasons, she decided to discontinue her current treatment (autonomy). Because her headaches improved, she is now able to care for her son, bring him to school, and help him with homework (happiness). Her decision to discontinue treatment (autonomy) is based on what she thinks is more important in her life (satisfaction with one's life), such as ability to care for her son rather than prolonging her life.

BORDERLINE CASE

Mrs. Jones is a 69-year-old woman who was diagnosed with extensive small cell lung cancer during late summer. Over the course of her disease, her symptoms have gotten progressively worse (failed perception of well-being). She finds it harder to tend to her garden (a regular daily activity that she loves to do). She was started on chemotherapy, which improved her condition so that she was able to tend her garden again (happiness). However, as the chemotherapy continued, so did her worsening fatigue. She then decided (autonomy) to take a break from her chemotherapy to regain some energy. Mrs. Jones used her final months to spend more time enjoying the company of family and friends, sharing stories of her life, success, and accomplishments despite the circumstance of her health (satisfaction withone's life).

CONTRARY CASE

Joe is a 50-year-old male, a vibrant painter with Stage III prostate cancer status after brachytherapy and external beam radiation 2 years ago. Currently, he is on monthly hormone therapy with which he is experiencing hot flashes and erectile dysfunction (failed perception of well-being). On his clinic visit today, he was very upset and angry about his laboratory results that showed a significant increase in his PSA level. He became more upset and angry when his nurse practitioner (NP) informed him that diagnostic examinations such as computerized tomography (CT) scans of chest, abdomen, and pelvis and a bone scan are needed to rule out possibility of disease progression. Despite the NP's explanation and offer to meet with his oncologist to discuss a management plan and any additional support that he may need, he refused to listen; instead, he stormed out of the examination room (failed autonomy and failed satisfaction with one's life). There is dissatisfaction and unhappiness, abrupt decision making (not consciously thought-out decision), and no general feeling of wellness (emotionally, psychologically, and physiologically).

ANTECEDENTS

The antecedents of QoL are mental consciousness and basic functional capacity. Life comes with the ability to grow, change, and experience life itself. It is not enough to be breathing and talking; rather, one must possess mental consciousness to perform an evaluation of or assess one's own life. QoL is a conscious experience. Without consciousness, an individual cannot discern or define what QoL is, nor can an individual decide what makes her satisfied or happy. Evaluation of one's life summarizes one's own experience. These experiences are judged or cognitively compared as to whether they make one's life happy or otherwise. The individual can change or modify those unfavorable experiences into favorable experiences. This ability to deal with life problems or unfavorable experiences may contribute to happiness and satisfaction (Veenhoven, 2012).

An individual should also have basic functional capacity. *Functional capacity* is the ability to effectively perform the basic functional competencies in daily living (Frisch, 2012). These basic activities of daily living include ability to have reasonable amount of sleep, ability to breathe easily, ability to eat, and ability to perform basic personal activities such as personal care. There can also be functional disability. Sleep disturbance, for example, negatively impacts QoL, as evidenced by a study done by Dickerson, Connors, Fayad, and Dean (2014) on sleep–wake disturbances in cancer patients. Gotze, Brahler, Gansera, Polze, and Kohler (2014) noted in their study that palliative care patients reported low QoL with low functional (physical, mental, and psychological) status.

CONSEQUENCES

Happiness and self-esteem are outcomes of QoL. *Happiness* denotes perception of something good (Veenhoven, 2012). An enjoyable outcome, effective coping with challenges in life, and/or the ability to deal with problems can provide instant or long-term happiness. The ability to be happy is central to adaptation and positive mental health. Happy individuals tend to be more self-controlled, social, charitable, cooperative, and productive members of the community (Lyubomirsky, Sheldon, & Schkade, 2005). It is, however, reasonable to keep in mind that every individual is unique, as she or he evaluates her or his own life and identifies what makes her or him happy or fulfilled.

Self-esteem is discerned when an individual is happy. Happiness, perception of general well-being, and self-worth/value or presence of self-esteem are key indicators of QoL (Apolone & Mosconi, 1998; Meeberg, 1993; Mandzuk & McMillan, 2005; Sarvimaki, 2000). An individual with QoL has an overall sense of happiness in life. Happiness and contentment mirror self-esteem. Self-worth, independence, and social engagement enhance self-esteem. These positive experiences improve QoL (Dugger, 2010). A patient who opted to discontinue her treatment to relieve her from symptoms or side effects of treatment for a better functional capacity, for example, defines QoL with self-esteem as well as happiness with her decision.

An individual who regains and improves functional capacity with symptom relief, such as controlled pain in a cancer patient, likewise experiences happiness and enhanced self-esteem. The ability to independently perform basic activities of daily living such as personal care raises the individual's self-esteem.

EMPIRICAL REFERENTS

Empirical referents refer to classes or categories of the actual phenomenon that by their presence demonstrate the occurrence of the concept. They indicate that the concept is present. Numerous wide-range measures of QoL are noted in the literature; however, recent research centers on two basic measurements. One focuses on subjective well-being, and the other focuses on objective measurements of quantifiable indicators such as economic production, literacy rate, and life expectancy, to name a few. Subjective well-being is concerned with self-reported happiness, pleasure, and fulfillment (Costanza et al., 2008).

A study by Marriage and Cummins (2004) on children ages 5 to 12 years, utilizing Comprehensive QoL Scale and Coopersmith Self-Esteem Inventory instruments, showed that self-esteem is not related to primary or secondary control in coping with everyday stress. This differs from adult literature showing that self-esteem and a sense of primary control are major predictors of subjective QoL. The meaning of QoL is variable from different individuals' perspectives. This may explain these differences in study results.

Observable or objective empirical referents can be challenging to identify. For example, a physical function deficit or material/monetary wealth does not necessarily mean that an individual has poor or good QoL, nor does it indicate that an individual is happy or unhappy. As QoL is mostly subjective, the best way to know is to ask an individual if she is happy and satisfied with her life. An individual who is happy and satisfied with life likely has high QoL (Figure 12.1).

SUMMARY

QoL is a multidimensional concept that encompasses multiple indicators of personal, social, environmental, economics, psychological, and emotional well-being. It is an integration of the subjective and objective indicators of an individual's life domains. It requires cognitive ability to discern what makes an individual happy as well as functional ability to perform basic activities of living. It is subjectively impacted by what an individual values and deems important in life.

It has been established that QoL is an important factor in medical care, especially with chronic diseases, the elderly with functional deficits, and individuals with serious or life-threatening conditions, to name a few. As individuals seek to be more involved in their medical care, for example, it is likely that their self-esteem and happiness will increase.

Indeed, QoL can be an elusive concept due to its variability and extent of multiple indicators. It cannot be measured solely from a subjective viewpoint, but rather should be measured by integrating both the subjective and objective indicators. It is meaningful and important to pursue research on QoL.

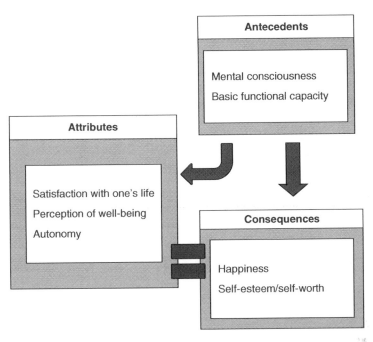

FIGURE 12.1 Quality of life.

REFERENCES

Apolone, G., & Mosconi, P. (1998). Review of the concept of quality of life assessment and discussion of present trend in clinical research. *Nephrology Dialysis Transplantation, 13*(Suppl. 1), 65–69.

Chinn, P. L., & Kramer, M. K. (1995). *Theory and nursing: A systematic approach* (4th ed.). St. Louis, MO: Mosby Year Book.

Costanza, R., Fisher, B., Ali, S., Beer, C., Bond, L., Boumans, R., … Snapp, R. (2008). An integrative approach to quality of life measurement, research, and policy. *Surveys and Perpectives Integrating Environment and Safety, 1*(1), 1–5. Retrieved from http://sapiens.revues.org/169

Dickerson, S. S., Connors, L. M., Fayad, A., & Dean, G. E. (2014). Sleep-wake disturbances in cancer patients: Narrative review of literature focusing on improving quality of life outcomes. *Nature and Science of Sleep, 6,* 85–100.

Dugger, B. R. (2010). Concept analysis of health-related quality of life in nursing home residents with urinary incontinence. *Urologic Nursing, 30*(2), 112–119.

Edgerton, J. D., Roberts, L. W., & von Below, S. (2012). Education and quality of life. In K. C. Land, A. C. Michalos, & J. M. Sirgu (Eds.), *Handbook of social indicators and quality of life research* (pp. 265–296). Dordrecht, The Netherlands: Springer. doi:1007/978-94-007-2421-1_12

Estebsari, F., Taghdisi, M. H., Mostafaei, D., Jamshidi, E., & Latifi, M. (2013). Determining the factors contributing to quality of life of patients at the last stage of life: A qualitative study. *Iranian Red Crescent Medical Journal, 15*(12), 1–6. doi:10.5812/ircmj.13594

Frisch, M. B. (2012). Quality of life well-being in general medicine, mental health, and coaching. In K. C. Land, A. C. Michalos, & M. J. Sirgy (Eds.), *Handbook of social indicators and quality of life research* (pp. 239–263). Dordrecht, The Netherlands: Springer. doi:1007/978-94-007-2421-1_11

Frisch, M. B. (2013). Evidence-based well-being/positive psychology assessment and intervention with quality of life therapy and coaching and the quality of life inventory. *Social Indicators Research, 114,* 193–227. doi:10.1007/s11205-012-0140-7

Gotze, H., Brahler, E., Gansera, L., Polze, N., & Kohler, N. (2014). Psychological distress and quality of life of palliative care patients and their caring relatives during home care. *Support Care Cancer, 22,* 2775–2782. doi:10.007/s00520-014-2257-5

Hacker, E. (2009). Exercise and quality of life: Strengthening the connection. *Clinical Journal of Oncology Nursing, 13*(1), 31–39.

Lyubomirsky, S. L., Sheldon, K. M., & Schkade, D. (2005). Pursuing happiness: The architecture of sustainable change. *Review of General Psychology, 9*(2), 111–131.

Mandzuk, L. L., & McMillan, D. E. (2005). A concept analysis of quality of life. *Journal of Orthopaedic Nursing, 9*(1), 12–18.

Marriage, K., & Cummins, R. A. (2004). Subjective quality of life and self-esteem in children: The role of primary and secondary control in coping with everyday stress. *Social Indicators Research, 66,* 107–122.

Mendlowicz, M. V., & Stein, M. B. (2000). Quality of life in individuals with anxiety disorders. *American Journal of Psychiatry, 157*(5), 669–682.

Osborne, L. A., Bindeman, N., Noble, G. J., & Reed, P. (2014). Different perspectives regarding quality of life in chronically ill and healthy individuals. *Applied Research Quality Life, 9,* 971–979. doi:10.1007/s11482-013-9280-4

Plummer, M., & Molzahn, A. E. (2009). Quality of life in contemporary nursing theory: A concept analysis. *Nursing Science Quarterly, 22*(2), 134–140.

Sanda, M. G., Dunn, R. L., Michalski, J., Sandler, H. M., Northouse, L., Hembroff, L, … Wei, J. T. (2008). Quality of life and satisfaction with outcome among prostate-cancer survivors. *New England Journal of Medicine, 358,* 1250–1261.

Sarvimaki, A. (2000). Quality of life in old age described as a sense of well-being, meaning and value. *Journal of Advanced Nursing, 32*(4), 1025–1033.

Schalock, R. L. (2004). The concept of quality of life: What we know and do not know. *Journal of Intellectual Disability Research, 48*(3), 203–216.

Veenhoven, R. (2012). Happiness, also known as "life satisfaction" and "subjective well-being." In K. C. Land, A. C. Michalos, & M. J. Sirgy (Eds.), *Handbook of social indicators and quality of life research* (pp. 63–77). Dordrecht, The Netherlands: Springer. doi:1007/978-94-007-2421-1_3

13

SELF-CARE STRATEGIES

Symptom management is a dynamic process that includes the interrelated steps of assessment, involvement in symptom management, and decision making (Fu, LeMone, & McDaniel, 2004). According to Dodd et al. (2001), the construct known as symptom management comprises the self-care prescribed by health care professionals and the self-care strategies used by patients themselves to manage symptoms. The purpose of this chapter is to present a concept analysis of the term *self-care strategies*.

It is documented that patients often make changes to the self-care strategies they use over time in response to the efficacy of symptom management strategies adopted (Fu et al., 2004). In addition, some patients depend on *self-taught* strategies, such as trial and error, which have helped them manage an earlier illness (Eller et al., 2005; Landers, McCarthy, Livingstone, & Savage, 2013; Teel, Meek, McNamara, & Watson, 1997). Therefore, the self-care strategies patients use to manage symptoms should be assessed by nurses on a regular basis. Conceptual clarification for a concept such as self-care strategies is needed to enable nurses to accurately assess the effectiveness of the self-care strategies patients use at home to manage problematic symptoms.

A review of the literature showed that the concept of self-care strategies was almost exclusive to nursing. In a study focusing on the alleviation of fatigue, self-care strategies were referred to as any intervention undertaken by a patient in an attempt to relieve this symptom and the effectiveness of that intervention (Borthwick, Knowles, McNamara, O'Dea, & Stroner, 2003). The term *self-care strategies* was described as the behaviors adopted by patients to manage symptoms associated with cancer treatment (Erickson, Spurlock, Kramer, & Davis, 2013), chronic conditions (Bliss, 2005; Hall, Rubin, Hungin, & Dougall, 2007), and the depressive symptoms in mental disease (Eller et al., 2002).

The review also highlighted that self-care strategies can be categorized into different groups. Following a review of the literature, Landers, Savage,

McCarthy, and Fitzpatrick (2011) grouped the self-care strategies that worked best for patients managing bowel symptoms into three categories: (a) functional self-care strategies, which were defined as those activities that focused on managing the bowel movement associated with symptoms of bowel dysfunction such as diarrhea; (b) social activity-related self-care strategies, which were the actions that patients took to manage bowel symptoms in social situations; and (c) alternative self-care strategies, which included complementary therapies. As already noted, patients' participation in their own after-care, by using self-care strategies, plays a significant role in the overall spectrum of symptom management. However, self-care strategies adopted by patients can also be classed as ineffective (Eller et al., 2002) or health damaging (Dodd et al., 2001; Humphreys et al., 2008). There is a lack of clarity as to what constitutes self-care strategies; hence the importance of making the meaning of the concept more explicit for research and practice.

DEFINING ATTRIBUTES

The defining attributes of self-care strategies are *self-care behavior, self-belief, self-taught, learned over time,* and *trial and error.*

The first attribute of the construct self-care strategies is self-care behaviors which are initiated by individual patients themselves. Erikson et al. (2013) investigated the self-care strategies to relieve fatigue in patients receiving radiation therapy. Self-care strategies were described as the self-care behaviors that patients adopted at home, following treatment, to relieve their fatigue.

Research showed that the self-care strategies adopted to manage bowel symptoms were individualistic and were chosen on the basis of what worked best for the person (Erikson et al., 2013; Landers, Savage, & McCarthy, 2012; Landers et al., 2013).

The second identifiable attribute is self-belief. Bandura (1995) proposes that individuals who possess self-belief have confidence in their ability to perform a task and are more likely to attempt it and deal with failure should they not succeed at the task.

A third attribute is trial and error. In a study underpinned by the symptom management theory, Eller et al. (2002) identified the self-care strategies used by people living with HIV to manage their depressive symptoms. Findings demonstrated that people living with HIV used multiple self-care strategies for the management of depressive symptoms. The study also highlighted that only 28% of self-care strategies used for the management of depressive symptoms were recommended by health care providers, whereas 31% of strategies used were learned through trial and error.

Linked to trial and error is the construct *self-taught*. Self-taught constitutes a fourth attribute. In a correlational study that investigated patients' bowel symptom experiences and self-care strategies following sphincter-saving surgery for rectal cancer, Landers et al. (2013) found that many strategies were self-taught.

The fifth attribute is *learned over time*. Findings from studies focusing on patients following sphincter-saving surgery showed that patients learned over time which strategies worked best for them in the management of specific bowel symptoms (Desnoo & Faithfull, 2006; Landers et al., 2013; Nikoletti et al., 2009).

DEFINITION

Self-care strategies are defined as the self-care behaviors that patients adopt to manage symptoms. Inherent in this definition is patients' self-belief in their ability to choose strategies to manage their symptoms. Thus, self-care strategies are self-taught and are learned over time through the process of trial and error.

MODEL CASE

The model case is an example of the concept (self-care strategies) that includes all the identified attributes: self-care behaviors, self-care ability, self-taught, trial and error, and learned over time. The model case used for this analysis was constructed by the author and was guided by the findings of a research study on patients' bowel symptom experiences and self-care strategies following sphincter-saving surgery for rectal cancer (Landers et al., 2012, 2013).

Mary, a 60-year-old female, had sphincter-saving surgery for rectal cancer 6 weeks ago. She is currently experiencing frequency of bowel movement. Mary has been invited to a social event and is worried about becoming incontinent. She decides to engage in a number of self-care behaviors, such as planning her diet in advance and cutting out fluids and foods that could exacerbate the problem and not eating prior to going out. Mary learned over time which foods and fluids help her to manage problematic bowel symptoms such as fecal incontinence. In this case, the patient is aware of the symptoms associated with sphincter-saving surgery. She knows which self-care behaviors might be helpful to her in preventing fecal incontinence. Through the process of trial and error, Mary has worked out the best strategies for her in the management of her bowel symptoms. Thus, strategies are self-taught and Mary has self-belief in her ability to choose strategies to manage her bowel symptoms. It is clear that this case is applicable to self-care strategies.

RELATED CASE

A related case does not contain all the defining attributes of the concept. However, it is an instance that is closely related to the concept. Mary, a 60-year-old female, had sphincter-saving surgery for rectal cancer 6 weeks ago. She is currently experiencing frequency of bowel movement. In this case, the patient is aware of the self-care behaviors that could help. Mary has been given an appointment to attend the colo-proctology clinic. She waits until her visit to the clinic (failed self-belief and self-taught) to collaborate with the clinical nurse specialist as to which foods to exclude from her diet to help her manage her symptoms.

In this case, Mary attends the colo-proctology clinic at the nearby hospital with the intention of collaborating with the clinical nurse specialist on which strategies to adopt. Thus, the decision on the self-care behaviors to use was based on the advice given by the clinical nurse specialist (failed learned over time and trial and error). It is clear that this related case is more applicable to self-management. As outlined earlier, self-management requires individuals to actively participate in the management of their illnesses, but under the supervision of a health care professional (Wilson, Kendall, & Brooks, 2006).

BORDERLINE CASE

Mary, a 60-year-old female, had sphincter-saving surgery for rectal cancer 6 weeks ago. She is currently experiencing frequency of bowel movement. She has been invited to a social event and is worried about becoming incontinent. She has engaged in a number of self-care behaviors in an effort to manage her symptoms. However, she is not confident that the strategies will be effective in managing her bowel symptoms (failed self-belief). Instead, she calls the clinical nurse specialist and requests a diet pamphlet developed for patients who have undergone sphincter-saving surgery for rectal cancer. This case is described as borderline because she failed the other attributes: self-taught, learned over time, and trial and error.

CONTRARY CASE

Since discharge from the hospital after sphincter-saving surgery for rectal cancer 6 weeks earlier, Mary, a 60-year-old female, has been experiencing frequency of bowel movement. Mary has been invited to a social event. However, she decides not to attend, as she feels she will not be able to manage the unpredictable bowel symptoms that she has been experiencing since her surgery. This case includes factors that are contrary to the defining attributes of self-care strategies. This example illustrates that Mary lacks self-belief in her ability to manage her bowel symptoms. She decides not to explore the self-care behaviors that could potentially alleviate her symptoms. This case does not include any of the defining attributes of self-care strategies. Thus, the example could be seen to depict an opposing concept.

ANTECEDENTS

Antecedents are patients experiencing and managing symptoms at home, the nature and presence of the symptoms, the symptom severity, duration of the symptom, and individual reaction to the symptom. Health care professionals are ultimately responsible for supporting patients in managing their symptoms. However, with more care now moving to the community

(Wilde & Garvin, 2007), the management of symptoms and the ensuing effects of treatments is being taken over by patients themselves (Dodd et al., 2001; Humphreys et al., 2008).

CONSEQUENCES

Consequences can be specific or more generalized, and can be both positive and negative. Alleviation or relief or the persistence of symptoms can be identified as the specific consequences of the adoption of self-care strategies. The effective management of a symptom through the use of appropriate self-care strategies should lead to a symptom status in which the symptom(s) is relieved, symptom distress is decreased, or symptom occurrence is prevented (Fu et al., 2004). Persistent or unrelieved symptom(s), worsening symptoms, or symptoms remaining distressing for patients were identified as negative consequences of the ineffective management of symptoms (Landers et al., 2012, 2013).

More generalized consequences of the effective management of a symptom should include overall improvement in health status, the ability to undertake activities of daily living, and resumption of a normal social life. However, Eller et al.'s findings (2002) highlighted that self-care strategies adopted can also be ineffective for patients. Disillusionment, social isolation, and depression were identified as long-term consequences when a strategy had little or no effect in alleviating symptoms (Annells & Koch, 2002, 2003; Eller et al., 2002; Landers et al., 2012; see Figure 13.1).

EMPIRICAL REFERENTS

The measurement of self-care strategies has the potential to involve the use of a number of empirical referents. However, valid and reliable instruments for the measurement of self-care strategies are not widely available.

A self-care strategy measure was developed for the purpose of a study on patients' experiences and self-care strategies following sphincter-saving surgery for rectal cancer (Landers et al., 2013). The measure was based on a review of existing literature concerning the symptom experiences and symptom management strategies of patients who suffer bowel symptoms following both sphincter-saving surgery and chronic bowel disease. The self-care strategy measure assessed three components. First, a measurement of patients' use of self-care strategies (e.g., number of self-strategies) was obtained. Second, the effectiveness of self-care strategies used (e.g., average effectiveness of strategies used) was calculated. Finally, patients were given the opportunity to identify any other self-care strategies that they used to manage bowel symptoms and the level of effectiveness achieved by using these strategies. The relevance and appropriateness of the content of the Self-Care Strategy Scale were confirmed by assessing the content validity of the items on this measure. However, the validity of the measure has yet to be established.

The Self-Care Diary was developed by Nail, Jones, Greene, Schipper, and Jensen (1991) to measure the incidence and severity of selected side effects of cancer treatment and the use and efficacy of self-care activities intended to manage those side effects (Nail et al., 1991). This instrument could be modified to include the term *self-care strategies*.

Patients' belief in their ability to choose self-care strategies to manage their symptoms could potentially be measured using a modified version of the Inflammatory Bowel Disease Self-Efficacy Scale (IBD-SES) developed by Keefer, Jennifer, Kiebles, and Taft (2011). In this scale, responses range from 10 (totally sure), to 5 (somewhat sure), to 1 (not sure at all).

SUMMARY

An analysis of the concept of self-care strategies has resulted in the tentative identification of antecedents, attributes, and consequences. As distinct from self-management, the analysis shows that the self-care-strategies adopted to manage symptoms are individualistic and are chosen on the basis of what works best for the person. The literature also shows that in the main, self-care strategies are not recommended by health care professionals. Patients tend to rely on self-taught strategies, learned through trial and error, that have helped them to cope with illness in the past. The working definition of self-care strategies formulated herein will aid in the development of concept-driven research to advance the concept toward greater accuracy and efficacy in nursing science.

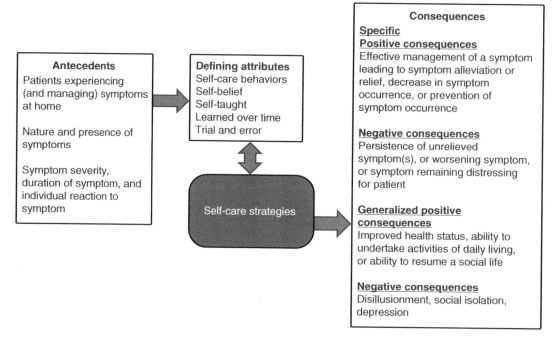

FIGURE 13.1 Self-care strategies.

REFERENCES

Annells, M., & Koch, T. (2002). Older people seeking solutions to constipation: The laxative mire. *Journal of Clinical Nursing, 11*(5), 613–612.

Annells, M., & Koch, T. (2003). Constipation and the preached trio: Diet, fluid intake, exercise. *International Journal of Nursing Studies, 40*(8), 843–852.

Bandura, A. (1995). *Self-efficacy in changing societies.* Cambridge, UK: Cambridge University Press.

Bliss, Z. D. (2005). Managing faecal incontinence: Self-care practices of older adults. *Journal of Gerontological Nursing, 31*(7), 35–44.

Borthwick, B., Knowles, G., McNamara, S., O'Dea, R., & Stroner, P. (2003). Assessing fatigue and self-care strategies in patients receiving radiotherapy for non-small cell lung cancer. *European Journal of Oncology Nursing, 7*(4), 231–241.

Desnoo, L., & Faithfull, S. (2006). A qualitative study of anterior resection syndrome: The experiences of cancer survivors who had undergone resection surgery. *European Journal of Cancer Care, 15*(3), 244–251.

Dodd, M. J., Jansen, S., Facione, N., Faucett, J., Froelicher, E. S., Humphreys, J., … Taylor, D. (2001). Advancing the science of symptom management. *Journal of Advanced Nursing, 33*(5), 668–678.

Eller, L. S., Corless, I., Bunch, E. H., Kemppainen, J., Holzemer, W., Nokes, K., … Nicholas, P. (2005). Self-care strategies for depressive symptoms in people with HIV disease. *Journal of Advanced Nursing, 51*(2), 119–130.

Erikson, J. M., Spurlock, L. K., Kramer, J. C., & Davis, M. A. (2013). Self-care strategies to relieve fatigue in patients receiving radiation therapy. *Clinical Journal of Oncology Nursing, 17*(3), 313–324.

Fu, M. R., Lemone, P., & McDaniel, R. W. (2004). An integrated approach to an analysis of symptom management in cancer patients. *Oncology Nursing Forum, 31*(1), 65–70.

Hall, N. J., Rubin, G. P., Hungin, A. P. S., & Dougall, A. (2007). Medication beliefs among patients with inflammatory bowel disease who report low quality of life: A qualitative study. *Gastroenterology, 7*(20), 1–8.

Humphreys, J., Lee, K. A., Carrieri-Kohlman, V., Puntiollo, K., Faucett, J., Janson, S., … The UCSF School of Nursing Symptom Management Faculty Group. (2008). The theory of symptom management. In M. J. Smith & P. R. Liehr (Eds.), *Middle range theory for nursing* (2nd ed., pp. 145–158). New York, NY: Springer.

Keefer, L., Jennifer, L., Kiebles, J. L., & Taft, T. H. (2011). The role of self-efficacy in inflammatory bowel disease management: Preliminary validation of a disease-specific measure. *Inflammatory Bowel Disease, 17*(2), 614–620.

Landers, M., McCarthy, G., Livingstone, V., & Savage, E. (2013). Patients' bowel symptom experiences and self-care strategies following sphincter-saving surgery for rectal cancer. *Journal of Clinical Nursing, 23*(15–16), 2343–2354.

Landers, M., Savage, E., & McCarthy, G. (2012). Bowel symptom experiences and management following sphincter saving-surgery for rectal cancer: A qualitative perspective. *European Journal of Oncology Nursing, 16*(3), 293–300.

Landers, M., Savage, E., McCarthy, G., & Fitzpatrick, J. (2011). Self-care strategies for the management of bowel symptoms following sphincter-saving surgery for rectal cancer. *Clinical Journal of Oncology Nursing, 5*(6), E105–E114.

Nail, L. M., Jones, L. S., Greene, D., Schipper, D. L., & Jensen, R. (1991). Use and perceived efficacy of self-care activities in patients receiving chemotherapy. *Cancer Oncology Nursing Forum, 18*(5), 883–387.

Nikoletti, S., Young, S., Levitt, M., King, M., Chidlow, C., & Hollingsworth, S. (2008). Bowel problems, self-care practices and information needs of colo-rectal survivors at 6 to 24 months after sphincter-saving surgery. *Cancer Nursing, 31*(5), 389–398.

Wilde, M. H., & Garvin, S. (2007). A concept analysis of self-monitoring. *Journal of Advanced Nursing, 57*(3), 339–350.

Wilson, P. M., Kendall, S., & Brooks, F. (2006). Nurses' responses to expert patients: The rhetoric and reality of self-management in long-term conditions: A grounded theory study. *International Journal of Nursing Studies, 43*(7), 803–818.

14

SELF-MOTIVATION

Self-motivation is a key concept relevant to professional practice in nursing and other disciplines. Self-motivation is a complex concept with multiple individual personal characteristics and external attributes. Self-motivation is an abstract concept independent of time and space (Reynolds, 1971). The meaning of self-motivation may be multifaceted and multidirectional. *Self-motivation* is the ability of individuals to satisfy a desire, expectation, or goal without being influenced by external forces (Ryan & Deci, 2000). Self-motivation is the key to behavioral changes along the course of the lifetime from childhood to adulthood. It evolves through the past, present, and future of each individual. Self-motivation depends on self-initiative drive and self-beliefs working toward accomplishing one's future goals (Murphy & Alexander, 2000).

Self-motivation is viewed as an internal personal drive, which comes from within the self, although it can be guided through external forces (deCharms & Muir, 1978). The internal and external powers blend into a unique strength of the self in conquering the present and future personal and social goals, basing them on past experiences (Guay, Vallerand, & Blanchard, 2000). Although this blend occurs daily in different situations, some people will be more intrinsic self-motivators and some will be extrinsic self-motivators (Guay et al., 2000). Positive energy enhances and strengthens self-motivation, producing an inner desire to grow and achieve higher aims in life (Kreps, 1997). Energy and motivation are seen as the same drive and ability to accomplish things (Ryan & Deci, 2000). However, *energy* may be interpreted as the physical ability to do activities and *motivation* as the emotional ability and desire to do things (Kreps, 1997). The spectrum of self-motivation lies between one end of a highly energetic force and another of a poor inner drive.

The self-perception theory foresees that intrinsic and extrinsic motivation do not bond additively, but rather interact (Zimmerman, Bandura, & Martinez-Pons, 1992). Studies have shown a significant interaction between intrinsic and extrinsic motivation for task fulfillment (Calder & Staw, 1975). The intrinsic self-motivators are guided by the inner satisfaction of performing a task, and they include having fun, pleasure, and interest (deCharms & Muir, 1978). Contrariwise, external forces or environmental factors influence extrinsic motivators. DeCharms defines intrinsic and extrinsic motivators based on their locus of control and causality (deCharms, 1968). Different people may be motivated by different intrinsic and extrinsic powers and triggers.

Other theories, have addressed the focus of self-motivation. The objective self-awareness (OSA) theory as a model of self-motivation assumes that diverse behaviors, such as accepting or denying responsibility for failure, originate from the same underlying dynamics (Silvia & Duval, 2004). Furthermore, cognitive theories of motivation focus on beliefs, values, expectations, and needs. Motivation depends on the degree to which people presume to be successful times the value they place on success (Gagné & Deci, 2005). According to Bandura's self-efficacy theory, individuals attain the ability to control their behaviors when doing a specific task or having a specific goal in mind (Bandura, 1997). Others foresee self-motivation as self-determination differentiating between goal setting and goal implementation (Zimmerman et al., 1992).

In the health belief model (HBM), motivation as an act to change behavior is equal to the perception of the reward achieved minus the perceived cost and barriers (Miller, 2000). The self-determination theory (SDT) explains and describes motivation as a predictor for well-being (Deci & Ryan, 2008). Other theorists such as Malone and Lepper, define *self-motivation* simply as what people would do without external influence (Mele, 1995). The majority of clinicians, psychologists, and theorists perceive self-motivation as an interaction between intrinsic and extrinsic motivations and conversely the split between intrinsic and extrinsic forces.

Self-motivation aligns itself through a spectrum of internal and external forces, which differ between individuals. Although there are variable forces that govern each individual's self-motivation, there are similar features that constitute self-motivation and its general attributes. Motivation is based on the inner drive, force, and energy that guide people toward achieving a personal or a professional goal. Often, self-motivation is aimed toward reaching desirable outcomes, such as increased power, increased safety, and self-esteem or pleasure and joy (Fletcher, 1999). However, self-motivation can be aimed toward reaching self-fulfillment and enrichment without any specific outcomes in mind (Murphy & Alexander, 2000). Additively, the intrinsic and extrinsic forces of self-motivation often lead to optimal outcomes. The purpose of this chapter is to present an in-depth analysis of the concept of self-motivation and explore it in the context of nursing practice and health, following Walker and Avant's framework (Walker & Avant, 2005).

DEFINING ATTRIBUTES

The defining attributes of self-motivation are *desire to do an action/behavior, inner drive and external force to achieve a goal,* and *desire to fulfill pleasure and joy.*

A desire to do an action/behavior is the first defining attribute because the inner desire to do specific activities and behaviors is the fundamental characteristic of self-motivation (Brush, Kirk, Gultekin, & Baiardi, 2011; Fletcher, 1999). Self-motivation is an intrinsic positive force that influences someone to do an action. The definition of *motivation* implies the condition of being eager to act or work and the circumstance of being motivated (Murphy & Alexander, 2000). Self is the identity of a person; motivation is defined as the drive to do things (Vallerand & Lalande, 2011).

An inner drive and external force to achieve a goal is the second defining attribute. Self-motivation may be triggered by specific goals. Self-motivation infers a conscious awareness to be successful and control behaviors while accomplishing short-term and long-term goals. The psychological definition of motivation is the method that guides and sustains goal-oriented behaviors (Miller, Deci, & Ryan, 1988). This includes the biological, emotional, social, and cognitive energies that stimulate behaviors (Miller et al., 1988).

A desire to fulfill pleasure and joy is a defining attribute, as the literature relates enjoyment leading to motivation. The extent of enjoyment after fulfilling a challenging task may promote responsible behavior in working situations and others (Isen & Reeve, 2005). Studies have shown that positive affect fosters intrinsic motivation and enjoyment while performing pleasurable tasks.

DEFINITION

Self-motivation is defined as an individual's desire to perform an action/ engage in a behavior, an inner drive and external force to achieve a goal, and a desire to fulfill pleasure and joy.

MODEL CASE

Daniel is a 45-year-old male admitted to the hospital with chest pain radiating to his left arm and jaw. He is currently a heavy smoker and for many years has smoked two packs daily. He had a cardiac workup in the hospital and was diagnosed with an acute myocardial infarction. Daniel had multiple discussions with his cardiologist and his primary care provider (PCP) about the critical effects of smoking on his overall health and cardiovascular condition. Both specialists and his family have reinforced the importance of quitting smoking and promoting his health and quality of life. Daniel, a highly motivated individual (a desire to perform an action/engage in a behavior) decided to take charge of his well-being. He was looking forward to spending time with his family without having smoking interfere with his activities (a desire to fulfill pleasure and joy outcomes). He decided to quit smoking and discussed the different options with his PCP. He enrolled in a community program and used a medication and support to reach his goal (an inner drive and external force to achieve a goal).

Daniel has gone faithfully to the support program and adhered to the medication regime. This has helped him to control his cravings. Daniel had no mood issues and he expressed his emotions freely (no mood or emotional disorder). He was very optimistic about his future goals without any negative thoughts or feelings. All defining attributes are present in this case.

RELATED CASE

Related cases have some of the defining attributes. An example is that of a 45-year-old male, mildly depressed, who had some marital issues with his wife that affected his children and the whole atmosphere at home. Alex had high self-esteem, but he had no desire to change his behavior (failed desire to do an action/behavior). Alex decided to communicate openly with his wife about the problems surrounding their marriage. Although he had no negative thoughts, he did not have any realistic goals in mind to alter the family situation (failed drive and external force to achieve a goal). Alex and his wife wanted to have joy and pleasure in their lives (desire to fulfill pleasure and joy outcomes), but he had mild depression that affected his life with his family.

BORDERLINE CASE

Borderline cases contain most of the attributes. Samantha is a 35-year-old female who has had diabetes for many years. She has been very driven and motivated in following her diabetes management (desire to do an action/behavior) and maintaining a strict diet, physical activity, and vigilant glucose monitoring. Recently, Samantha has been busy socially and she has cheated slightly on her diet. However, she continued to have positive thoughts without any mood changes. Samantha went to a follow-up visit with her PCP, who did a blood test while discussing any changes in her life. She admitted to her PCP that her lifestyle has changed and she is going out on multiple dinners throughout the week. She honestly told her PCP that she has eaten different types of food usually not included in her diet in the past 4 weeks. She has eaten more without any adjustment of her medications and had less drive to monitor her condition to achieve positive outcomes, self-satisfaction, and joy (failed desire to fulfill pleasure and joy outcomes). Samantha felt guilty about her recent changes when discussing them with her PCP. As she discussed her recent social life with him, she realized that she has to forgo her recent dietary changes and resume her strict vigilant monitoring of her diet, exercise, and glucose follow-up. She notified her PCP that she would return to her usual routines to maintain control of her diabetes. She had inner drive and environmental forces, including support from her health care provider, that promoted reaching her goals of better dietary control (drive and external force to achieve a goal). She recognized the importance of her quality of life and health and their superiority to her social life without any emotional or mood changes.

CONTRARY CASE

Eric, a young patient who was in a very depressed state of mind, was evaluated by his neurologist during a follow-up visit. For several years now, Eric has had multiple sclerosis (MS), which is a chronic progressive and degenerative neurological disease. He had no ambition or desire to change his behaviors (failed desire to do an action/behavior) and manage his disease optimally. He has been depressed for many years and has negative thoughts and drives leading to amotivation. Eric did not have any personal or social interests or pleasure during his daily activities (failed desire to fulfill pleasure and joy outcomes). Eric admitted to his neurologist and his family that he has no personal goals or desires (failed drive and external force to achieve a goal). He did not care for himself and did not follow any of the medical instructions to promote his health and wellness. Eric had no pleasure or joy (failed desire to fulfill pleasure and joy outcomes) in his life and he did not adhere to his medical and nursing instructions to enhance his quality of life. Eric's MS and depression have continued to worsen and affect his daily activities. His emotional and physical condition has deteriorated, negatively influencing his family, vocational, and social life. This example does not exemplify the concept, as it does not have any of the defining attributes.

ANTECEDENTS

The antecedents of self-motivation are: (a) sense of self-discipline and self-responsibility, (b) sense of self-determination and confidence, (c) willpower and self-efficacy, and (d) having certain values and beliefs (Fletcher, 1999).

The cognitive evaluation theory emphasizes the importance of the antecedents of motivation. This theory proposes that autonomy, competence, and social relatedness are the three keystones of intrinsic motivation leading to positive behaviors and attitudes promoting health and wellness (Deci & Ryan, 2008).

CONSEQUENCES

The consequences of self-motivation are the outcomes of the activities and behaviors. These consequences include sense of control and autonomy; joy, pleasure, and satisfaction; sense of achievement and success; and sense of pride, self-worth, and integrity (Fletcher, 1999).

EMPIRICAL REFERENTS

Empirical referents are measurable methods to determine the occurrence of the concept (Walker & Avant, 2005). Self-motivation varies considerably among individuals; however, this concept has mutual characteristics that can be measured and assessed. Self-motivation is a concept that lies on a continuum of constructs between those that can be measured and those that are abstract. The more abstract a concept, the less it can be directly measured (Chinn & Kramer, 1999). On this continuum, self-motivation may be placed on the more abstract end, because of its intangible and subjective nature; however, it can be measured (based on its shared attributes) mainly by self-report instruments.

The Echelle de Motivation en Education (EME) is a French motivation instrument that is based on the SDT (Vallerand et al., 1992). The EME is comprised of 28 items subdivided into 7 subscales assessing 3 types of intrinsic motivation: intrinsic motivation to know, to accomplish things, and to experience stimulation; and three types of extrinsic motivation: external, introjected, and identified regulation; and amotivation (Vallerand et al., 1992). The EME was translated into English through appropriate methodological procedures, and named the Academic Motivation Scale (AMS). The internal consistency of the instrument was high ($r = 0.81$) and the reliability (test–retest correlation) of the AMS tool was $r = 0.79$. The AMS has adequate validity and reliability for its use in evaluating motivation in many arenas (Vallerand & Lalande, 2011; Vallerand et al., 1992).

The Situational Motivation Scale (SIMS) is another instrument that measures the state of motivation. The SIMS is designed to assess the constructs of intrinsic motivation, identified regulation, external regulation, and amotivation in communities and laboratory settings (Miller et al., 1988; Rigby, Deci, Patrick, & Ryan, 1992). The SIMS has been validated as a motivation measure in clinical settings. Overall, the SIMS exemplifies a brief and multipurpose self-report instrument of situational intrinsic motivation, internal regulation, external regulation, and amotivation. The Academic Motivation and the Situational Motivation self-report tools are essential in evaluating motivation in corporations, nursing, and health care (Figure 14.1).

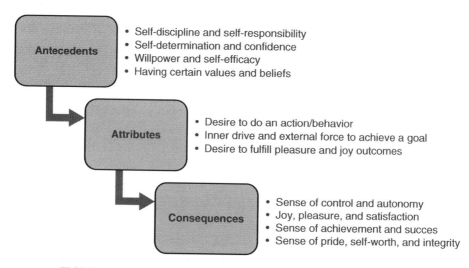

FIGURE 14.1 Schematic representation of self-motivation concept.

SUMMARY

Self-motivation is important for attaining success in personal and social life. People have inner motives driving them into certain behaviors toward accomplishing their life goals. According to Maslow, people have an internal drive motivating them toward self-actualization (Watson, 1996). Motivation is composed of individual and interpersonal factors leading to certain behaviors and actions. The individual factors include challenge, curiosity, control, and fantasy, and the interpersonal factors include competition, cooperation, and recognition. Deci and Ryan have contemplated that internal locus of control may lead to motivation (Deci & Ryan, 2008). However, locus of causality determines if people are self-determined and intrinsically motivated. People may be intrinsic or extrinsic motivators based on their character, their personality, and their short-term and long-term life goals.

REFERENCES

Bandura, A. (1997). Theoretical perspectives. In A. Bandura (Ed.) *Self-efficacy: The exercise of control* (pp. 1–35). New York, NY: Freeman.

Brush, B. L., Kirk, K., Gultekin, L., & Baiardi, J. M. (2011). Overcoming: A concept analysis. *Nursing Forum, 46*(3), 160–168.

Calder, B. J., & Staw, B. M. (1975). Self-perception of intrinsic and extrinsic motivation. *Journal of Personality and Social Psychology, 31*(4), 599–605.

Chinn, P. L., & Kramer, M. K. (1999). *Theory and nursing: Integrated knowledge development* (5th ed.). St. Louis, MO: Mosby.

deCharms, R. (1968). *Personal causation: The internal affective determinants of behavior.* Ann Arbor, MI: Academic Press.

deCharms, R., & Muir, M. S. (1978). Motivation: Social approaches. *Annual Review of Psychology, 29*, 91–113.

Deci, E. L., & Ryan, R. M. (2008). Self-determination theory: A macrotheory of human motivation, development, and health. *Canadian Psychology/Psychologie Canadienne, 49*, 182–185.

Fletcher, A. B. (1999). A concept analysis of motivation. *Journal of Cultural Diversity, 6*(4), 130.

Gagné, M., & Deci, E. L. (2005). Self-determination theory and work motivation. *Journal of Organizational Behavior, 26*, 331–362.

Guay, F., Vallerand, R. J., & Blanchard, C. (2000). On the assessment of situational intrinsic and extrinsic motivation: The Situational Motivation Scale (SIMS). *Motivation and Emotion, 24*, 175–213.

Isen, A. M., & Reeve, J. (2005). The influence of positive affect on intrinsic and extrinsic motivation: Facilitating enjoyment of play, responsible work behavior, and self-control. *Motivation and Emotion, 29*, 297–325.

Kreps, D. M. (1997). Intrinsic motivation and extrinsic incentives. *American Economic Review, 87*, 359–364.

Mele, A. R. (1995). Motivation: Essentially motivation-constituting attitudes. *Philosophical Review, 104*, 387.

Miller, J. F. (2000). *Coping with chronic illness: Overcoming powerlessness* (3rd ed.). Philadelphia, PA: F.A. Davis.

Miller, K. A., Deci, E. L., & Ryan, R. M. (1988). Intrinsic motivation and self-determination in human behavior. *Contemporary Sociology, 17*, 253.

Murphy, P., & Alexander, P. (2000). A motivated exploration of motivation terminology. *Contemporary Educational Psychology, 25*, 3–53.

Reynolds, P. D. (1971). *A primer in theory construction* (p. 184). Indianapolis, IN: Bobbs-Merrill.

Rigby, S. C., Deci, E. L., Patrick, B. C., & Ryan, R. M. (1992). Beyond the intrinsic-extrinsic dichotomy: Self-determination in motivation and learning. *Motivation and Emotion, 16*, 165–185.

Ryan, R. M., & Deci, E. L. (2000). Intrinsic and extrinsic motivations: Classic definitions and new directions. *Contemporary Educational Psychology, 25*, 54–67.

Silvia, P. J., & Duval, T. S. (2004). Self-awareness, self-motives, and self-motivation. In R. A. Wright, J. Green, & S. Brehm (Eds.), *Motivational analyses of social behavior: Building on Jack Brehm's contributions to psychology* (pp. 57–75). Mahwah, NJ: Lawrence Erlbaum.

Vallerand, R. J., & Lalande, D. R. (2011). The MPIC model: The perspective of the hierarchical model of intrinsic and extrinsic motivation. *Psychological Inquiry, 22*, 45–51.

Vallerand, R. J., Pelletier, L. G., Blais, M. R., Briere, N. M., Senecal, C., & Vallieres, E. F. (1992). The Academic Motivation Scale: A measure of intrinsic, extrinsic, and amotivation in education. *Educational and Psychological Measurement, 52*, 1003–1017.

Walker, L. O., & Avant, K. (2005). *Strategies for theory construction in nursing* (4th ed.). Upper Saddle River, NJ: Pearson Education.

Watson, T. J. (1996). Motivation: That's Maslow, isn't it? *Management Learning, 27*, 447–464.

Zimmerman, B. J., Bandura, A., & Martinez-Pons, M. (1992). Self-motivation for academic attainment: The role of self-efficacy beliefs and personal goal setting. *American Educational Research Journal, 29*, 663–676.

DONALD GARDENIER

15

STIGMATIZATION

The stigmatization of populations and individuals is a ubiquitous social phenomenon that has been recognized for some time (Goffman, 1963). Stigmatization affects the provision and utilization of health care and may therefore adversely affect the health of the stigmatized person or group. Despite its pervasiveness, stigmatization is not well understood and often not recognized, even by those directly involved. Thus, an improved understanding of stigmatization and its potential effect on the health of individuals and populations is of central importance to improving health outcomes and therefore to nursing (Kim, Ohan, & Dear, 2015).

Though widely discussed and understood to adversely affect the care of individuals and groups, a consistent definition of *stigmatization* is not readily available in the literature (Scheff, 2014). The attributes of stigma are more consistent but not always cited, leading to literature in which stigma is named as a factor and to greater or lesser extent explored, though not concisely defined. Analysis and clarification of the concept of stigmatization are therefore necessary in order to enhance understanding of it. Improved understanding in turn will lead to more consistent recognition and measurement of stigmatization.

Stigmatization has been widely recognized to occur in the care of marginalized populations, such as incarcerated individuals, those living with HIV/AIDS, the mentally ill, socioeconomically disadvantaged individuals, and other underserved groups. A key attribute of stigma is poor understanding either of its antecedents, or how to address the presenting problem, or both. The groups mentioned previously are frequently named in the literature as being stigmatized. However, among the attributes of stigma is the potential for the health care provider not to recognize it. It is therefore important to remember, in considering the influences of stigma on health care, that any health care provider can be a perpetrator of stigma and any individual or group can become a target of stigmatization. The stigmatization of less readily identified individuals and groups, such as the wealthy, or of an individual whom the health care provider or society venerates or otherwise holds in higher esteem, can be more difficult to recognize and understand. It is therefore of particular utility to analyze stigma at the conceptual level in order to better deal with its effects in the context of the delivery of health care (Keene & Padilla, 2014).

DEFINING ATTRIBUTES

The defining attributes of stigmatization are *separation, labeling,* and *misunderstanding.*

Separation from general society is experienced by stigmatized groups in a variety of ways. In some cases, physical separation itself becomes a source of the stigmatization. When a marginalized group is isolated socioeconomically, for example, it is also likely to be isolated geographically. Disparities in a wide variety of social provisions, including the availability of healthy foods, health care services, and the provision of public safety services, for example, as well as disparities in the quality of housing and their attendant health consequences, result in stigmatization or its reinforcement. Also referred to in the literature as "spatial stigma" (Keene & Padilla, 2014), the physical and social separation of groups that are traditionally subject to stigmatization is particularly associated with health disparities, including higher incidence of asthma, increased rates of obesity and metabolic disease, tobacco addiction, substance use, and mental health issues, as well as decreased utilization of preventive services such as colorectal and breast cancer screening (Keene & Padilla, 2014).

Labeling of stigmatized groups occurs frequently and in most cases reinforces the attendant stigma. Many lay definitions of stigma include physical signs of difference. This definition has carried over into health care, where physical exam signs are taken as evidence of underlying disease, such as the palmar erythema associated with cirrhosis of the liver. Stigmatized groups or individuals may or may not have physical signs or may be misunderstood to carry physical signs, thus leading to labeling, either correctly or incorrectly. Persons with HIV/AIDS, for example, may have no outward signs of their disease and thus be judged by others not to have HIV/AIDS (often referred to as "clean") and therefore not subjected to stigmatization. Conversely, individuals perceived because of some attribute to be members of groups disparately affected by HIV/AIDS, such as men who have sex with men, may be perceived to have HIV/AIDS because they possess the attribute, and therefore are stigmatized not because they have HIV/AIDS but because they are thought to have an attribute that many people with HIV/AIDS have. They may thus be subject to stigmatization despite not living with HIV/AIDS; in fact, the perception of possession of an attribute has the same stigmatizing effect as actual possession of the attribute (Ventura, dosSantos, Mendes, & Trevizan, 2014).

Misunderstanding, which can be characterized as either an incomplete or an incorrect understanding, is inherent in stigma and stigmatization and also gives rise to stigmatization. In particular, judging conditions such as obesity or alcohol or tobacco dependence to be choices that are largely under the control of the stigmatized individual is rooted in an incomplete understanding of the etiology and pathology of these conditions. Nonadherence to health care provider recommendations is another source of stigma that has its origins in misunderstanding. If an individual knows that following the regimen that the health care provider has recommended will improve his or her health, why would that individual not follow that recommendation? The answer to that question is poorly understood. Similarly, lack of understanding of the transmission of infectious diseases can lead to physical and social isolation, such as occurred early in the HIV/AIDS pandemic and more recently in the Ebola outbreaks in West Africa. Stigma substitutes for factual knowledge in those scenarios. By contrast, gaining an understanding of disease states tends to lessen stigma. Thus, lack of understanding can be seen as a defining attribute of stigma (Scheff, 2014).

DEFINITION

Stigmatization is the labeling and separation applied by a larger group to an individual or group perceived to be of a lesser status based on misunderstanding that the attributes of that individual or group are undesirable, potentially harmful, shameful, and/or repugnant.

MODEL CASE

A person with a prior history of injection drug use presents to the clinic to discuss her recently diagnosed chronic hepatitis C virus (HCV) infection. She had discussed treatment previously with her peers and a counsellor at her methadone maintenance program, but decided not to pursue treatment at that time because she did not know where she might access treatment (misunderstanding). She also had some peers who underwent treatment and had a very difficult time with side effects and even then were not cured. She has no idea how much liver damage has already taken place. Additionally, none of her family members knows she has HCV, and she is concerned that they might find out if she had obvious side effects during treatment that she could not otherwise explain (labeling). Currently, she helps care for her grandchildren and she does not want her son to think his children may be at risk for catching it from her. She thinks they probably cannot, but she is not sure. She is anxious to go back to work but is concerned that her history and current methadone therapy would be obstacles. She has also not worked for many years and worries that she will no longer be able to (separation). She also lives in public housing that is tied to her low income status and is concerned that she might no longer qualify for her housing if she got a job.

RELATED CASE

A patient presents to the emergency room with shortness of breath and chest pain. He is diagnosed with a pulmonary embolus and his team recommends admission to the hospital for treatment. He agrees but insists that he must go home first to make arrangements for his pet and secure his belongings (misunderstanding). He says he will return later the same day. After some negotiation with his team he signs himself out, goes home, and then returns late that same night as planned. Upon his return, security guards meet him in the waiting room and instruct him to leave the emergency room immediately (separation). He advocates for himself but he is unsuccessful in convincing the security guards of the prior plan and is physically removed (misunderstanding), sustaining minor injuries in the process. He contacts his emergency room physician from his mobile phone and makes a plan to meet him at the door, and he is eventually readmitted to the emergency room and then to the hospital. The emergency room physician explained that there had been a problem earlier with another individual who fit his physical description and he was mistaken for the other individual (misunderstanding, failed labeling).

BORDERLINE CASE

An individual with metabolic disease and obesity goes to the outpatient clinic for follow-up care. His 8-year-old granddaughter has the day off from school and is with him. He takes a number of medications to treat his various conditions and has spoken to the nurse practitioner at past visits about diet and exercise that, in addition to medication, are needed to manage his conditions. He says he tries to walk every day but the weather has been too cold. His blood pressure is at or near goal when checked. His cholesterol is improved, but he has not lost much weight and his blood sugar, though better than previously, continues to be out of control (misunderstanding). On monitoring, his kidneys continue to function normally but his liver enzymes have increased slightly, showing early signs of fatty liver disease. He has heard from friends that cholesterol medicine is bad for the liver and so took it upon himself to stop taking the medication since the last visit (misunderstanding). Most recently, he has been suffering from joint pains and, after taking more than his allotment of days off, has gone on disability from his job as a security guard because it includes more walking and standing than he is able to do (separation). When asked about his diet, he reports that he eats very little and in fact denies eating anything over the past 24 hours. When his granddaughter asked why he did not report the chips he ate while they were waiting in the waiting room, he quickly instructed her to be quiet (failed labeling).

CONTRARY CASE

A young adult who recently immigrated to the United States from her home country of Mongolia presents to an outpatient clinic. She was diagnosed in Mongolia with chronic hepatitis B infection. She was informed that there was no treatment available, but that most of the time people did not have problems and so treatment was not really needed and she should not worry. She was advised at the time of diagnosis to consider not telling anyone that she was infected, since there was a lot of misunderstanding regarding hepatitis B and people might believe that they could also become infected and that this would have a negative impact on her. In fact, as a blood borne disease, casual contact was not a risk. In the United States, she was a student who was also working part time, and she took it upon herself to do some research. She learned that in fact there was treatment for chronic hepatitis B that could help her avoid the complications that she was at risk for (failed misunderstanding). Unfortunately, she did not have access to health care in the United States, so she was still not able to be treated. While talking with a friend who was also a fellow student (failed separation), she learned of a program available to individuals like them who did not have health coverage to gain access to evaluation and treatment. She contacted the clinic (absence of internalization, status loss, shame), made an appointment, and began treatment (failed labeling). Her disease is under control and she is doing well.

ANTECEDENTS

The antecedents of stigmatization include perception of inequality and misperception of social circumstances.

Stigma requires certain circumstances before it can occur. Social inequality, which exists to greater or lesser extent in most places, is a required antecedent, because loss of status would not otherwise be possible. In order for one group to stigmatize another, one group must occupy a social position favorable to that of the other group. For stigmatization to result in health disparities, there must also be the potential for such disparities in the first place. In a complex system such as that of the United States, where access to care varies from none to ready access, disparities are relatively common and expected. However, in a cohort of injection drug users in Brazil, where access to health care is universal, disparities still exist, in part because of the perceptions of the individuals who perceive that their right to health care is different because of their injection drug use (Ventura et al., 2014).

Another antecedent of stigma is a misperception of the social condition of the individual or group. For example, poverty or homelessness can lead one individual or group to stigmatize another. These misperceptions can be isolated (an individual's alcohol use) or widely held (racism). They may be historically rooted (sexism) or related to more current events (Ebola, preventive vaccination) and may or may not have a sense of urgency.

CONSEQUENCES

There are a number of consequences of stigma relevant to nursing and the delivery of health care. In most instances, the effects of stigma are negative. *Shame* is experienced by the stigmatized individual as she or he comes to understand the object or reason for the stigmatization as being defiling or repulsive. The individual's understanding is derived from societal perceptions of and reactions to the individual's possession of the trait that is the source of the stigmatization. In many stigmatized groups, such as persons who inject drugs or persons with HIV/AIDS, individuals experiencing self-stigmatization identify with and may be drawn to others with similar attributes and thus feelings of repulsion become shame (Scheff, 2014).

Status loss may be a perceptual result when a stigmatizing condition or attribute becomes known, or status loss may be attendant to the stigmatizing condition. In the former case, an individual who might otherwise be held in high regard by others is revealed to inject drugs, abuse alcohol, or be living with HIV/AIDS. Perception of that individual by others, as well as by society, will change strictly based on the new knowledge and loss of status, including income and family relationships, is likely to occur. In other cases, being sentenced to prison after the commission of a crime places one in a stigmatized group and simultaneously causes the loss of employment, social position, and changes in family relationships. Thus, status loss, as a result of both actual and perceived change, is attendant to stigma and stigmatization (Keene & Padilla, 2014).

Internalization occurs when the stigmatized individuals or group take on the external perception of them and the quality or qualities that they possess which has led to the stigma that they experience. This process and the resulting state are also known as *self-stigmatization*. Among users of illegal drugs, for example, it has been found that the individuals themselves may perceive that their human rights, including their right to receive health care, are different from those of mainstream society. At the outset of the movement to achieve marriage equality in the United States, a majority of gays and lesbians themselves were not in favor of marriage equality and voiced that not getting married was part of who they were, thus showing evidence of internalization of stigma. Thus, it can be surmised that stigmatization as a phenomenon comprises both external stigmatization of an individual or group by society as a whole and self-stigmatization by the stigmatized individuals or groups of themselves (Keene & Padilla, 2014).

Stigma leads to a decline in health care quality, decreased access to care, and subsequently to poor outcomes. Because stigma is often preceded by suboptimal socioeconomic attributes, stigmatized groups are often faced with suboptimal care and decreased access to care at baseline, and then further stigma in the provision of health care leads to further stigmatization, creating a downward cycle.

A better understanding of stigma can lead to a more successful approach to a stigmatized population that creates improved health outcomes and better quality of care. Improved care often means less burden on society, including improved population health, decreased poverty, and cost savings at the societal level. Interventions targeted at access can decrease downstream costs of secondary and tertiary care, improved economic productivity, and better integration into society.

EMPIRICAL REFERENTS

A number of validated instruments are cited in research in which stigma has been studied. Literature characterizing stigma among individuals with HIV/AIDS is often measured using the HIV Stigma Scale (Berger, 2001; Bunn, 2007).

Preville et al. (2015) utilized the STIG scale, a modified version of the perceived stigma subscale of the Depression Stigma Scale (Griffiths, 2008), to measure perceived social stigma in an older adult population with mental health problems. Brener, Horwitz, von Hippel, Bryant, and Treloar (2015) utilized a 12-item scale in two parts and a yes/no question to measure perceived stigma in their comparative study of stigmatization conducted with HCV-infected individuals with injection drug histories and health care workers. Stigma may also be measured qualitatively (Ventura et al., 2014; Figure 15.1).

SUMMARY

A ubiquitous and complex phenomenon, stigma may be found in many health care environments and affects the delivery of care to both individuals and populations. The perpetration of stigma can occur by one individual or group toward another, or by an individual or group toward itself. The latter condition, known as self-stigmatization, is usually preceded by pervasive social stigma during which the stigmatized group assimilates the characteristics that are being assigned to it by the stigmatizing group or society at large. Stigma has been characterized in social science research for some time and has been conceptualized and studied in a number of health care environments. Stigma is relevant to nursing given its effect on the delivery of care. Understanding stigma has the capacity to help nurses formulate better understandings of patients' circumstances, particularly their disease states, and to

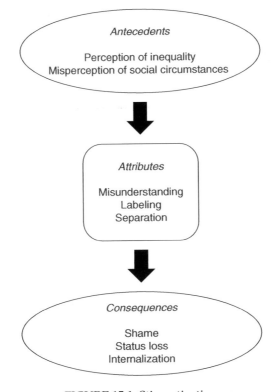

FIGURE 15.1 Stigmatization.

inform nursing care planning. Incorporating the conceptual models of stigma in various disease states can result in improved clinical models and, in turn, more efficacious care of historically stigmatized populations. Better understanding of the process of stigmatization can also assist the nurse in recognizing stigma early and potentially avoiding some of its adverse effects on health.

Stigma plays a greater role in underserved populations than in the general population. As the largest group of health care providers, and with nurses' expertise in caring for underserved individuals and populations, effective nursing care requires an increased ability to recognize and understand stigma and its role in the delivery of nursing care to all individuals and populations. A better awareness and understanding of stigma has the potential to enhance nursing care for all individuals.

REFERENCES

Berger, B. E. (2001). Measuring stigma in people with HIV: Psychometric assessment of the HIV stigma scale. *Research in Nursing & Health, 24*(6), 518–529.

Brener, L., Horwitz, R., von Hippel, C., Bryant, J., & Treloar, C. (2015). Discrimination by health care workers versus discrimination by others: Countervailing forces on HCV treatment interventions. *Psychology Health and Medicine, 20*(2), 148–153.

Bunn, J. Y. (2007). Measurement of stigma in people with HIV: A reexamination of the HIV stigma scale. *AIDS Education and Prevention, 19*(3), 198–208.

Goffman, E. (1963). *Stigma.* Englewood Cliffs, NJ: Prentice Hall.

Griffiths, K. C. (2008). Predictors of depression stigma. *BioMed Central Psychiatry, 8*, 25.

Keene, D. E., & Padilla, M. B. (2014). Spatial stigma and health inequality. *Critical Public Health, 24*(4), 392–404.

Kim, E., Ohan, J. L., & Dear, G. (2015). The stigmatisation of the provision of services for alcohol and other drug users: A systematic literature review. *Drugs Education Prevention and Policy, 22*(1), 19–25.

Preville, M., Tahiri, S. D., Vasiliadis, H.-M., Quesnel, L., Gontijo-Guerra, S., Lamoureux-Lamarche, C., & Berbiche, D. (2015). Association between perceived social stigma against mental disorders and use of health servcies for psychological distress symptoms in the older adult population: Validity of the STIG scale. *Aging and Mental Health, 19*(5), 464–474.

Scheff, T. (2014). Toward a concept of stigma. *International Journal of Social Psychiatry, 60*(7), 724–725.

Ventura, C. A., dos Santos, J. C., Mendes, I. A., & Trevizan, M. A. (2014). The perception of drug users about their human rights. *Archives of Psychiatric Nursing, 28*(6), 372–376.

PART II   CAREGIVER-FOCUSED CONCEPTS

CATRINA HEFFERNAN

16

ANXIETY

Anxiety is a global health problem (Oliveira, Chianca, & Hussein Rasool, 2008). The prevalence rates of anxiety disorders vary across the world; however, in America 20% of the population is affected at any given time (National Alliance on Mental Illness [NAMI], 2012). In Ireland, 13.7% of the adult population is known to experience anxiety, which accounts for one in eight adults. In the United Kingdom, one in six adults experience anxiety, which accounts for 10% of the population (Social Anxiety Ireland, 2014). According to Dowbiggin (2009), reported levels of anxiety have risen alarmingly in successive birth cohorts and from one country and culture to another. Anxiety predisposes individuals to many physical illnesses, mental health issues, behavioral disturbances, and inappropriate reactions (Frazier et al., 2003; NAMI, 2012; Ramos, Jaccard, & Guilamo-Ramos, 2008; World Health Organization [WHO], 2008).

In professions such as nursing, the work environment can increase anxiety levels. It is well established that nursing practice produces considerable anxiety (Chiffer, Buen, Bohan, & Maye, 2010; Gao et al., 2013; Hegney et al., 2013; Kuroda, Kanoya, Sasaki, Katsuki, & Sato, 2009; Larijani, Aghajani, Baheiraei, & Neiestanak, 2010; Menzies, 1960; Morrissey, Boman, & Mergier, 2013; O'Kane, 2011; Polat, Alemdar, & Gurol, 2013; Yada et al., 2014). There is an abundance of research investigating the sources of anxiety (Chang & Hancock, 2003; Duchsler, 2001; McKenna & Green, 2004; Thomka, 2001) and the management of anxiety (Alanazi, 2014; Nooryan, Gasparyan, Sharif, & Zolad, 2012). Despite this evidence and attention, there is still a paucity of published papers examining anxiety in registered nurses. Understanding registered nurses' anxiety in the clinical setting will help nurse managers to develop a supportive environment that is conducive to caring for patients.

During a search of the literature, three concept analyses of anxiety were identified (Bay & Algase, 1999; Hsu & Chen, 2008; Whitley, 1992). One concept analysis was published in the Chinese language (Hsu & Chen, 2008) and therefore a review of this is not included. Whitley (1992) undertook a concept analysis on anxiety based on the Walker and Avant (1988) framework.

Although this analysis is older, it is included due to the limited number of published concept analysis papers on anxiety. Bay and Algase (1999) examined the concept of anxiety using a modified simultaneous concept analysis method described by Haase, Kline Leidy, Coward, Brit, and Penn (1992). Even though this analysis included two concepts (anxiety and fear), the findings specifically related to anxiety were included, as it is useful to examine the perspective offered by Bay and Algase (1999).

DEFINING ATTRIBUTES

Three attributes of anxiety have been identified in the literature: *a subjective unpleasant feeling, unknown source,* and *emotional response.*

The first attribute is a subjective unpleasant feeling that cannot be observed or measured directly. Whitley (1992) described the presence of a vague, uneasy feeling of discomfort or dread as an attribute of anxiety when used as a nursing diagnosis; Bay and Algase (1999) identified the vague uneasiness or increasing tension experienced by the individual. When patients experience psychological distress, it may be manifested by change, for example, from a stable baseline emotional state to one of anxiety (Massee, 2000). There is an acceptance by Whitley (1992) that the description of anxiety proposed describes psychological or subjective components of the anxiety experience. This is true for anxiety experienced by nurses also.

The second attribute identified is an unknown source of the anxiety. This is likened to the attribute identified by Bay and Algase (1999) and Whitley (1992) that neither the source nor cause of the felt danger is known. This attribute is the one characteristic that differentiates anxiety from fear. *Fear* and *anxiety* are sometimes used interchangeably and in ways that confuse the differentiation of the two concepts. The source of fear, generally, is known and specific to the individual, unlike anxiety, where the source is unknown and not specific.

The third attribute consists of observable and nonobservable emotional response *either subjective or objective* that is unique to the individual. Firstly, observable responses are objective and include any response that manifests as a behavior that is measurable. Bay and Algase (1999) describe transformation into relief behaviors as a response to anxiety. These behaviors result in objective behaviors such as restlessness, voice quivering, and cardiovascular excitation, which can enhance the mental state of alertness or increase arousal (Whitley, 1992). The degree of excitation is more subjective and is known only to the person, for during anxiety there is a greater focus on the self. Some of these behaviors manifest in the early stages of anxiety. Another important early sign may be depicted when a person avoids certain scenarios (Twamas & Bangi, 2003). An example of this in nursing may be the registered nurse who communicates with the patient for the sole purpose of acquiring the minimum information for a nursing diagnosis. Whitley (1992) identifies "objective signs" as an attribute. Objective signs, which may be classified as physiologic, psychological, and/or behavioral or cognitive, are the result of the transformation of the energy into relief behaviors and the responses present in the individual (Whitley, 1992).

Second, nonobservable emotional responses are subjective: They can manifest in psychological or behavioral responses and thus may or may not be measurable. Bay and Algase (1999) and Whitley (1992) subscribe to the notion of describing subjective responses as those that act as "energizers" and cannot be observed directly. The responses can be described as the signs and symptoms of anxiety. In terms of understanding anxiety in nursing, this means that the signs and symptoms experienced by each individual nurse may not be the same and they can be either state or trait. Spielberger, Gorsuch, Lushene, Vagg, and Jaobs (1983) distinguish between *state anxiety* (a temporal condition experienced in specific situations, e.g., in a specific unit in the hospital setting) and *trait anxiety* (a general tendency of the nurse to perceive situations as threatening).

DEFINITION

Anxiety is defined as a subjective unpleasant feeling that cannot be observed or measured directly, where there is an unknown source that manifests in an emotional response.

MODEL CASE

Annette graduated as a registered nurse 6 months ago from a university in California. She has been working as a registered nurse in a private residential home since her graduation. Today is Annette's first day as a registered nurse on a medical unit in a city hospital in Arizona. She has just been introduced into the staff working in the unit. The nurse manager is inducting Annette into the unit when a loud bell is heard ringing. Staff nurses run toward a room at the end of the corridor. The nurse manager apologizes to Annette and tells her that she will not be too long as she walks hurriedly in the direction of the room. Annette stands still, unsure what to do next as she is feeling uneasy (subjective unpleasant feeling). She hears another bell ringing. She walks in the direction of the ringing bell and a patient in a bed beckons Annette over to her. She walks toward the patient. There are a lot of pumps around the patient. Some are bleeping. The bell is still ringing. Annette finds the bell and turns it off. Annette can hear more bells ringing. Her palms are sweaty and her mouth is dry (unknown source). She finds it hard to smile at the lady in the bed as she says in a quivering voice, "What can I do for you?" (emotional response). This case fully portrays all the defining attributes of anxiety. Annette perceived an unpleasant feeling and was unsure of the source or the reason for this unpleasant feeling. This may be a culmination of her first day on the ward, moving to a new area, working in a hospital, the bells ringing, her boyfriend, and so on, but Annette does not know—it is nonspecific. The source or cause of the anxiety was nonspecific. She felt uneasy. In responding to this nonspecific danger, Annette demonstrated a change in behavior both objectively and subjectively. She responded objectively with a quivering voice and subjectively with increased apprehension.

RELATED CASE

Related cases have some of the defining attributes. John, a nurse manager in the emergency department, and the staff are busy preparing and updating policies in anticipation of an external audit. Five student nurses have commenced a 3-week placement in the department. It has been noted that John was abrupt (emotional response) with the students on several occasions, which is out of character for John. On another occasion, John was noted to have a fine tremor (emotional response) when double-checking medication with a registered nurse. While chatting with John during a lunch break, he states that he is worried about the upcoming external audit (unpleasant feeling) but does not fully understand why (failed unknown source). This case illustrates many of the attributes of anxiety. John is demonstrating objective and subjective response through his abrupt tone and his trembling hand. John clearly states that the upcoming audit is a source of distress for him. John was aware of an unpleasant feeling; however, in this instance the source of the unpleasant feeling is known—that is, anticipation of the audit. Therefore, this case is an example of the concept of fear and not anxiety. The specific fear was identified (the anticipation of the audit). Fear is a concept that is closely related to, and often interchanged with, the concept of anxiety.

BORDERLINE CASE

Borderline cases contain most of the attributes. Emma is a registered nurse. She is working in a surgical unit, which she enjoys. There is a high turnover of patients and it has been noted that Emma spends time with the patients and "puts them at ease" prior to surgery. Of late, she is observed as spending only the minimum amount of time with patients in order to get the required paper-work done (emotional response). When questioned by the nurse manager, Emma says that she does not know why she is spending less time with the patients and she states that she normally enjoys being with them (unknown source). This is a borderline case, as it contains most of the defining attributes of anxiety but not all of them. It contains two of the three attributes: an emotional response and a feeling for which the source is unknown. Emma is not experiencing the unpleasant feeling, uneasiness, or increasing tension that is consistent with anxiety. This case helps further define anxiety.

CONTRARY CASE

Mary is working in the intensive care unit (ICU). Mary is caring for a patient on a ventilator when a man, named Josh, abruptly interrupts, saying that both he and his family want to talk to her right now. Josh is a relative of a patient that Mary is caring for. Mary informs Josh that she will be with him as soon as she finishes caring for her patient. Mary meets with Josh and his family in a quiet room. Mary is observed pouring coffee for Josh and his family and chatting with them. Mary's body posture is relaxed; she is sitting squarely, with an open posture, leaning toward Josh and his family and maintaining good eye contact with all family members. The family members are nodding and smiling at Mary.

This case reflects an absence of the attributes of anxiety. Mary recognized that Josh was upset; however, she did not neglect her duty of care, even though it was an uncomfortable situation to be confronted by a relative. However, Mary showed none of the attributes of anxiety (failed a subjective unpleasant feeling, failed an unknown source, and failed emotional response) in managing the situation and caring for her patient. This example does not exemplify the concept of anxiety, as it does not have any of the defining attributes.

ANTECEDENTS

The first antecedent to anxiety is a capacity to feel and experience emotions. The second antecedent identified is a perception of potential threat to the individual. Bay and Algase (1999) believe that there must be a perceived threat by the individual in order to experience anxiety. This perceived threat activates the fight-or-flight response (Seyle, 1974). Walker and Avant (2005) identified the parallel of antecedents in concept analysis with etiologies in a nursing diagnosis. It is important to apply "perception of threat" in a nursing context. This is explained within the nursing diagnosis framework, where anxiety has 11 etiologies. They are threat to self-concept; unmet needs; situational crises; threat to or change to role functioning, role status, interaction patterns, environment, or socioeconomic status; unconscious conflict about essential values; interpersonal transmission; and death (North American Nursing Diagnoses Association [NANDA], 2014).

CONSEQUENCES

The consequences of anxiety are similar according to both Bay and Algase (1999) and Whitley (1992). Personal growth for the individual has been cited as being one of the consequences of anxiety identified (Bay & Algase 1999; Whitley, 1992). Miles, Holditch-Davis, Burhinal, and Nelson (1999) reported that mothers of severely ill infants often achieved personal growth from the experience of having a sick infant. Physical illness and acting-out behavior are other consequences outlined by Bay and Algase (1999). Consequences may include permanent damage to a person (Murray & Huelskoetter, 1983), temporary damage to a person, and/or personal growth for the person (Miles et al., 1999). Whitley (1992) explains the consequences of anxiety as a change in behavior which may be positive or negative. It is important to note that the consequences of anxiety vary from person to person, and that anxiety can lead to other types of ill health (Maisel, 2003). Interventions directed toward assisting individuals in positive adaptations that result in growth and learning are essential. Based on the analyses reviewed and the literature, the following consequences have been identified for anxiety: personal growth, positive change in behavior, physical illness, and negative change in behavior.

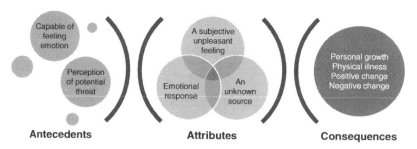

FIGURE 16.1 Anxiety.

EMPIRICAL REFERENTS

Empirical referents are classes or categories of actual phenomena that by their existence or presence demonstrate the occurrence of the concept itself (Walker & Avant, 2011). There are many valid and reliable instruments that measure anxiety, such as the State Trait Anxiety Inventory (STAI; Spielberger et al., 1983) and the Hospital Admission Depression Scale (HADS; Zigmond & Snaith, 1983). However, the majority of instruments were developed to measure anxiety in a patient. Considering the cases presented and moving forward, it is essential to accurately assess anxiety in nurses and provide the necessary support mechanisms.

SUMMARY

Anxiety is depicted through an array of symptoms that range from behavioral to psychological. The presentation of attributes related to the concept of anxiety, along with its antecedents and consequences, may enable registered nurses to identify anxiety when present in self and/or colleagues and thus provide the necessary support. The presentation of case studies has differentiated between anxiety and other closely related concepts such as fear. An analysis of the concept of anxiety within the context of registered nurses has resulted in the identification of antecedents, attributes, and consequences (Figure 16.1).

REFERENCES

Alanazi, A. A. (2014). Reducing anxiety in preoperative patients: A systematic review. *British Journal of Nursing*, *23*(7), 387–394.

Bay, E. J., & Algase, D. L. (1999). Fear and anxiety: A simultaneous concept analysis. *Nursing Diagnosis*, *10*(3), 103–111.

Chang, E. M., & Hancock, K. (2003). Role stress and role ambiguity in new nursing graduates in Australia. *Nursing & Health Sciences*, *5*(2), 155–163.

Chiffer-McKay, K. A., Buen, J. A., Bohan, K. J., & Maye, P. (2010). Determining the relationship of acute stress, anxiety, and salivary amylase level with performance of student nurse anesthetists during human-based anesthesia simulator training. *AANA Journal*, *78*(4), 301–309.

Dowbiggin, I. R. (2009). High anxieties: The social construction of anxiety disorders. *Canadian Journal of Psychiatry*, *54*(7), 429–436.

Duchsler, J. (2001). Out in the real world: Newly graduated nurses in acute-care speak out. *Journal of Nursing Administration, 31*(9), 426–439.

Frazier, S. K., Moser, D. K., Daley, L. K., McKinley, S., Riegel, B., Garvin, B. J., & An, K. (2003). Critical care nurses' beliefs about and reported management of anxiety. *American Journal of Critical Care, 12*(1), 19–27.

Gao, Y.-Q., Pan, B.-C., Sun, W., Wu, H., Wang, J. N., & Wang, L. (2013). Anxiety symptoms among Chinese nurses and the associated factors: A cross-sectional study. *BMC Psychiatry, 12*(141), 2–9.

Haase, J., Kline Leidy, N., Coward, D., Brit, T., & Penn, P. E. (1993). Simultaneous concept analysis: A strategy for developing multiple interrelated concepts. In B. L. Rodgers & K. A. Knafl (Eds.), *Concept development in nursing: Foundations, techniques and applications* (pp. 175–192). Philadelphia, PA: Saunders.

Hegney, D. G., Craigie, M., Hemsworth, D., Osseiran-Moisson, R., Aoun, S., Francis, K., & Drury, V. (2013). Compassion satisfaction, compassion fatigue, anxiety, depression and stress in registered nurses in Australia: Study 1 results. *Journal of Nursing Management, 22*, 506–518.

Hsu, W., & Chen, H. (2008). A concept analysis of anxiety (Chinese). *Tzu Chi Nursing Journal, 7*(3), 65–70.

Kuroda, T., Kanoya, Y., Sasaki, A. O., Katsuki, T., & Sato, C. (2009). Relationship between educational programs offered at midsize hospitals in Japan and novice nurses' anxiety levels. *Journal of Continuing Education in Nursing, 40*(3), 132–137.

Larijani, T. T., Aghajani, M., Baheiraei, A., & Neiestanak, N. S. (2010). Relation of assertiveness and anxiety among Iranian university students. *Journal of Psychiatric and Mental Health Nursing, 17*, 893–899.

Maisel, E. (2003). *The Van Gogh blues: The creative person's path through depression.* New Emmaus, PA: Rodale.

Massee, R. (2000). Qualitative and quantitative analyses of psychological distress: Methodological complementarity and ontological incommensurability. *Qualitative Health Research, 10*(3), 411–423.

McKenna, L., & Green, C. (2004). Experiences and learning during a graduate nurse program: An examination using a focus group approach. *Nurse Education in Practice, 4*, 258–263.

Menzies, L. I. (1960). Social systems as a defense against anxiety. An empirical study of the nursing service of a general hospital. *Human Relations, 13*, 95–121.

Miles, M. S., Holditch-Davis, D., Burhinal, P., & Nelson, D. (1999). Distress and growth outcomes in mothers of medically fragile infants. *Nursing Research, 48*(3), 129–140.

Morrissey, L., Boman, P., & Mergier, A. (2013). Nursing a case of the blues: An examination of the role of depression in predicting job-related affective well-being in nurses. *Issues in Mental Health Nursing, 34*, 158–168.

Murray, R. B., & Huelskoetter, M. W. (1983). *Psychiatric and mental health nursing: Giving emotional care.* East Norwalk, CT: Appleton and Lange.

National Alliance on Mental Illness. (2012). *Mental health by the numbers.* Retrieved from https://www.nami.org/Learn-More/Mental-Health-By-the-Numbers

North American Nursing Diagnoses Association. (2014). *Nursing diagnoses. Definitions and classifications.* Philadelphia, PA: Author.

Nooryan, K., Gasparyan, K., Sharif, F., & Zolad, M. (2012). Controlling anxiety in physicians and nurses working in intensive care units using emotional intelligence items as an anxiety management tool in Iran. *International Journal of General Medicine, 5*, 5–10.

O'Kane, C. E. (2011). Newly qualified nurses' experiences in the intensive care unit. *Nursing in Critical Care, 17*(1), 44–51.

Oliveira, N., Chianca, C. M., & Hussein Rasool, G. (2008). A validation study of the nursing diagnosis anxiety in Brazil. *International Journal of Nursing Terminologies and Classifications, 19*(3), 102–110.

Polat, S., Alemdar, D. K., & Gurol, A. (2013). Paediatric nurses' experience with death: The effect of empathic tendency on their anxiety levels. *International Journal of Nursing Practice, 19*, 8–13.

Ramos, B., Jaccard, J., & Guilamo-Ramos, V. (2008). Dual ethnicity and depressive symptoms: Implications of being black and Latino in the United States. *Journal of Behavioural Science, 25*, 147–173.

Seyle, H. (1974). *Stress without distress*. Philadelphia, PA: J.B. Lippincott.

Social Anxiety Ireland. (2014). *Overview*. Retrieved from http://socialanxietyireland.com/social-anxiety/how-common-is-social-anxiety

Spielberger, C. D., Gorsuch, R., Lushene, P., Vagg, P., & Jaobs, G. (1983). *Manual for state-trait anxiety inventory (STAI)*. Palo Alto, CA: Consulting Psychologists Press.

Thomka, L. (2001). Graduate nurses' experiences of interactions with professional nursing staff during transition to the professional role. *Journal of Continuing Education in Nursing, 32*(1), 15–19.

Twamas, G., & Bangi, A. (2003). *Women's mental health research*. New York, NY: Routledge.

Walker, L., & Avant, K. (1988). *Strategies for theory construction in nursing* (2nd ed.). Norwalk, CT: Appleton and Lange.

Walker, L., & Avant, K. (2005). *Strategies for theory construction in nursing* (4th ed.). Upper Saddle River, NJ: Pearson/Prentice Hall.

Walker, L., & Avant, K. (2011). *Strategies for theory construction in nursing* (5th ed.). Upper Saddle River, NJ: Pearson/Prentice Hall.

Whitley, G. (1992). Concept analysis of anxiety. *Nursing Diagnosis, 3*(3), 107–116.

World Health Organization. (2008). *International classification of disease* (11th ed.). Geneva, Switzerland: Author.

Yada, H., Abe, H., Omori, H., Matsuo, H., Masaki, O., Ishida, Y., & Katoh, T. (2014). Differences in job stress experienced by female and male Japanese psychiatric nurses. *International Journal of Mental Health Nursing, 23*, 468–476.

Zigmond, A., & Snaith, R. (1983). The hospital anxiety and depression scale. *Acta Psychiatric Scandinavia, 67*, 361–370.

17

CAREGIVER BURDEN IN MENTAL ILLNESS

Caregiver burden is a negative effect associated with caregiving experience (Pinquart & Sörensen, 2007). Historically, the concept of burden in caregiving was demonstrated by Breuer and Freud in 1893 in their case study of Elisabeth Von R (Sörensen, Duberstein, Gill, & Pinquart, 2006). They identified the adverse effects associated with caring for individuals with an illness as consisting of both physical and emotional elements, such as constant worrying, neglecting self-needs, and trouble sleeping. Caregiver burden has become a subject of interest to many researchers due to the deinstitutionalization of individuals with mental illness in early 1970s (Chan, 2011). In many cases, individuals with severe mental illness require long-term care; thus, responsibility for patient management has been placed on caregivers or family members.

Although other terms, such as *stress, distress, strain,* and *burnout,* have been used interchangeably in the literature to represent burden, these terms have not been clearly distinguished (Rombough, Howse, & Bartfay, 2006). Some researchers use the term *caregiver stress* to refer to caregiver burden (Brannan & Heflinger, 2001). This has resulted in a lack of conceptual clarity and difficulty with interpretation and generalization of research findings (Bastawrous, 2012). Given these inconsistencies, the purpose of this chapter is to examine the concept of caregiver burden in mental illness and specifically to identify the main attributes, antecedents, and consequences of the concept.

DEFINING ATTRIBUTES

The defining attributes of caregiver burden are *caregiver's subjective perception, hardship,* and *change over time.*

The first attribute for caregiver burden is a caregiver's subjective perception. Caregiver burden is always conceptualized as a personal and individual experience for those encountering it (Chou, 2000). Different people often perceive the same crisis in their lives differently. In a study among female caregivers in Mexico, Mendez-Luck, Kennedy, and Wallace (2008) reported that most participants conceptualized burden as a feeling of tiredness, sadness, and frustration. However, in a qualitative study to describe everyday experiences of mothers ($N = 16$) of a child with severe mental illness, Johansson, Anderzen-Carlsson, Ahlin, and Andershed (2010) found that most participants were always in a state of constant stress and uncertainty.

A second attribute of caregiver burden is hardship. Burden as experienced by an individual is commonly triggered by unexpected events, such as illness and financial constraints (Sörensen et al., 2006). In relation to caregiver burden, a vast amount of research has focused on burden among caregivers of individuals with physical (Ågren, Evangelista, & Strömberg, 2010; Bevans & Sternberg, 2012), emotional (Rodrigo, Fernando, Rajapakse, De Silva, & Hanwella, 2013), or cognitive disabilities (Al-Krenawi, Graham, & Al Gharaibeh, 2011). A review of qualitative literature suggested that caregivers with higher levels of burden were in constant stress as reflected by the following subthemes: uncertainty (Chang & Horrocks, 2006; Huang, Hung, Sun, Lin, & Chen, 2009; Johansson et al., 2010; Seloilwe, 2006), stigma perceived by the caregivers and individual with mental illness (Seloilwe, 2006), embarrassment (Chang & Horrocks, 2006, Seloilwe, 2006), and a constant sadness (Johansson et al., 2010).

Burden is considered by most authors as dynamic in nature, yet changing over time as diseases or other causes progress. Previous studies have reported high levels of burden among caregivers when they are caring for patients who are at the early stages of an illness (Gaugler et al., 2010; Zauszniewski, Bekhet, & Suresky, 2008). As time progresses, adaptation and coping eventually occur and, as a result, most patients or caregivers report lower levels of burden. For example, in a study examining the perceived burden among family members ($N = 66$) of adults with serious mental illnesses, the researchers found a higher level of burden reported during earlier stages of the diagnosis (Zauszniewski et al., 2008); however, resilience eventually developed as caregivers adapted to the caregiving role. Another dynamic characteristic of burden has been demonstrated in a study by Gaugler et al. (2010). That study sought to examine the effect of temporal change on patients' behavior problems as contributing to the rise in caregiver burden, as well as in nursing home admission time among caregivers ($N = 4,545$) who looked after patients with dementia. Findings suggested that patient behavior problems are different across disease trajectories. Therefore, caregivers experience different levels of burden at different points of a patient's illness.

DEFINITION

Caregiver burden can be defined as a caregiver's subjective perception of hardship in providing necessary direct care to an ill individual which will change over time.

MODEL CASE

This model case demonstrates all of the defining attributes of the caregiver burden concept (Walker & Avant, 2005). Jane is a 55-year-old female who cares for her son with schizophrenia. When Jane is asked about any difficulties in caring for her son, she becomes tearful, as nobody has ever asked her about her feelings before (caregiver's subjective perception). Jane believes that caring for her son is like carrying a heavy load because sometimes she cannot cope with the demands of caregiving and as a result, she always feels overworked, stressed, angry, and dissatisfied (hardship). She also suffers a great deal of embarrassment and shame associated with her son's behavior problems. Jane herself was diagnosed with arthritis 2 years ago and is currently unemployed due to her disability; thus, her income is restricted. Jane feels that the burden intensified after her husband passed away a few years ago and since then there has been nobody to assist her with caregiving tasks (change over time).

RELATED CASE

Sofia is a 22-year-old college student who lives with her parents and two siblings in a small apartment near the city center. Her younger brother is diagnosed with paranoid schizophrenia and frequently shows psychotic symptoms. At one time, Sofia overheard him talking and arguing in an agitated manner even though there was no one around. As a result, Sofia feels stressed (hardship) and is reluctant to go home after class. Sofia has always been a high achiever, but now she is struggling to maintain her academic achievements. Her friends have noticed that Sofia has changed from a cheerful and optimist student to a quiet and stressed one (change over time). In this example, Sofia has only two attributes of caregiver burden, namely the hardship and change over time, but failed caregiver's subjective perception. Sofia's behavioral and emotional changes are more applicable to the concept of psychological distress.

BORDERLINE CASE

The borderline case contains most of the attributes but not all of them (Walker & Avant, 2005). Sally, a 30-year-old female, accompanied her mother, who has major depression, to a clinic follow-up. Sally has been taking care of her mother for 2 years. Sometimes she feels stressed by caregiving tasks, but she believes it is her responsibility as a child to take care of her mother (caregiver's subjective perception). Her mother is able to function quite independently (failed hardship), but most of the time she needs to be consistently reminded of her personal hygiene, medication, and meals. Sally is now learning new skills and attending a support group in order to meet the demands of caregiving. Consequently, Sally is able to recognize that her burden level has changed over time, as she is experiencing a lower level of caregiver burden than before. Now, Sally is more confident in taking care of her mother. In this case, Sally only has two attributes of caregiver burden: caregiver's subjective perception and change over time; the attribute of hardship is not present.

CONTRARY CASE

The contrary case is a clear example of what the concept is not (Walker & Avant, 2005). John, a 50-year-old male, is caring for his wife with bipolar disorder. His wife is able to manage her personal hygiene and household chores, as well as take medications independently. In the past 2 days, though, his wife has had trouble sleeping, her activity level has increased, and she is showing excessive irritability. John admits that his wife might be in a manic phase of bipolar, so he takes his wife to a psychiatrist for further examination and evaluation. He also speaks with his children about their mother's behavior. Thus, in this example, John has experienced unexpected changes in his wife's behaviors, but he has been able to recognize the reasons of these behavior problems and immediately seek help. Therefore, the three attributes of caregiver's subjective perception, hardship, and change over time do not apply here.

ANTECEDENTS

The antecedents of burden are unexpected events/illnesses, imbalance between demands and resources, and negative coping. Burdens are commonly caused by an unexpected event or illness that disrupts the balance or equilibrium of a person's life (Wynaden, 2007). In health care, for example, illnesses or diseases are common events that contribute to burden in various contexts. From a caregiver's perspective, burden is associated with caregiving activities in either practical or emotional forms. Involvement in practical support, such as doing household chores and finances, as well as shopping and other daily errands, somehow contributes to the burden of caregivers. As most illnesses happen unpredictably, the majority of the caregivers do not expect to assume this role. Limited support during this transitional phase eventually leads to deteriorating mental health and quality of life among caregivers (Blum & Sherman, 2010). A correlational study was conducted to determine the burden experienced by partners ($N = 135$) of patients with chronic heart failure (Ågren et al., 2010). Findings suggested that in the case of chronic heart failure, partners, rather than other family members, are often responsible for providing assistance, care management, and psychological support for the patient. In addition, partners' mental health status and the patient's physical conditions correlate with the level of burden experienced by the partners. In addition, involvement in caregiving activities requires additional hours and commitment and often leads caregivers to sacrifice their jobs. Consequently, a higher level of burden is experienced by unemployed caregivers and leads to more patient comorbidities (Saunders, 2008).

The second antecedent of caregiver burden is imbalance between demands and resources. Burden experienced by an individual is commonly caused by either increased demands in daily life or insufficient resources to balance the demands, or a combination of both. For example, when new demands are introduced or become intensified, individuals who experience them employ strategies to meet these demands; failure to cope with the demands leads to a feeling of burden. Using structural equation modeling, Sherwood, Given, Given, and Von Eye (2005) studied a cohort of 488 family caregivers in order to analyze the relationship between a care recipient's mental and physical status and the recency of care demands, burden, and depressive symptoms. In this study, the care recipient's mental and physical status increased the demand on caregivers. Findings indicate that both variables were predictors of caregiver burden and depressive symptoms. Thus, it can be concluded that increases in demand contribute to increased levels of burden. Similarly, the findings of this study were supported by findings from a study that examined burden and coping strategies among caregivers (N = 150) of persons with schizophrenia (Tan et al., 2012). Tan et al. (2012) reported that individuals who have other commitments, suffer from a lack of resources, or have insufficient financial resources demonstrated a high level of burden. A qualitative, grounded theory study conducted by Wynaden (2007) provided a better interpretation of how the imbalance between demand and resources causes burden. Wynaden (2007) studied 20 caregivers to understand their experience in caring for individuals with mental illness. The aim of this study was to construct a theory that provided a better understanding of the burden associated with caregiving. Two dimensions of burden were identified: namely, "being consumed" and "seeking balance." When dealing with increased demand, the initial stage faced by an individual is commonly the disruption of established lifestyle which then progresses to "sustained threat to self-equilibrium." This is the stage in which individuals experience an increase in care demand in the form of, for example, day-to-day caring activities, grief and loss, and personal cost of caring. During the "seeking balance" phase, individuals try to cope with and adapt to the demand by means of knowledge and available resources. Insufficient resources, such as lack of practical and emotional support, may cause burden in this process.

Another antecedent for burden is negative coping. In some cases, when individuals adopt a negative pattern of coping, this may progress to burden. *Negative coping* can be defined as the degree with which negative methods are used by an individual to control burden (Lim & Ahn, 2003). Liu, Lambert, and Lambert (2007) reported a negative correlation between burden and coping patterns among parental caregivers (N = 97). Caregivers of children with mental disability reported feeling ashamed of the situation and thus were reluctant to invite their friends and relatives to their home. However, this negative coping diminished their social support and thus contributed to higher levels of burden in caregiving activities. In addition, Mu (2005) also reported that coping patterns are important predictors of depression among parents of children with epilepsy. The findings from Lim and Ahn's study (2003) among caregivers (N = 57) of patients with schizophrenia in Korea indicate that negative coping can mediate the relationship among caregiver's knowledge, duration of caregiving, and patient's relationship with the caregiver. In addition, lack of knowledge and experience may directly influence a caregiver's utilization of effective coping strategies, and consequently contribute to high level of burden.

CONSEQUENCES

The consequences are psychological and physical morbidity, and coping and adaptation. An individual who experiences burden also reports increased physical and psychological morbidity; for example, an insufficient cellular immune system (Thompson et al., 2004), more illness symptoms and number of chronic diseases (Chang, Chiou, & Chen, 2010), and a lower self-perceived health score (Chang et al., 2010; Pinquart & Sörensen, 2007). Caregivers for those with debilitating diseases report having to modify their lifestyles to accommodate the patient's need, thus limiting their leisure activities and interaction with close friends and family members. Because most caregivers prioritize the needs of patients over their own, numerous health-related problems such as sleep disturbances, fatigue (Bevans & Sternberg, 2012), and poor mental health (Moller & Folden, 2009) have been reported by caregivers.

Coping and adaptation are a possible outcome of burden for some people. A study by Casado and Sacco (2012) set out to identify factors associated with burden among family members ($N = 146$) of disabled older adults. Findings indicate that family members experience lower levels of burden or are able to cope with burden if they have a larger support network and greater self-efficacy. In this study, family members employed coping strategies by getting assistance from other people, as well as mastering care management of the illness. However, different people may utilize different coping techniques when dealing with burden. Basically, in relation to burden, the coping responses are facilitated by an individual's prior exposure to, knowledge of, or experience with a particular burden (Wynaden, 2007). Another study reported that coping and adaptation were significantly associated with burden. Papastavrou, Kalokerinou, Papacostas, Tsangari, and Sourtzi (2007) conducted a study to examine the consequences of caring for individuals with dementia and strategies used by family members ($N = 172$) to cope with burden associated with caregiving. Even though a higher level of burden was reported in this study (68%), a lower level of burden was reported by individuals who used more problem-solving approaches to adapt to their burden. Conversely, a higher level of burden was reported by those using emotional-focused coping strategies. The findings indicate that though some people experience a high level of burden, with the appropriate coping techniques, coping and adaptation are possible. In contrast, failure to adopt an effective coping technique to meet demand may lead to a negative coping approach (Papastavrou et al., 2007). As discussed in the previous section, negative coping can be an antecedent to burden. This unique cycle of burden shows that this concept unfolds over time and it is not a static phenomenon.

EMPIRICAL REFERENTS

The concept of caregiver burden, although subjective in nature, is measurable via existing measurement scales such as the Zarit Burden Interview (Zarit, Reever, & Bach-Peterson, 1980), the Caregiver Strain Index (Robinson, 1983), the Caregiver Burden Inventory (Novak & Guest, 1989), the Caregiver Burden Scale (Biegel, Milligan, Putnam, & Song, 1994), and the Burden Assessment Schedule (Thara, Padmavati, Kumar, & Srinivasan, 1998). Scales developed to measure burden can capture the burden experienced by caregivers either subjectively or objectively or a combination of both. Most studies reported a high internal consistency of the scales used. However, although burden is multidimensional (Bastawrous, 2012; Chou, 2000; Etters, Goodall, & Harrison, 2008), most of the earlier scales, such as the Zarit Burden Interview (Zarit et al., 1980) and the Caregiver Strain Index (Robinson, 1983), were developed to measure burden focusing only on the subjective dimension. The more recent scales, such as the Caregiver Burden Inventory (Novak & Guest, 1989), the Caregiver Burden Scale (Biegel et al., 1994), and the Burden Assessment Schedule (Thara et al., 1998), were developed to measure burden from both objective and subjective dimensions of caregiver burden (Figure 17.1).

SUMMARY

Caregiver burden is a common negative consequence experienced by people who are involved in caring for individuals with health problems. These phenomena are shared by caregivers from various cultural backgrounds, although the contributing factors might be different from one population to another. This concept analysis has established caregiver burden as a distinct concept relevant to nursing practice. The discussion of attributes related to the concept, together with identification of antecedents and consequences, should assist health care providers to recognize the presence of burden in caregivers. A clear understanding of the concept of caregiver burden enables nurses and other health care providers to plan for specific interventions or programs targeting the groups at high risk of caregiver burden.

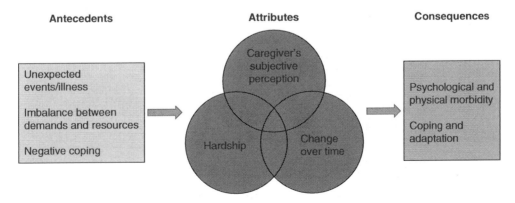

FIGURE 17.1 Caregiver burden in mental illness.

REFERENCES

Ågren, S., Evangelista, L., & Strömberg, A. (2010). Do partners of patients with chronic heart failure experience caregiver burden? *European Journal of Cardiovascular Nursing, 9*(4), 254–262.

Al-Krenawi, A., Graham, J. R., & Al Gharaibeh, F. (2011). The impact of intellectual disability, caregiver burden, family functioning, marital quality, and sense of coherence. *Disability & Society, 26*(2), 139–150.

Bastawrous, M. (2012). Caregiver burden: A critical discussion. *International Journal of Nursing Studies, 50*(3), 431–441.

Bevans, M., & Sternberg, E. M. (2012). Caregiving burden, stress, and health effects among family caregivers of adult cancer patients. *JAMA: Journal of the American Medical Association, 307*(4), 398–403.

Biegel, D., Milligan, S., Putnam, P., & Song, L.-Y. (1994). Predictors of burden among lower socioeconomic status caregivers of persons with chronic mental illness. *Community Mental Health Journal, 30*(5), 473–494.

Blum, K., & Sherman, D. W. (2010). Understanding the experience of caregivers: A focus on transitions. *Seminars in Oncology Nursing, 26*(4), 243–258.

Brannan, A. M., & Heflinger, C. A. (2001). Distinguishing caregiver strain from psychological distress: Modeling the relationships among child, family, and caregiver variables. *Journal of Child and Family Studies, 10*(4), 405–418.

Casado, B., & Sacco, P. (2012). Correlates of caregiver burden among family caregivers of older Korean Americans. *Journals of Gerontology Series B: Psychological Sciences & Social Sciences, 67B*(3), 331–336.

Chan, S. W. (2011). Global perspective of burden of family caregivers for person with schizophrenia. *Archives of Psychiatric Nursing, 25*(5), 339–349.

Chang, H.-Y., Chiou, C.-J., & Chen, N.-S. (2010). Impact of mental health and caregiver burden on family caregivers' physical health. *Archives of Gerontology and Geriatrics, 50*(3), 267–271.

Chang, K. H., & Horrocks, S. (2006). Lived experiences of family caregivers of mentally ill relatives. *Issues and Innovation in Nursing Practice, 53*, 435–443.

Chou, K.-R. (2000). Caregiver burden: A concept analysis. *Journal of Pediatric Nursing, 15*(6), 398–407.

Etters, L., Goodall, D., & Harrison, B. E. (2008). Caregiver burden among dementia patient caregivers: A review of the literature. *Journal of the American Academy of Nurse Practitioners, 20*(8), 423–428.

Gaugler, J. E., Wall, M. M., Kane, R. L., Menk, J. S., Sarsour, K., Johnston, J. A., … Newcomer, R. (2010). The effects of incident and persistent behavioral problems on change in caregiver burden and nursing home admission of persons with dementia. *Medical Care, 48*(10), 875–883.

Huang, X. Y., Hung, B. J., Sun, F. K., Lin, J. D., & Chen, C. C. (2009). The experiences of carers in Taiwanese culture who have long-term schizophrenia in their families: A phenomenological study. *Journal of Psychiatric and Mental Health Nursing, 16*, 874–883.

Johansson, A., Anderzen-Carlsson, A., Ahlin, A., & Andershed, B. (2010). Mothers' everyday experiences of having an adult child who suffers from long-term mental illness. *Issues in Mental Health Nursing, 31*, 692–699.

Lim, Y. M., & Ahn, Y. (2003). Burden of family caregivers with schizophrenic patients in Korea. *Applied Nursing Research, 16*(2), 110–117.

Liu, M., Lambert, C. E., & Lambert, V. A. (2007). Caregiver burden and coping patterns of Chinese parents of a child with a mental illness. *International Journal of Mental Health Nursing, 16*, 86–95.

Mendez-Luck, C., Kennedy, D., & Wallace, S. (2008). Concepts of burden in giving care to older relatives: A study of female caregivers in a Mexico City neighborhood. *Journal of Cross-Cultural Gerontology, 23*(3), 265–282.

Moller, T., & Folden, G. E. (2009). The experience of caring in relatives to patients with serious mental illness: Gender differences, health and functioning. *Scandinavian Journal of Caring Sciences, 23*, 153–160.

Mu, P. (2005). Parental reactions to a child with epilepsy: Uncertainty, coping strategies and depression. *Journal of Advanced Nursing, 49*(4), 367–376.

Novak, M., & Guest, C. (1989). Application of a multidimensional caregiver burden inventory. *Gerontologist, 29*, 798–803.

Papastavrou, E., Kalokerinou, A., Papacostas, S. S., Tsangari, H., & Sourtzi, P. (2007). Caring for a relative with dementia: Family caregiver burden. *Journal of Advanced Nursing, 58*(5), 446–457.

Pinquart, M., & Sörensen, S. (2007). Correlates of physical health of informal caregivers: A meta-analysis. *Journals of Gerontology Series B: Psychological Sciences and Social Sciences, 62*(2), P126–P137.

Robinson, B. C. (1983). Validation of a caregiver strain index. *Journal of Gerontology, 38*(3), 344–348.

Rodrigo, C., Fernando, T., Rajapakse, S., De Silva, V., & Hanwella, R. (2013). Caregiver strain and symptoms of depression among principal caregivers of patients with schizophrenia and bipolar affective disorder in Sri Lanka. *International Journal of Mental Health Systems, 7*(1), 2.

Rombough, R. E., Howse, E. L., & Bartfay, W. J. (2006). Caregiver strain and caregiver burden of primary caregivers of stroke survivors with and without aphasia. *Rehabilitation Nursing, 31*(5), 199–209.

Saunders, M. M. (2008). Factors associated with caregiver burden in heart failure family caregivers. *Western Journal of Nursing Research, 30*(8), 943–959.

Seloilwe, E. S. (2006). Experiences and demands of families with mentally ill people at home in Botswana. *Journal of Nursing Scholarship, 38*(3), 262–268.

Sherwood, P. R., Given, C. W., Given, B. A., & Von Eye, A. (2005). Caregiver burden and depressive symptoms: Analysis of common outcomes in caregivers of elderly patients. *Journal of Aging & Health, 17*(2), 125–147.

Sörensen, S., Duberstein, P., Gill, D., & Pinquart, M. (2006). Dementia care: Mental health effects, intervention strategies, and clinical implications. *Lancet Neurology, 5*(11), 961–973.

Tan, S. C. H., Yeoh, A. L., Choo, I. B. K., Huang, A. P. H., Ong, S. H., Ismail, H., … Chan, Y. H. (2012). Burden and coping strategies experienced by care of persons with schizophrenia in the community. *Journal of Clinical Nursing, 21*, 2410–2418.

Thara, R., Padmavati, R., Kumar, S., & Srinivasan, L. (1998). Burden assessment schedule: Instrument to assess burden on caregivers of chronically mentally ill. *Indian Journal of Psychiatry, 40*(1), 21–29.

Thompson, R. L., Lewis, S. L., Murphy, M. R., Hale, J. M., Blackwell, P. H., Acton, G. J., … Bonner, P. N. (2004). Are there sex differences in emotional and biological responses in spousal caregivers of patients with Alzheimer's disease? *Biological Research for Nursing, 5*(4), 319–330.

Walker, L., & Avant, K. (2005). *Strategies for theory construction in nursing* (4th ed). Upper Saddle River, NJ: Prentice Hall.

Wynaden, D. (2007). The experience of caring for a person with a mental illness: A grounded theory study. *International Journal of Mental Health Nursing, 16*(6), 381–389.

Zarit, S. H., Reever, K. E., & Bach-Peterson, J. (1980). Relatives of the impaired elderly: Correlates of feeling of burden. *Gerontologist, 26,* 260–266.

Zauszniewski, J. A., Bekhet, A. K., & Suresky, M. J. (2008). Factors associated with perceived burden, resourcefulness and quality of life in female family members of adults with serious mental illness. *Journal of the American Psychiatric Association, 14*(2), 125–135.

18

CLINICAL AUTONOMY

The purpose of this concept analysis is to create clarity around the understanding of the concept of clinical autonomy. It is useful to consider a number of theoretical perspectives on autonomy. While there appears to be a belief that autonomy relates to self-determination (Blöser, Scöpf, & Willaschek, 2010; MacDonald, 2002), autonomy is based on the expectation that one has the ability, authority, and capacity for self-determination (MacDonald, 2002; Neuhouser, 2011). Simple understandings of autonomy do not account for an individual's participation in a wider society or community (MacDonald, 2002; Neuhouser, 2011). This belief has relevance for nursing as a profession because nurses form part of a wider society involving other professional groups, patients/clients/service users, and legislators. For individuals to be autonomous, they must have some control over their actions and the capacity for rational and critical thinking (Blöser et al., 2010; MacDonald, 2002; Nickel, 2007). Blöser et al. (2010) believe that the exercise of autonomy involves complex mental activity surrounding reflection and the shaping of decisions. There is a belief that autonomy is not merely the absence of restriction but also the application of the freedom espoused in autonomy (Nickel, 2007). The complexity of autonomy is reflected in the literature; it is apparent that, while there are differing viewpoints regarding the concept, they represent a congruent whole rather than divergent views (Blöser et al., 2010; Nickel, 2007).

There appears to be the same divergence in views regarding the level of independence involved in the understanding of autonomy in nursing (Kramer, Maguire, & Schmalenberg, 2006; Lewis, 2006; McParland et al., 2000; Seago, 2006; Weston, 2008). Definitions of autonomy in nursing espouse a freedom to practice within accepted boundaries for the profession and that autonomy is not an absolute in terms of freedom from restriction to practice. Nevertheless, there is confusion in the literature about autonomy in nursing, with differing terms being used to describe autonomy at different levels (Weston, 2008). Of most relevance to the profession is autonomy in clinical practice or clinical autonomy (Kramer et al., 2006; Weston, 2008). Kramer et al. (2006) differentiate clinical autonomy from job/organizational autonomy in terms of the knowledge and skills required to exercise each realm of autonomy. They identify organizational knowledge and skills as necessary for job/organizational autonomy, whereas clinical skills and good clinical judgment ability are required for clinical autonomy. Weston (2008) summarizes this by stating that clinical autonomy relates to decision making in clinical nursing practice.

DEFINING ATTRIBUTES

The following are the defining attributes of clinical autonomy in nursing practice: *practicing within a professional context, capacity to exercise clinical judgment, authority to make patient care decisions*, and *context of interdisciplinary collaboration*.

Practicing within a professional context refers to practice that is self-regulating through a professional regulatory body. A statutory body sets, monitors, and maintains the standards for, and regulation of, nursing practice. To practice as a nurse and to exercise autonomy as a nurse, the nurse must possess and maintain registration as a nurse. The regulation of the profession nursing ensures that patient and public safety are upheld though professional registration, regulation, and standard setting (An Bord Altranais, 2000). This does not detract from the autonomy of nurses in clinical practice; rather, it instills a confidence in the profession among the communities that nurses serve in the robustness of nurses' clinical decision making. A recognized "sphere" of nursing practice provides the context for clinical autonomy among nurses (Kramer et al., 2006).

Practicing within a professional context also relates to the practice setting in which nurses practice. Specific practice contexts require nurses to possess particular competencies and skills in order to engage in clinical practice; an example is nurses working in critical care areas such as the emergency department (ED). A practice setting that supports the professional development of nurses will contribute to greater clinical involvement and by association greater clinical autonomy among nurses (Hinno, Partanen, Vehvilainen-Julkunen, & Aaviksoo, 2009; Kramer et al., 2007).

Capacity to exercise clinical judgment is key to the effective exercise of clinical autonomy in nursing. This is based on a nurse's knowledge and skills to function within the scope of practice. Autonomy is based on the ability and authority to make decisions, and a capacity for decision making is viewed as central to autonomy in any context (Blöser et al., 2010). According to Nickel (2007), the capacity for decision making is largely dependent on the individual's ability for critical thinking. Although clinical autonomy is determined by capacity for clinical judgment, there needs to be an acknowledgment of boundaries, recognizing that autonomy in nursing may be limited to the realm of nursing practice (Lewis, 2006), even if at times it extends beyond.

The third attribute is the authority to make patient care decisions regarding clinical nursing care. Maas, Specht, and Jacox (1975) recognized that the exercise of autonomy requires authority to do so. In understanding autonomy, there needs to an acknowledgment that *authority and sanction* for clinical autonomy are required. The role of the organization in which nurses practice in authorizing the clinical autonomy of nurses has been highlighted in the literature (Kramer & Schmalenberg, 2003). This has been identified as nurses having a voice in terms of clinical care decision making (Stewart, Stansfield, & Tapp, 2004) with the influence of organizational management identified as having a significant role to play (Mrayyan, 2004).

The fourth attribute is practicing in the context of interdisciplinary collaboration. Weston (2008) supports the idea of interdisciplinary and *collaborative practice* in health care by observing that nurses work in interdisciplinary teams where all activities are integrated, and therefore autonomy must be viewed in this context. Kramer et al. (2006) refer to interdisciplinary overlap and interdependence. Being able to make practice decisions within one's own sphere of practice does not assume that collaboration or interaction outside of nursing in spheres of practice that overlap with other professions cannot occur. Indeed, collaboration with, for example, physicians has been found to have a positive influence on the clinical autonomy of nurses (Cotter & McCarthy, 2014).

DEFINITION

Clinical autonomy is defined as practicing within a professional nursing context, having the capacity to exercise clinical judgment and the authority to make patient care decisions in the context of interdisciplinary collaboration.

MODEL CASE

David is a registered general nurse who is employed in an emergency department (practicing within a professional nursing context). During his assessment of a patient who presented with an injury to his right knee, David discovers that the patient is suffering from moderate pain and decides that he would benefit from some analgesia (capacity to exercise clinical judgment). The organization in which David works has authorized nurses who work in triage to administer analgesia, based on their own clinical judgment, to patients without the need for a prescription from a doctor (the authority to make patient care decisions). David administed oral analgesia as well as supplying crutches to the patient to aid with mobilization while in the emergency department. David discussed his assessment and management of the patient with the physician on duty in the emergency department, who sought David's opinion on the level of priority that should be assigned to the patient's care (the context of interdisciplinary collaboration.

RELATED CASE

Sarah a recently registered nurse, was participating in a hospital-wide induction program for all new recruits (context of interdisciplinary collaboration). She was permitted to escort well patients between units but not provide unsupervised care (failed practicing within a professional nursing context and failed the authority to make patient care decisions). During her placement in the emergency department, she was asked by David, one of the staff nurses, to escort a patient to the rehabilitation ward. During the journey to the ward, she noticed that the patient appeared to become unwell (capacity to exercise clinical judgment). She told Hannah, the staff nurse on the rehabilitation ward, that she thought there was something wrong with the patient and then left the unit to return to the emergency department. This case has some of the defining attributes but not all.

BORDERLINE CASE

While working on a rehabilitation unit, Hannah, a registered nurse (practicing within a professional nursing context) received a new patient from an acute hospital following a stroke. Hannah had completed specialist postgraduate education in rehabilitation nursing (capacity to exercise clinical judgment) and during her assessment of the patient determined that the patient would benefit from a walking frame to aid mobilization. However, the hospital did not allow nurses to prescribe walking frames for patients (failed the authority to make patient care decisions). Hannah contacted the physiotherapist, who was permitted to prescribe walking aids within the hospital, and discussed the case with her. It was agreed between them that a walking aid was appropriate in this case (context of interdisciplinary collaboration) and it was prescribed for the patient by the physiotherapist.

CONTRARY CASE

Martha is a clerical assistant working in a surgical outpatient department (failed practicing within a professional nursing context). One of the patients complained to her that she had been advised that her dressing should not be changed every day but rather every third day. The patient asked Martha if this was appropriate. Martha is unaware that the dressing being used for the patient is most effective when changed every third day and is ineffective if changed more frequently; she states that in her opinion, the dressing should be changed more frequently (failed capacity to exercise clinical judgment). When asked by the patient if she would change the dressing, Martha stated that she did not have the authority to change dressings (failed the authority to make patient care decisions) and that the patient should visit the wound care nurse specialist. The patient asked Martha if she would discuss the patient's dressing with the wound care nurse specialist and arrive at an agreed plan for the management of her wound. Martha informed the patient that while she was friendly with the nurse specialist, she did not have a clinical relationship with her such that she could be involved in clinical decision making (failed context of interdisciplinary collaboration).

ANTECEDENTS

The antecedents to clinical autonomy among nurses are nursing knowledge and skills, ability to achieve and maintain professional registration or license, desire for autonomy, collaborative interprofessional relationships, and organization that values and supports nursing practice.

Nursing knowledge and skills are the tools of clinical judgment for any nurse who practices clinically. For nurses to exercise clinical autonomy, they must have the knowledge and skills to engage in clinical reasoning and clinical judgment. However, knowledge and skills in and of themselves do not automatically lead to increased clinical autonomy (Cotter & McCarthy, 2014). The application of clinical judgment in an autonomous manner in clinical practice requires a number of other antecedents.

Professional registration or licensing is a requirement to practice as a nurse in all countries where the profession is organized and regulated. It therefore follows that for a nurse to practice clinically with any autonomy, she or he must first be registered/licensed (Keenan, 1999).

The nurses themselves must have a desire to exercise autonomy in practice. Not every nurse will want the same level of decision making or influence over clinical patient care. Among the themes generated from semistructured interviews with 15 nurses in Canada, in a study by Gagnon, Bakker, Montgomery, and Palkovits (2010), were that autonomy is an unspoken workplace opportunity developed through professional and personal growth acquired over time and illustrating autonomous behaviors.

The value of good interprofessional collaboration has been highlighted as having a positive influence over levels of autonomy among nurses, especially strong relationships with physicians (Hinno et al., 2009; Gagnon et al., 2010; Maylone, Raneire, Griffin, McNulty, & Fitzpatrick, 2010; Papathanassoglou et al., 2012). The definition offered for clinical autonomy in this concept analysis embraces influence over care and care decisions beyond the recognized nursing practice realm, and therefore it is obvious that good professional relationships with other professions are required to facilitate this.

The organization in which nurses work has a significant influence over the clinical autonomy of nurses. A qualitative study by Gagnon et al. (2010) sought to explore oncology nurses' perception and demonstration of autonomy in practice in Canada. The researchers conducted semistructured interviews and observation of participants in practice on a sample of 15 oncology nurses. Among the findings from this study was the importance of the support from managers in facilitating autonomy. Mrayyan (2004) conducted a comparative descriptive study examining the role of nurse managers in enhancing the autonomy of hospital-based staff nurses. Mrayyan accessed a large sample of nurses in the United States, Canada, and the United Kingdom ($N = 3615$) and collected data via an electronic survey. Supportive management was seen as the most significantly positive factor in enhancing autonomy among nurses in clinical practice, whereas autocratic management was viewed as the most negative influence on autonomy of nurses in practice. In a study of 100 emergency department staff nurses, Cotter and McCarthy (2014) found a significant relationship between the organizational influence on nursing practice and participants' level of clinical autonomy.

CONSEQUENCES

There are a number of consequences of clinical autonomy among nurses. These include: job satisfaction, nurse retention, accountability for care decisions, and improved patient care and safety.

A number of studies have examined the relationship between autonomy in nursing practice and job satisfaction (Finn, 2001; Hayhurst, Saylor, & Stuenkel, 2005; Iliopoulou & While, 2010; Zurmehly, 2008). One example that illustrates this relationship is found in a descriptive study by Finn (2001), who sought to establish baseline data on autonomy and job satisfaction among nurses. Using a convenience sample of 320 nurses (with a response of 178 nurses) working in a large teaching hospital in Brisbane, Australia, Finn measured importance of work components using a modified version of the Index of Work Satisfaction Instrument (Stamps & Piemonte, 1986). The single most important component for nurses in terms of job satisfaction was autonomy. Finn found support for this finding in the results of previous studies (Goodell & Coeling, 1994; Stamps & Piemonte, 1986).

Nurse retention is also linked with levels of autonomy among nurses in clinical practice (Brunetto, Farr-Wharton, & Shacklock, 2011; Mosely & Paterson, 2008). In a review of 38 papers, Mosely and Paterson (2008) found that there was a link between autonomy in clinical practice and retention of nurses. Similarly, in a study of 900 nurses in Australia, Brunetto et al. (2011) also found a significant link between autonomy among nurses and their intention to leave their current position.

When describing autonomy in nursing, Blegen et al. (1993) highlighted the issue of accountability for care decisions. Increased autonomy in patient care leads to increased decision making, which naturally comes from accountability for practice.

Ultimately, improvements in patient care and safety are the goal of any progressive health system and of the professions working within that system. Clinical autonomy among nurses has been found to positively affect patient care and safety (Institute of Medicine, 2004; Shang, Friese, Wu, & Aiken, 2012; Zurmehly, 2008).

EMPIRICAL REFERENTS

Empirical referents are the means by which a concept may be demonstrated (Walker & Avant, 2005). There is some divergence over the usage of autonomy in nursing, and therefore a number of generic instruments used to measure the concept have been shown not to be valid measures of clinical autonomy (Weston, 2009). One instrument that measures practice behaviors of autonomy among nurses is the Dempster Practice Behaviours Scale (DPBS) (Dempster, 1990). Measures proporting to measure clinical autonomy among nurses need to focus on autonomous acts in the provision of direct patient care rather than on other understandings of autonomy such as professional autonomy or organizational autonomy. Clinical autonomy is concerned with direct provision of patient care (Figure 18.1).

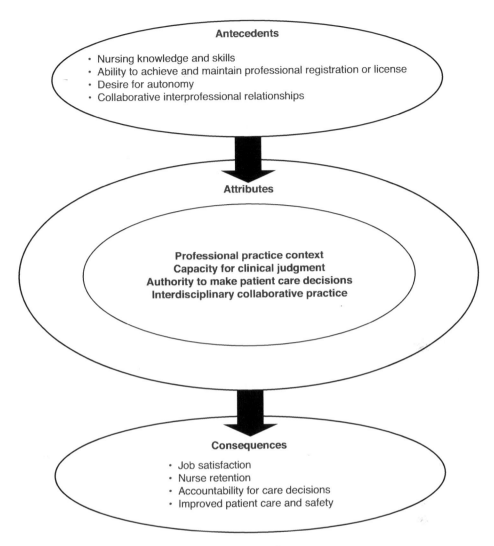

FIGURE 18.1 Clinical autonomy.

SUMMARY

There appear to be a number of understandings of autonomy in the general usage of the term, and the nursing profession is no different in its usage of the term. What is evident from the literature is that autonomy in clinical practice or clinical autonomy is of most importance to nurses. This concept analysis aims to create some clarity around the concept and to differentiate it from other understandings of the concept in nursing. The definition, identification of defining attributes, and identification of antecedents are focused on the clinical act of providing care. Also of importance is the recognition that nursing does not happen in a vacuum; the importance of a professional context for practice, the role of the organization, and collaboration are highlighted. The model case present the defining attributes in context, while the other cases provide contrasting perspectives to reinforce the understanding of clinical autonomy conveyed in this concept analysis.

REFERENCES

An Bord Altranais. (2000). *The code of professional conduct for each nurse and midwife.* Dublin, OH: Author.

Blegen, M. A., Goode, C. J., Johnson, M., Maas, M., Chen, L., & Moorehead, S. (1993). Preferences for decision-making. *Journal of Nursing Scholarship, 25,* 339–344.

Blöser, C., Schöpf, A., & Willaschek, M. (2010). Autonomy, experience and reflection. On a neglected aspect of personal autonomy. *Ethical Theory and Moral Practice, 13,* 239–253.

Brunetto, Y., Farr-Wharton, R., & Shacklock, K. (2011). Supervisor-subordinate communication relationships, role ambiguity, autonomy and affective commitment for nurses. *Contemporary Nurse, 39*(2), 227–239.

Cotter, P., & McCarthy, G. (2014). Clinical autonomy and nurse/physician collaboration in emergency nurses. *International Emergency Nursing, 22*(4), 253.

Dempster, J. S. (1990). Autonomy in practice: Conceptualization, construction, and psychometric evaluation of an empirical instrument. *Dissertation Abstract International, 50,* 3320A.

Finn, C. P. (2001). Autonomy: An important component for nurses' job satisfaction. *International Journal of Nursing Studies, 38,* 349–357.

Gagnon, L., Bakker, D., Montgomery, P., & Palkovits, J.-A. (2010). Nurse autonomy in cancer care. *Cancer Nursing, 33*(3), 21–28.

Goodell, T., & Coeling, H. (1994). Outcomes of nurses' job satisfaction. *Journal of Nursing Administration, 24*(11), 36–41.

Hayhurst, A., Saylor, C., & Stuenkel, D. (2005). Work environmental factors and the retention of nurses. *Journal of Nursing Care Quality, 20*(3), 283–288.

Hinno, S., Partanen, P., Vehvilainen-Julkunen, K., & Aaviksoo, A. (2009). Nurses' perceptions of the organizational attributes of their practice environment in acute care hospitals. *Journal of Nursing Management, 17,* 965–974.

Iliopoulou, K. K., & While, A. E. (2010). Professional autonomy and job satisfaction: Survey of critical care nurses in mainland Greece. *Journal of Advanced Nursing, 66*(11), 2520–2531.

Institute of Medicine. (2004). *Keeping patients safe: Transforming the work environment of nurses.* Washington, DC: National Academy Press.

Keenan, J. (1999). A concept analysis of autonomy. *Journal of Advanced Nursing, 29*(3), 556–552.

Kramer, M., Maguire, P., & Schmalenberg, C. (2006). Excellence through evidence: The what, when, and where of clinical autonomy. *Journal of Nursing Administration, 36*(10), 479–491.

Kramer, M., Maguire, P., Schmalenberg, C., Andrews, B., Burke, R., Chmielewski, L., … Tachibana, C. (2007). Excellence through evidence: Structures enabling clinical autonomy. *Journal of Nursing Administration, 37*(1), 41–52.

Kramer, M., & Schmalenberg, C. (2003). Magnet hospital staff nurses describe clinical autonomy. *Nursing Outlook, 51*(1), 13–19.

Lewis, F.M. (2006). Autonomy in nursing. *Ishikawa Journal of Nursing, 3*(2), 1–6.

Maas, M., Specht, J., & Jacox, A. (1975). Nurse autonomy: Reality not rhetoric. *American Journal of Nursing, 75*(12), 2201–2208.

MacDonald, C. (2002). Nurse autonomy as relational. *Nursing Ethics, 9*(2), 194–201.

Maylone, M. M., Raneire, L. A., Griffin, M. T. Q., McNulty, R., & Fitzpatrick, J. J. (2010). Collaboration and autonomy: Perceptions among nurse practitioners. *Journal of the American Academy of Nurse Practitioners, 23,* 51–57.

McParland, J., Scott, P. A., Arnt, M., Dassen, T., Gasull, M., Lemonidou, C., … Leino-Kilpi, H. (2000). Autonomy and clinical practice 1: Identifying areas of concern. *British Journal of Nursing, 9*(8), 507–513.

Mosely, A., & Paterson, J. (2008). The retention of the older nursing workforce: A literature review exploring factors that influence the retention of older nurses. *Contemporary Nurse, 30,* 46–56.

Mrayyan, M. T. (2004). Nurses' autonomy: Influence of nurse managers' actions. *Journal of Advanced Nursing, 45*(3), 326–336.

Neuhouser, F. (2011). Jean-Jacques Rousseau and the origins of autonomy. *Inquiry, 54*(5), 478–493.

Nickel, J. (2007). Interests and purposes in conceptions of autonomy. *Paideusis: Journal of the Canadian Philosophy of Education Society, 16*(1), 29–40.

Papathanassoglou, E. D. E., Karanikola, M. N. K., Kalafati, M., Giannakopoulou, M., Lemonidou, C., & Albarran, J. W. (2012). Professional autonomy, collaboration with physicians, and moral distress among European intensive care nurses. *American Journal of Critical Care, 21*(2), e41–e52.

Seago, J. A. (2006). Autonomy: A realistic goal for the practice of hospital nursing? *Aquichan, 6*(1), 92–103.

Shang, J., Friese, C. R., Wu, E., & Aiken, L. H. (2012). Nursing practice environment and outcomes for oncology nursing. *Cancer Nursing, 36*(3), 206.

Stamps, P., & Piemonte, E. (1986). *Nurses and work satisfaction: An index for measurement.* Ann Arbor, MI: Health Administration Press.

Stewart, J., Stansfield, K., & Tapp, D. (2004). Clinical nurses' understanding of clinical autonomy: Accomplishing patient goals through interdependent practice. *Journal of Nursing Administration, 34*(10), 443–450.

Walker, L. O., & Avant, K. C. (2005). *Strategies for theory construction in nursing* (4th ed.). Upper Saddle River, NJ: Pearson/Prentice Hall.

Weston, M. J. (2008). Defining control over nursing practice and autonomy. *Journal of Nursing Administration, 38*(9), 404–408.

Weston, M. J. (2009). Validity of instruments for measuring autonomy and control over nursing practice. *Journal of Nursing Scholarship, 41*(1), 87–94.

Zurmehly, J. (2008). The relationship of educational preparation, autonomy and critical thinking to nursing job satisfaction. *Journal of Continuing Education in Nursing, 39*(10), 453–460.

19

COMPASSION FATIGUE

Lynch and Lobo (2012) provide a review of the historical development of the concept of compassion fatigue, noting that the term was first devised in the 1980s to explain the emotional challenges facing health care professionals. Ray, Wong, White, and Heaslip (2013) noted that compassion fatigue was first used to more aptly describe the phenomenon of burnout for nursing professionals. Specifically, Joinson (1992) was among the first to use the term *compassion fatigue* when she was studying burnout among nurses in the emergency room. Even though compassion fatigue had been utilized to understand the experiences of nurses since the early 1990s, Ray and colleagues argue that it was not until 2001, with the development of the Compassion Stress/Fatigue Model by Figley (2001), that the true nature of compassion fatigue in nursing was illuminated. In 2002, Figley defined compassion fatigue in nurses as a state of tension and preoccupation with traumatized patients evidenced by reliving the traumatic events coupled with avoidance and numbing of reminders and persistent arousal associated with traumatized patients (Figley, 2002, p. 1435). This leads to a situation in which the nurse bears the suffering of others which, in turn, can cause emotional exhaustion and the inability to care (Hinderer et al., 2014). Authors from South Africa have defined compassion fatigue as being present when the nurse lacks recovery power, as the restorative processes are less than the compassionate energy used when caring for patients (Coetzee & Klopper, 2010). These authors indicated than compassion fatigue is the end result of a progressive process following prolonged stressful intense contact with patients with lack of sufficient rest to recover from these situations.

In the health care fields, compassion fatigue has been defined by a number of related terms. Potter et al. (2013) provide some insight into the current uses of the concept, noting that compassion fatigue is viewed as the combination of burnout and secondary traumatic stress. *Burnout*, according to these authors, refers to "a state of physical, emotional, and mental exhaustion caused by a depletion of a person's ability to cope with one's environment";

they describe *secondary traumatic stress* as the stress resulting from helping or wanting to help a traumatized suffering person (p. 180). In a related study, Slocum-Gori, Hemsworth, Chan, Carson, and Kazanjian (2013) further note that compassion fatigue has been conceptualized in the context of emotional stress experienced by the health care worker, rendering him or her unable to provide care. These situations are often ones that are difficult to predict, as compassion is typically an integral component of the caring and helping professions and also varies in level from person to person (Slocum-Gori et al., 2013).

Craig and Sprang (2010) argue that compassion fatigue typically results as a byproduct of the working environment for health care specialists. Professionals in these fields are continually brought into contact with individuals who have experienced some type of trauma or distress (Craig & Sprang, 2010). The emotional relationship between the caregiver professional and the client or patient requiring service results in the development of emotional tension or stress for the professional, leading to an erosion of coping capabilities over time (Craig & Sprang, 2010). The end result of this process is the development of symptoms that mirror burnout; however, the root cause of burnout in these cases is often difficult to predict or prevent.

From this study, it is also important to note that compassion fatigue is seen as resulting from indirect exposure to trauma, or vicarious traumatization (Craig & Sprang, 2010). This continued exposure to suffering dramatically affects the psychological and emotional state of the health care professional, resulting in significant changes in identity and world view as well as alterations in behavior (e.g., loss of empathy, poor performance, and disengagement; Craig & Sprang, 2010). In most instances, the health care professional is unaware of these changes, as they gradually result from daily exposure to vicarious trauma. Thus, compassion fatigue, while resulting in outcomes similar to those of burnout, often has a more rapid onset that may be difficult to detect.

DEFINING ATTRIBUTES

The critical attributes of compassion fatigue are emotional exhaustion, erosion of coping capabilities, and a decline in work performance.

Emotional exhaustion has been defined as a state of feeling overwhelmed and exhausted with evidence of being emotionally overextended by work (Wright & Cropanzano, 1998; Zohar, 1997). The nurse feels that there are excessive work demands on her physically and emotionally. She is unable to give anything of herself. She feels drained and empty and under constant intense stress. These feelings lead her to think that she is a failure, as she knows she is not providing high-quality nursing care to her patients, but due to the emotional exhaustion she has no concern about this.

Erosion of coping capabilities occurs when there is a depletion in a person's ability to cope with the environment. Lazarus and Folkman (1984) developed a model identifying two types of coping, emotional-focused coping and physical-focused coping. The type of coping strategies used will depend on the source of the stressors; for example, the nurse may employ emotional coping strategies to deal with stressors outside her control. However, when there is compassion fatigue, the nurse will notice that coping strategies that usually work well are not working and that even when new coping strategies are employed there is increasing evidence of erosion of coping capabilities.

A decline in work performance is an attribute in the nurse that may first be evident to the nurse manager. It may be the first outward sign that all is not right with the registered nurse who usually exhibits high performance levels. The nurse herself may feel disengaged and be aware that her performance is not up to her usual standard as time goes on, especially as she becomes more emotionally exhausted.

DEFINITION

Compassion fatigue is defined as emotional exhaustion coupled with the erosion of coping capabilities and a decline in work performance.

MODEL CASE

John is a palliative care nurse who works in the oncology department of a local hospital. Each day, he provides care for dying patients and their families, making recommendations to ensure that patients are made comfortable in their final days and weeks of life. John loves his job and the ability to provide such a valuable service to families in need. He has always had very good feedback from his patients about the care they receive from him. Over the past few weeks, however, John finds that he is physically exhausted, though he has not made any changes in his schedule. He is emotionally insensitive to patient's needs (emotional exhaustion) in spite of his compassion for their unfortunate situation. He provides for the patients' needs in a robotic way and gives the minimum of himself (declined work performance). He is unable to concentrate or make basic decisions. John is unable to sleep at night and often re-experiences the intense feelings of grief that are common among the family members of dying patients. He is often heard making cynical comments about his patients and is having a difficult time coping with his daily routine (erosion of coping capabilities).

RELATED CASE

Louise is an advanced practice palliative care nurse providing care in patients' homes. She works very long hours to make sure she completes all her patient visits every day. Often there are long driving commutes from one patient to the next. Louise is exhibiting the signs of the classic case of burnout, with the presence of exhaustion at the physical and emotional levels (emotional exhaustion) due to lack of proper staffing. In her case, several nurses have recently left the oncology department, leaving Louise as the sole community palliative care nurse. His workload in recent weeks has more than tripled, making it difficult for her to provide effective care for her patients. Although Louise is physically overwhelmed by her responsibilities, she is providing adequate standards of care by working longer hours, as it takes her longer than usual to meet each patient's needs (failed decline in work performance, failed erosion of coping capabilities).

BORDERLINE CASE

Adam is a registered nurse who works in the surgical intensive care unit. The acuity levels of his assigned patients are very high and it is not unusual for some of his patients to die. Adam works hard to care for his patients and to meet the needs of the families as best he can during these trying times. However, due to the constant heavy intense workload, Adam is experiencing mild levels of physical, emotional, and mental exhaustion (emotional exhaustion). Often he does not seem that interested and lacks some follow-up abilities (decline in work performance); however, he may still be able to compensate for these deficits by making sure he takes his assigned breaks and by engaging additional support from social workers to combat the stress that he is feeling. Although Adam is experiencing symptoms of compassion fatigue, these symptoms have not directly affected his ability to care for his patients and their families, due to the coping strategies he has employed (failed erosion of coping capabilities).

CONTRARY CASE

Alexis is a registered nurse working in the coronary care unit. Despite having an emotionally challenging job, she enjoys her current position and looks forward to going to work every day. Alexis feels that she is able to provide effective/safe care that demonstrates respect and compassion for both patients and their families (failed emotional exhaustion). Her patients and their families are very satisfied with the high standard of care she provides (failed decline in work performance). She regularly seeks the help of other nurses to discuss her emotions, and to help her cope with the emotional demands of her job. She exercises regularly and has many diverse interests outside of work to help her deal with the emotional and physical aspects of her job (failed erosion of coping capabilities). Alexis has a positive outlook on her work and her ability to help so many patients in need.

ANTECEDENTS

The antecedents for compassion fatigue are *continuous exposure to traumatic stress* and *overuse of emotional reserve*. Compassion fatigue has been seen to arise when the nurse is continually exposed to vicarious or secondary trauma through the suffering of his or her patients and their families (Hinderer et al., 2014). Increasingly in today's health care, patients in hospital are more critically ill than in the past and may have multiple comorbidities. Length of hospital stay is shorter and nurses are under pressure to care for the patients, get them well, and have them ready for discharge in a short span of time. The exposure of the nurse to the stress of the high-pressure environment, in tandem with the traumatic stresses of the illness and suffering of the patients, sets the stage for compassion fatigue.

Overuse of emotional reserve is a critical antecedent to compassion fatigue and one that the nurse must vigilantly guard against. The demands of caring in nursing can place a toll on the nurse, particularly if she or he becomes emotionally overinvolved with patients and their families. This overinvolvement can negatively affect the nurse's health and relationships, eventually leading to compassion fatigue. To minimize this overuse of emotional reserve, the nurse may participate in critical incident debriefing sessions at the end of a shift (Pickett, Brennan, Greenberg, Licht, & Worrell, 1994). It is also important for the nurse to involve the interdisciplinary team members in the emotional aspects of patient care.

CONSEQUENCES

The consequences of compassion fatigue are *physical illness manifestations* and *emotional detachment*. Nurses experiencing compassion fatigue may develop physical illnesses as a result of not being able to provide safe care and the stress they feel related to this failure. These illnesses may include obesity, depression, diabetes and heart disease, headaches, asthma, and anxiety. Berger, Polivka, Smoot, and Owens (2015), in their study on compassion fatigue in pediatric nurses, asked the sample to recount a situation where they had compassion fatigue. The nurses described consequences of compassion fatigue such as overeating, crying, and grieving (Berger et al., 2015).

Compassion fatigue in which the nurse is unable to provide safe care for his or her patient results in the development of emotional detachment from the caring environment. Nurses in this situation experience overwhelming negative feelings, anger, irritability, and emotional breakdown. Generally speaking, compassion fatigue appears to involve an automatic coping mechanism that is intended to prevent further harm from vicarious victimization, though the consequences for the nurse are quite significant and systemic.

EMPIRICAL REFERENTS

The attributes of compassion fatigue—emotional exhaustion, the erosion of coping capabilities, and declined work performance—can potentially be measured quantitatively. The emotional exhaustion nine-item subscale of the Maslach Burnout Inventory (Maslach & Jackson, 1981) can be used to measure emotional exhaustion. This subscale has good reliability. Items are on a seven-point Likert scale with scores ranging from 0 (never) to 6 (always).

The erosion of coping capabilities can be measured using the well validated and reliable Ways of Coping questionnaire devised by Folkman and Lazarus (1985, 1988). Work performance can be assessed by the nurse manger and any decline in work performance can be tracked over time.

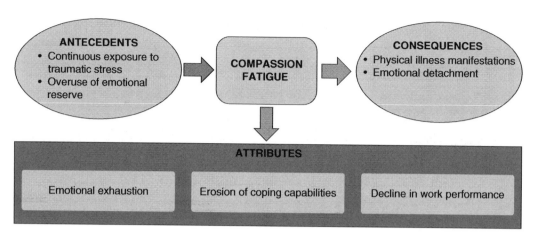

FIGURE 19.1 Compassion fatigue.

Another indicator of decline in work performance is a negative change in patient satisfaction scores. Also, feedback from patients' families may indicate a decline in the nurse's work performance (Figure 19.1).

SUMMARY

In this chapter, compassion fatigue is defined. The attributes, antecedents, and consequences of this concept related to nurses are identified. Case studies demonstrating the presence and absence of the attributes are provided. Nurses need to have a clear conceptual understanding of compassion fatigue if they are to avoid or minimize its presence. They can develop compassion fatigue programs using the antecedents and consequences as an educational framework. Empirical referents for the concept are identified and can be used to measure the presence or absence of the concept.

REFERENCES

Berger, J., Polivka, B., Smoot, E. A., & Owens, H. (2015). Compassion fatigue in pediatric nurses. *Journal of Pediatric Nursing.* doi:10.1016/j.pedn.2015.02.005

Coetzee, S. K., & Klopper, H. C. (2010). CF within nursing practice: A concept analysis. *Nursing and Health Sciences, 12,* 235–243. doi:10.1111/j.1442-2018.2010.00526.x

Craig, C. D., & Sprang, G. (2010). Compassion satisfaction, compassion fatigue, and burnout in a national sample of trauma treatment therapists. *Stress & Coping, 23*(3), 319–339.

Figley, C. R. (2001). Compassion fatigue as secondary traumatic stress: An overview. In C. R. Figley (Ed.), *Compassion fatigue: Coping with secondary traumatic stress disorder* (2nd ed., pp. 1–20). New York, NY: Bruner/Mazel.

Figley, C. R. (2002). Compassion fatigue: Psychotherapists' chronic lack of self care. *Journal of Clinical Psychology/In Session, 58,* 1433–1441.

Folkman, S., & Lazarus, R. S. (1985). If it changes it must be a process: Study of emotion and coping during three stages of a college examination. *Journal of Personality and Social Psychology, 48,* 150–170.

Folkman, S., & Lazarus, R. S. (1988). *The ways of coping questionnaire.* Palo Alto, CA: Consulting Psychologists Press.

Hinderer, K. A., VonRueden, K. T., Friedmann, E., McQuillan, K. A., Gilmore, R., Kramer, B., & Murray, M. (2014). Burnout, compassion fatigue, compassion satisfaction and secondary traumatic stress in trauma nurses. *Journal of Trauma Nursing, 21*(4), 160–169.

Joinson, C. (1992). Coping with compassion fatigue. *Nursing, 22*, 116–121.

Lazarus, R. S., & Folkman, S. (1984). *Stress, appraisal, and coping.* New York, NY: Springer Publishing Company.

Lynch, S. H., & Lobo, M. L. (2012). Compassion fatigue in family caregivers: A Wilsonian concept analysis. *Journal of Advanced Nursing, 68*(9), 2125–2134.

Maslach, C., & Jackson, S. (1981). The measurement of experienced burnout. *Journal of Organizational Behavior, 2*, 99–113.

Pickett, M., Brennan, A. M., Greenberg, H. S., Licht, L., & Worrell, J. D. (1994). Use of debriefing techniques to prevent compassion fatigue in research teams. *Nursing Research, 43*, 250–252.

Potter, P., Deshields, T., Berger, J. A., Clarke, M., Olsen, S., & Chen, L. (2013). Evaluation of a compassion fatigue resiliency program for oncology nurses. *Oncology Nursing Forum, 40*(2), 180–187.

Ray, S. L., Wong, C., White, D., & Heaslip, K. (2013). Compassion satisfaction, compassion fatigue, work life conditions, and burnout among frontline mental health care professionals. *Traumatology, 19*(4), 255–267.

Slocum-Gori, S., Hemsworth, D., Chan, W. W., Carson, A., & Kazanjian, A. (2013). Understanding compassion satisfaction, compassion fatigue and burnout: A survey of the hospice palliative care workforce. *Palliative Medicine, 27*(2), 172–178.

Wright, T. A., & Cropanzano, R. (1998). Emotional exhaustion as a predictor of job performance and voluntary turnover. *Journal of Applied Psychology, 83*(3), 486–493.

Zohar, D. (1997). Predicting burnout with a hassle-based measure of role demands. *Journal of Organizational Behavior, 18*(2), 101–115.

KAREN BAUCE

20

CULTURAL COMPETENCE

Cultural competence is described in the health care literature as an essential component of contemporary nursing practice, given the increased cultural diversity of patients. It has also been suggested that cultural competence is fundamentally nursing competence, because it reflects the nurse's ability to provide individualized patient care regardless of the patient's social or cultural background (Dreher & MacNaughton, 2002). Cultural competence implies the ability to understand the patient's point of view (Spector, 2013). This requires nurses to be sufficiently knowledgeable about cultural variations, particularly health beliefs and practices, to plan and implement culturally appropriate interventions. The assumption that cultural competence can be learned (Schim, Doorenbos, Benkert, & Miller, 2007) has resulted in a proliferation of training programs designed to teach and improve the cultural competence of health care providers (Beach et al., 2005). Standards of practice for culturally competent nursing care have been established (Douglas et al., 2009), as have regulatory and institutional mandates for cultural and linguistic competence (Spector, 2013).

Enhancing practitioner cultural competence has become a strategy to address racial/ethnic disparities in health and health care (Betancourt, Green, Carrillo, & Ananeh-Firempong, 2003) and to change health outcomes (Brach & Fraser, 2000). Differences in patient–provider cultural backgrounds and health-related beliefs, practices, and preferences have been identified as barriers to care (Betancourt et al., 2003). Culturally competent education and training are used to improve communication, treatment, and understanding, which may result in improved outcomes for minority group members (Brach & Fraser, 2002).

Several models of cultural competence have emerged since Leininger (Leininger & McFarland, 2002) first theorized that humans are cultural beings inseparable from their cultural background, and linked care with culture. Each framework provides a different theoretical perspective of cultural competence, resulting in conceptual ambiguity and a lack of consensus as to how to operationalize culture for purposes of quantifying and assessing practitioner cultural competence. An additional source of confusion is the synonymous use of the term *cultural competence* with closely related terms such as *cultural sensitivity, cultural responsiveness,* and *cultural awareness.* Despite definitional differences, common themes associated with cultural competence are that it is associated with individual characteristics and reflects an ongoing process (Dudas, 2012; Suh, 2004).

DEFINING ATTRIBUTES

The defining attributes of cultural competence are cultural awareness, cultural sensitivity, cultural knowledge, and cultural skill.

Cultural awareness is a cognitive construct which includes knowledge and recognition of diversity among individuals and the various factors that contribute to differences in and between groups (Schim et al., 2007). Awareness also involves an examination of the ways in which one's own cultural values, beliefs, and attitudes, including prejudices and biases, influence behavior (Leininger & McFarland, 2002). Without cultural awareness, the potential exists for health care workers to impose their own belief systems on those from different cultural backgrounds (Purnell, 2005). In addition, ethnocentrism, or believing in the superiority of one's beliefs, can lead to stereotyping members of other cultures, cultural clashes, and negative outcomes (Leininger & McFarland, 2002).

Cultural sensitivity is an affective construct that refers to attitude about oneself and others and willingness to become more culturally knowledgeable (Schim et al., 2007). Cultural sensitivity requires accepting and respecting cultural differences (Purnell, 2005) and adopting an attitude of openness and cultural humility in every encounter with patients (Leininger & McFarland, 2002). Culturally sensitive providers avoid language that might offend patients from different backgrounds and recognize that culturally appropriate language changes over time and within groups (Purnell, 2005).

Cultural knowledge refers to the educational foundation used to understand other cultures (Suh, 2004). Knowledge of the patient's emic (within the culture) perspective facilitates the integration of health-related cultural beliefs and practices into care (Leininger & McFarland, 2002; Purnell, 2005). While it is unrealistic to have complete knowledge of the cultural characteristics of every group, it is possible to gain sufficient knowledge of differences and similarities while recognizing that patients have unique life experiences (Meleis, 1999).

Cultural skill is required for effective and empathic communication (Balcazar, Suarez-Balcazar, & Taylor-Ritzler, 2009). Performing accurate "culturatological" care assessments is a means of learning beliefs and practices that are important to the patient and family (Leininger & McFarland, 2002). Becoming a culturally skillful communicator may include learning new languages and methods of dealing with communication gaps (Berry-Caban & Crespo, 2008), effectively using interpreters, and understanding the patient's nonverbal communication (Zander, 2007).

DEFINITION

Cultural competence is defined as the process of developing the cultural awareness, cultural knowledge, cultural sensitivity, and cultural skill that are required for the provision of individualized patient care.

MODEL CASE

A nurse working in the intensive care unit of a large urban teaching hospital has been taking care of an elderly man from a far-eastern country. He is in an isolation room because it was the last bed available when he was admitted. His wife and children understand that he is near death and become increasingly concerned about what will be done to his body after he dies. The nurse is aware (cultural awareness) that cultural and religious beliefs concerning postmortem care vary and she asks the son, whom she has observed to be the spokesperson for the family (cultural knowledge), to describe their customary practices (cultural skill). The patient's son states that after death, the body must remain undisturbed for 3 days so that the soul can journey to a higher level. A window must be open for the soul to leave and candles must be lit to illuminate the path. The nurse knows the hospital's safety policies prohibit the use of candles and the opening of windows in patient rooms. In addition, it is an unspoken policy of the intensive care unit to provide postmortem care quickly in order to make beds available for new admissions. The nurse explains the hospital's safety policies to the family, but also reassures them that she understands how important it is for the patient's soul to make a safe journey (cultural sensitivity). She discusses the situation with her nurse manager, and, working together with hospital administration, the nurse develops a plan for postmortem care that is acceptable to the patient's family. After the patient dies, the door to his room is closed and his body remains undisturbed for 3 days. A maintenance supervisor unlocks the window and leaves it open 6 inches. Several electric candles are used to provide a source of light. The family expresses gratitude to the nurse for helping the patient's soul on its journey. All of the defining attributes are present.

RELATED CASE

A student nurse doing a clinical rotation on a medical unit in a large urban teaching hospital was assigned to care for an 80-year-old Orthodox Jewish woman with diverticulitis. The student had grown up in a small homogeneous community and assumed that people were all alike (failed cultural awareness). The student's preceptor informed her that there are Orthodox Jewish dietary practices (cultural knowledge) that must be incorporated into care planning, and the student was eager to learn her patient's preferences (cultural sensitivity). When the patient stated she would not eat hospital food, the student reported the information to her preceptor (failed cultural skill). The student nurse in this case had cultural knowledge of religious dietary beliefs and demonstrated cultural sensitivity in her desire to learn them. There is failed cultural skill related to care provision and failed cultural awareness as to cultural variations.

BORDERLINE CASE

A nurse working in the intensive care unit of an internationally known cancer center requested to be assigned a patient who had just been admitted for complications related to recent abdominal surgery. The patient was a 40-year-old man who had travelled from Germany specifically for treatment at this hospital. He spoke no English and appeared to be quite apprehensive. The nurse had lived in Germany for several years (cultural knowledge) as a child and believed she could still remember a few words of German. She felt she could help the patient overcome his fears by speaking to him in his native language (cultural sensitivity) and also wanted to understand any specific care preferences (cultural awareness). When the nurse introduced herself to the patient in German, he expressed relief that he was finally able to speak with someone who understood him. He then asked a question which the nurse did not understand. He repeated the question several times, and in an effort to demonstrate that she understood him the nurse nodded affirmatively and smiled. The patient immediately became agitated (failed cultural skill); assuming that he was uncomfortable from his recent surgery, the nurse administered pain medication. The nurse discovered later that the patient had asked if he was going to need a second surgery, and she had smiled and nodded yes. This case illustrates all of the defining attributes with the exception of failed cultural skill due to ineffective intercultural communication.

CONTRARY CASE

A nurse working on a medical unit in a large urban teaching hospital has just admitted a 25-year-old male newly diagnosed with non-Hodgkin's lymphoma. The patient's wife of 2 months enters the room, visibly upset, and begins to pray at her husband's bedside. The patient smiles at his wife as she is praying and strokes her hand. The wife then asks the nurse if she can leave the container of holy water she has brought with which to anoint her husband.

The nurse becomes annoyed (failed cultural sensitivity) because she believes the patient's condition is too serious to be helped by anything other than modern medicine (failed cultural knowledge); she tells the patient's wife that she cannot leave the holy water and should stop praying because it is useless (failed cultural awareness). When giving shift report to the oncoming nurse, she describes the patient's wife as a "religious nut" and mockingly imitates her praying (failed cultural skill). None of the defining attributes are present in this case.

ANTECEDENTS

The antecedents of cultural competence are cultural encounter and cultural commitment. Cultural encounter, or an interaction between a nurse and patient from different cultural backgrounds (Grey & Thomas, 2006), has been determined to be an environmental precondition for cultural competence (Suh, 2004, p. 98). During cultural encounters, the nurse is exposed to both dominant beliefs of cultural groups and variations that exist within those groups. These encounters help nurses to gain a greater understanding of the cultural basis of their own values (Montuori & Fahim, 2004) and to reexamine existing beliefs that may be stereotypical.

The author proposes that a second antecedent required for cultural competence is cultural commitment, or the dedication to engage in lifelong learning from encounters with diverse groups or individuals. Cultural commitment requires more than a willingness to work with diversity; inherent is intentional cultural learning through experience, self-reflection, and critical thinking about one's cultural orientation and behaviors in professional practice. Cultural commitment provides the stimulus for experiential learning in cultural encounters.

CONSEQUENCES

The consequences of cultural competence include both client-based and provider-based outcomes. At the patient/client level, it has been suggested that culturally competent practice results in health promoting, maintaining, and/or regaining behavior (Kagawa-Singer & Kassim-Lakha, 2003), as well as satisfaction with the caregiver relationship (Paez, Allen, Beach, Carson, & Cooper, 2009; Napoles-Springer, Santoyo, Houston, Perez-Stable, & Stewart, 2005). In addition, higher scores of self-reported cultural competence among primary care providers (physicians, nurse practitioners, and physician assistants) in outpatient HIV care settings were associated with more equitable care, medication self-efficacy, and viral suppression across racial/ethnic groups (Saha et al., 2013). A corollary to culturally responsive care is the promotion of the patient's subjective good and respect for patient autonomy (Leever, 2011).

At the provider level, consequences of cultural competence have included dimensions of psychological empowerment among acute care nurses (Bauce, Kridli, & Fitzpatrick, 2014); improved knowledge, attitudes, and skills of health professionals (Beach et al., 2005; Salman et al., 2007; Schim, Doorenbos, & Borse, 2006); and increased cultural self-efficacy of registered nurses (Smith, 2001). A short-term immersion experience in a different culture has been shown to increase the cultural sensitivity and competency of both nursing faculty and students (Wood & Atkins, 2006).

EMPIRICAL REFERENTS

The primary empirical referents for measuring cultural competence are self-assessment instruments that measure at the provider level. The instruments vary in the specific domains that are measured, but there is some overlap (Loftin, Hartin, Branson, & Reyes, 2013). A significant limitation to the use of self-reporting of cultural competence is the possibility of socially desirable responding. Additional concerns with current empirical referents are related to the absence of linkages to the client's experience with and evaluation of care or to identifiable client outcomes (Bauce et al., 2014).

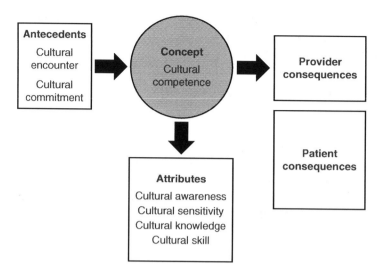

FIGURE 20.1 Cultural competence.

Eleven instruments have been identified that assess constructs of cultural competence in nurses and nursing students (Loftin et al., 2013). At least two of the instruments, such as the Cultural Competence Assessment (CCA) (Schim, Doorenbos, Miller, & Benkert, 2003) and Cultural Awareness Scale (CAS) (Rew, Becker, Cookston, Khosropour, & Martinez, 2003), are based on an identified model or theoretical framework. The CCA is currently the only assessment instrument developed for use by health care providers and staff with diverse roles, education, and backgrounds (Doorenbos, Schim, Benkert, & Borse, 2005). Further development is required for cultural competence empirical referents that incorporate direct observation of provider behaviors, patient evaluations of care, and patient and family outcomes (Figure 20.1).

SUMMARY

Cultural competence continues to be an important construct in contemporary nursing practice. The results of this concept analysis suggest that cultural competence is an ongoing developmental process with four defining attributes. Cases were developed to illustrate the concept with all, some, or none of its defining attributes. Antecedents and consequences were identified, as well as current and potential empirical referents.

REFERENCES

Balcazar, F. E., Suarez-Balcazar, Y., & Taylor-Reitzler, T. (2009). Cultural competence: Development of a conceptual framework. *Disability and Rehabilitation, 31*(4), 1153–1160. doi:10.1080/09638280902773752

Bauce, K., Kridli, S. A., & Fitzpatrick, J. J. (2014). Cultural competence and psychological empowerment among acute care nurses. *Online Journal of Cultural Competence in Nursing and Healthcare, 4*(2), 27–38. doi:10.9730/ojccnh.org/v4n2a3

Beach, M. C., Price, E. G., Gary, T. L., Robinson, K. A., Gozu, A., Palacio, A., . . . Cooper, L. A. (2005). Cultural competency: A systematic review of health care provider educational interventions. *Medical Care, 43*(4), 356–373.

Berry-Caban, C. S., & Crespo, H. (2008). Cultural competency as a skill for health care providers. *Hispanic Health Care International, 6*(3), 115–121. doi:10.1891/1540-4153.6.3.115

Betancourt, J. R., Green, A. R., Carrillo, J. E., & Ananeh-Firempong, O. (2003). Defining cultural competence: A practical framework for addressing racial/ethnic disparities in health and health care. *Public Health Reports, 118*, 293–302.

Brach, C., & Fraser, I. (2000). Can cultural competency reduce racial and ethnic health disparities? A review and conceptual model. *Medical Care Research and Review, 57*, 181–207. doi:10.1177/1077558700574009

Brach, C., & Fraser, I. (2002). Reducing disparities through culturally competent health care: An analysis of the business case. *Quality Management in Health Care, 10*(4), 15–28.

Doorenbos, A. Z., Schim, S. M., Benkert, R., & Borse, N. N. (2005). Psychometric evaluation of the cultural competence assessment instrument among healthcare providers. *Nursing Research, 54*(5), 324–331.

Douglas, M. K., Pierce, J. U., Rosenkoetter, M., Callister, L. C., Hattar-Pollara, M., Lauderdale, J., … Pacquiao, D. (2009). Standards of practice for culturally competent nursing care: A request for comments. *Journal of Transcultural Nursing, 20*(3), 257–269. doi:10.1177/1043659609334678

Dreher, M., & MacNaughton, N. (2002). Cultural competence in nursing: Foundation or fallacy? *Nursing Outlook, 50*(5), 181–186. doi:10.1067/mno.2002.125800

Dudas, K. I. (2012). Cultural competence: An evolutionary concept analysis. *Nursing Education Perspectives, 33*(5), 317–321. doi:10.5480/1536-5026-33.5.317

Grey, P. D., & Thomas, D. J. (2006). Critical reflections on culture in nursing. *Journal of Cultural Diversity, 13*(2), 76–82.

Kagawa-Singer, M., & Kassim-Lakha, S. (2003). A strategy to reduce cross-cultural miscommunication and increase the likelihood of improving health outcomes. *Academic Medicine, 78*(6), 577–587.

Leever, M. G. (2011). Cultural competence: Reflections on patient autonomy and patient good. *Nursing Ethics, 18*(4), 560–570. doi:10.1177/0969733011405936

Leininger, M., & McFarland, M. R. (2002). *Transcultural nursing: Concepts, theories, research, & practice* (3rd ed.). New York, NY: McGraw Hill.

Loftin, C., Hartin, V., Branson, M., & Reyes, H. (2013). Measures of cultural competence in nurses: An integrative review. *Scientific World Journal*, 1–10. doi:10.1155/2013/289101

Meleis, A. I. (1999). Culturally competent care. *Journal of Transcultural Nursing, 10*(1), 12.

Montuori, A., & Fahim, U. (2004). Cross-cultural encounter as an opportunity for growth. *Journal of Humanistic Psychology, 44*, 243–264. doi:10.1177/0022167804263414

Napoles-Springer, A. M., Santoyo, J., Houston, K., Perez-Stable, E. J., & Stewart, A. L. (2005). Patients' perceptions of cultural factors affecting the quality of their medical encounters. *Health Expectations, 8*, 4–17.

Paez, K. A., Allen, J. K., Beach, M. C., Carson, K. A., & Cooper, L. A. (2009). Physician cultural competence and patient ratings of the patient-physician relationship. *Journal of General Internal Medicine, 24*(4), 495–498. doi:10.1007/s11606-009-0919-7

Purnell, L. (2005). The Purnell model for cultural competence. *Journal of Multicultural Nursing & Health, 11*(2), 7–15.

Rew, L., Becker, H., Cookston, J., Khosropour, S., & Martinez, S. (2003). Measuring cultural awareness in nursing students. *Journal of Nursing Education, 42*(6), 249–257.

Saha, S., Korthuis, P. T., Cohn, J. A., Sharp, V. L., Moore, R. D., & Beach, M. C. (2013). Primary care provider cultural competence and racial disparities in HIV care and outcomes. *Journal of General Internal Medicine, 28*(5), 622–629. doi:10.1007/s11606-012-2298-8

Salman, A., McCabe, D., Easter, T., Callahan, B., Goldstein, D., Smith, T. D., . . . Fitzpatrick, J. J. (2007). Cultural competence among staff nurses who participated in a family-centered geriatric care program. *Journal for Nurses in Staff Development, 23*(3), 103–111. doi:10.1097/01.NND.0000277179.40206.be

Schim, S. M., Doorenbos, A., Benkert, R., & Miller, J. (2007). Culturally congruent care: Putting the puzzle together. *Journal of Transcultural Nursing, 18*(2), 103–110. doi:10.1177/1043659606298613

Schim, S. M., Doorenbos, A. Z., & Borse, N. N. (2006). Cultural competence among hospice nurses. *Journal of Hospice and Palliative Nursing, 8*(5), 302–307. doi:10.1097/00129191-200609000-00016

Schim, S. M., Doorenbos, A., Miller, J., & Benkert, R. (2003). Development of a cultural competence assessment instrument. *Journal of Nursing Measurement, 11*(1), 29–40. doi:10.1891/jnum.11.1.29.52062

Smith, L. S. (2001). Evaluation of an educational intervention to increase cultural competence among registered nurses. *Journal of Cultural Diversity, 8*(2), 50–63.

Spector, R. E. (2013). *Cultural diversity in health and illness* (8th ed.). Upper Saddle River, NJ: Pearson.

Suh, E. E. (2004). The model of cultural competence through an evolutionary concept analysis. *Journal of Transcultural Nursing, 15*(2), 93–102. doi:10.1177/1043659603262488

Wood, M. J., & Atkins, M. (2006). Immersion in another culture: One strategy for increasing cultural competence. *Journal of Cultural Diversity, 13*(1), 50–54.

Zander, P. E. (2007). Cultural competence: Analyzing the construct. *Journal of Theory Construction & Testing, 11*(2), 50–54.

MARY T. QUINN GRIFFIN, DEBORAH
J. STILGENBAUER, AND GERMAINE NELSON

21

DECISION MAKING BY NURSE MANAGERS

The purpose of this concept analysis is to define the concept of decision making by nurse managers. Health care is extremely complex and continuously changing. According to Aitken (2003), effective decision making can potentially facilitate improvements in health care. Decision making is the essence of leadership and not a new concept for nurse managers. Taylor (1978) described the effectiveness of nurse leaders as their ability to render the right decision to various problems. Managers and leaders are expected to make decisions, which are the visible outcome of their leadership and management process (Clancy, 2006). Decision making is also a behavior exhibited in making a selection and implementing a course of action from alternative courses of action to address a situation or problem (Clancy, 2006). Guo (2008) defined *decision making* as a procedure for choosing the best alternative to realize the organizational or individual goals.

Throughout history, great thinkers have contemplated the concept of decision making: Plato and Aristotle in the 4th century BC, Francis Bacon's introduction of inductive thinking, and René Descartes's framework for the scientific method. In the 20th century, Chester Barnard identified the difference between personal and organizational decision making; strength, weakness, opportunity, and threat (SWOT) analysis was developed; and the beginning of computer-based decision-making tools were created at the Carnegie Institute (Buchanan & O'Connell, 2006).

Hammond's cognitive continuum theory (Hammond, 1988, 1996, 2000) is useful in helping to define decision making as related to nurse managers. In this theory, decision making has six cognitive modes on a continuum going from intuitive judgment to scientific experiment (Hamm, 1988). The type of nurse manager task influences decision making. Well-structured routine tasks require a different type of decision making than tasks that arise in emergency situations and may not have been seen with new specific task elements before (Harbison, 2001). Hammond's cognitive continuum theory (Hammond, 1988, 1996, 2000) has a role in nurse manager decision making, as it potentially applies to many different types of decision making. In decision making, the perception of complexity and uncertainty is influenced by prior knowledge and previous experience of the particular type of decision being made (Tversky & Kahneman, 1982). Complexity and rapid change in the health care environment require nurse managers to keep pace with the changes if they are to be effective decision makers. They must modify their styles, skills, and behaviors, and understand the need to be flexible and change as an organization changes (Shearer, 2012). The levels of complexity and uncertainty may be reduced by using a structured decision-making approach.

The acute care setting provides the nurse manager with many competing priorities and constant opportunities for decision making. Acutely ill patients, shorter lengths of stay, technological advances, the focus on patient and employee satisfaction scores, quality indicators, and financial performance are all challenges the nurse manager must address daily. Other challenges for the nurse manager focus on patient outcomes and affect reimbursement, such as the outside influences of the regulatory agencies, the Affordable Care Act, Centers for Medicare and Medicaid, Hospital Consumer Assessment of Health Care Provider and Systems (HCAHPS), and value-based purchasing. Nurse managers are making decisions every day based on their experience, available options, and innovative ideas for improving care and reducing expenses. The good news is that decision making is a skill that can be improved, leading to more positive outcomes (Guo, 2008).

Nurses have always been aware that their decisions have important implications for the patient's recovery and final outcomes (Effken, Verran, Logue, & Hsu, 2010). Increasingly, nurse managers are active decision makers involved in clinical, administrative, and financial decisions for their units. Many of these decisions related to the work environment are complex, and major strategic decisions are made with reference to the overall organization. Nurse managers must have a clear understanding of the concept of decision making by nurse managers, and the definitions of the key attributes involved. This clear, succinct presentation of the concept can guide their decision making.

DEFINING ATTRIBUTES

Decision making is defined by the following attributes: *information gathering, critical thinking,* and *use of a defined process.* These attributes were identified following a review of the literature.

Information gathering is critical to decision making. Information should be obtained from a variety of sources and analyzed according to importance (Frank, 2006). To be valuable, the information must have relevance and be timely (Porter-O'Grady & Malloch, 2015). It is paramount that an effective system to obtain and record information be utilized to make a sound decision (Robbins, 2005). Risk is inherent in all decision making and cannot be totally eliminated. Gathering too much information will not reduce risk, but will reduce the timeliness of any action taken (Porter-O'Grady & Malloch, 2015). However, shortening the process of information gathering may initially save time but may lead to challenges and other problems further down the road.

Critical thinking, the second defining attribute, involves a process of assessment, exploration of alternatives, intervention, and reevaluation (Cirocco, 2007). It is not memorization of lists or steps; rather, it is a process that allows the formulation of judgments about a situation and is integral to good decision making (Cirocco, 2007). According to Frank (2006), critical thinking skills enhance the quality of problem solving and decision making. Porter-O'Grady and Malloch (2015) identify eight elements of critical thinking: analyzing language, making assumptions, formulating problems, weighing evidence, evaluating conclusions, discriminating between arguments, justifying claims, and clarifying values.

Use of a defined process is the third defining attribute of decision making. Nurses are taught to use the steps of the nursing process to guide the provision of care. The nursing process is a systematic and dynamic approach with five steps (Pokorski, Moraes, Chiarelli, Costanzy, & Rabelo, 2009). Using decision-making models can help the nurse manager make more effective decisions (Guo, 2008). There are many formalized decision-making models: decision tree, cost-benefit analysis, cause-and-effect charts, DECIDE, and evidence-based decision-making (EBD) model. The nurse manager can also use simpler processes as well, such as "pro" and "con" lists. The choice of a model should be determined by the complexity or importance of the problem. However, the process of making judgments and choosing between two or more alternatives is not always straightforward, and is often characterized by a personal and professional struggle to determine what is best for patients (Goethals, Dierckx de Casterle, & Gastmans, 2013).

Electronic decision-making tools may also be available. Many staffing and scheduling systems have productivity modules to provide data for nurse leaders to use in decision making. The decision-making process should include stakeholders in order to promote acceptance, collaboration, and sense of being valued (Grahm-Dickerson et al., 2013).

DEFINITION

Decision making is defined as information gathering, the use of critical thinking, and use of a defined process.

MODEL CASE

CK has been a nurse manager for 10 years and has recently chosen to manage a medical/surgical amenities unit that hosts many international and high-profile patients. The patient and employee satisfaction scores, as well as Hospital Consumer Assessment of Healthcare Providers and Systems (HCAHPS) scores have steadily improved, increasing by 10 to 20 points. The unit on average has been over budget by 7%. CK decided she wanted to "master finance." She identified a problem: the unit was consistently over budget. She began reviewing reports and staffing data, and meeting with the Director of Nursing Finance monthly (information gathering). CK began to understand the basic elements of finance and how her prior decisions had influenced expenses resulting in an unfavorable outcome (critical thinking).

CK then focused on systematic changes, creating a balanced schedule, rigorous daily attention to staffing, and census information. She involved, educated, and empowered her staff to make staffing decisions based on acuity, census, pending, and discharges. She also shared reports with the staff to engage them in the goal of having a favorable variance (use of a defined process). Last year was the first year the unit had a year-end favorable variance and the favorable variance continued into first quarter of this year. In this example, the nurse leader engaged in decision making to turn around the financial performance of the unit.

RELATED CASE

HS is a new manager of a cardiac telemetry unit. She has been in the position 6 months and is highly motivated to do a good job. She was a skilled clinician and involved in day-to-day problem-solving issues as a charge nurse. HS has identified an issue related to the unit having an unfavorable variance. She reviews the monthly finance reports and identifies an unfavorable overtime variance, but fails to review and analyze all contributing aspects of all expenses (failed information gathering). She has implemented a moratorium on overtime as a way to decrease expense (use of a defined process). Although this moratorium will be effective in reducing overtime, there may be consequences to banning overtime (failed critical thinking). HS needs to analyze the reasons for the current use of overtime. To successfully manage a budget, all contributing aspects of expense must be thoroughly analyzed. HS will have a decrease in overtime; however, HS is using problem-solving techniques rather than embracing the three attributes of decision making by nurse managers.

BORDERLINE CASE

MB has been the nurse manager for an intensive care unit (ICU) for 5 years. He is smart and motivated by his inquisitive nature to understand topics of interest to him. The unit has seasonal fluctuations related to occupancy. Position control (vacancy replacement) is always important; however, it is critical to managing the budget on this unit because of the fluctuating census. Allowing positions to stay vacant during low-occupancy periods and filling vacant positions in anticipation of the high-occupancy swing is paramount to avoid unfavorable variances.

MB is knowledgeable of the unit trends and understands the need to manage vacancies related to census fluctuations (information gathering). The unit has a blended acuity unit, a combination of ICU beds and step-down beds. MD understands that adjusting daily staffing targets based on the number of step-down to ICU beds is a strategy to control expense (critical thinking). MB is aware that controlling vacancies is a strategy because of seasonal fluctuations in census. Positions are left vacant during lower-occupancy months; however, they remain vacant too long when the volume increases. The unit must then rely on expensive supplemental staff to care for patients, resulting in unfavorable variances (failed use of a defined process).

CONTRARY CASE

RT is the nurse manager of a bone marrow transplant (BMT) unit. This patient population is a combination of two types of BMT: allo and auto. The number of allo transplants has decreased and there has been an increase in auto transplants. The auto transplant patients require less intensive nursing care than the allo patients and have lower nursing care hours (NCHs).

The nurse manager does not incorporate the concept of adjusting staffing to acuity and decreasing related expense. Because the unit is on budget, she does not perceive that there is a problem. Although the unit is not over budget, changes in patient population (lower acuity) should result in monthly expenses lower than the projected budget. RT collects data on patient numbers but does not collect data on case type (failed information gathering). She does not analyze the data by correlating the lower-acuity case type with less nursing care requirements and adjusting staffing levels accordingly (failed critical thinking). RT makes her staffing decisions based on census alone, not considering acuity; she does not use a systematic decision-making model to make an informed decision (failed use of a defined process).

ANTECEDENTS

The antecedents to decision making by nurse managers are *identification of a problem, knowledge,* and *organizational initiatives.* Identification of a problem is an activity that the nurse leader does before decision making takes place. The nurse leader must be able to recognize or identify that there is a problem: either a clinical practice problem or an administration problem. According to Clancy (2006), decision making may or may not be the result of an immediate problem. Depending upon the answer to the question, the nurse leader considers the complexity of the issue and the consequences of taking action or not. Deciding to act or not is the beginning of the decision-making process.

Knowledge, both nursing and non-nursing knowledge, is the second key antecedent to decision making by nurse managers. Nurse managers today are managing nurses working in increasing complex technological environments with acutely and seriously ill patients who have complex conditions. Nurse managers need to have up-to-date knowledge about the patients' conditions, the nursing care required, patient acuity, and technological knowledge about equipment used. Also essential for the nurse manager is in-depth financial knowledge to manage and balance the budget, and the knowledge required to ensure a safe, high-quality work environment. Staff mix and staff ratios, length-of-stay data, and insurance companies' requirements are among some of the other areas with which the nurse manager needs to be knowledgeable.

Organizational initiatives are critical antecedents to decision making. A second reason to engage in decision making is to operationalize organizational goals or initiatives (Clancy, 2006). Health care is in a constant state of change, which means nurse managers need to adapt and develop new approaches to the challenges of the role. Operationalizing organizational goals requires a thoughtful approach, taking into consideration how the idea will affect all of the stakeholders. The nurse manager may or may not consider including the stakeholders in the decision-making process. Transparency with regard to the operational initiatives, and the ability to identify them as antecedents to the decision making by nurse managers will influence the concept and will help the nurse manager identify the best decision-making process to use to achieve a decision.

CONSEQUENCES

There are two consequences of decision making by nurse managers: *elimination of the problem* and *acceptance by stakeholders*. The result of all decision making is a consequence of one type or another. Strategic thinkers anticipate many factors, alternatives, and potential outcomes. One outcome of decision making is elimination of the problem at hand (Clancy, 2006). A second consequence of decision making is acceptance by the stakeholders; staff who feel involved in the decision-making process feel empowered (Grahm-Dickerson et al., 2013). According to Taylor (1978), the acceptance of a decision is as important to its success as the quality of the decision. Clancy articulates that leadership decision making focuses on choices that advance the group's goal (Clancy, 2006). The nurse leader must be flexible and able to adapt to the outcomes that are a result of the decision-making process.

EMPIRICAL REFERENTS

Information gathering is a defining attribute that has no measurement for how much is appropriate. As stated by Porter-O'Grady and Malloch (2015), the key is not the quantity of information but whether there is enough to make a decision. The complexity and magnitude of the problem or goal will determine how much information should be gathered. While one is gathering information, additional questions may require further examination.

Urgency to make a decision, one's own interpretation of the facts, and jumping to conclusions may affect the nurse manager's decision-making ability. A document listing the information that must be gathered will provide assurance that all of the information is considered and included in the decision-making process.

Critical thinking is a defining and professional attribute integral to good decision making; however, there is no clear way to measure it (Cirocco, 2007). Although strategies have been identified to improve critical thinking, the effectiveness is anecdotal (Staib, 2003). There are a number of instruments to measure critical thinking: the Watson-Glaser Critical Thinking Appraisal (Watson & Glaser, 1980); the Ennis-Weir Critical Thinking Essay Test (Ennis & Weir, 1985); and, most recently, the Halpern Critical Thinking Assessment Using Everyday Situations (Halpern, 2007). Porter-O'Grady and Malloch (2015) identify eight components of critical thinking: analyzing language, making assumptions, formulating problems, weighing evidence, evaluating conclusions, discriminating between arguments, justifying claims, and clarifying values. These eight components can be used as a tool to ensure all necessary information is included in the analysis.

Use of a defined process is the third defining attribute and the easiest to measure. There are numerous well-defined decision-making strategies adapted to suit the complexity of the problem or goal to be implemented. All decision-making processes include a step-by-step approach (Clancy, 2006). Nurse managers should choose a strategy with which they are comfortable and allow the steps to guide the process. The measurement of use of a defined process validates that all of the steps were included in the decision making.

Simulation is a new, innovative method to validate that the nurse manager is using a defined process when making decisions. This method will use scenarios with different problems requiring decisions by nurse managers. Nurse managers will be asked to identify the decision-making model or process they plan to use to make a decision related to each simulation scenario. These simulation decision-making interactions with the nurse manager can be videotaped, and with the aid of a grading rubric the presence or absence of the steps involved in the defined process can be assessed (Figure 21.1).

SUMMARY

Decision making by nurse managers is a key aspect of their leadership and involves implementing a course of action after considering alternatives (Clancy, 2006). In this chapter, the antecedents of decision making have been identified. There are three defining attributes of decision making by nurse managers: information gathering, critical thinking, and use of a defined process. Decision making is a key component of leadership and focuses on choices to eliminate a problem or gain stakeholders' acceptance.

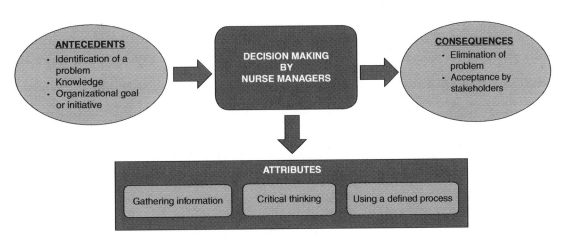

FIGURE 21.1 Decision making by nurse managers.

REFERENCES

Aitken, L. M. (2003). Critical care nurses' use of decision-making strategies. *Journal of Clinical Nursing, 12*, 476–483.

Buchanan, L., & O'Connell, A. (2006). A brief history of decision making. *Harvard Business Review, 84*(1), 32–41. Retrieved from http://dx.doi.org/unpan1.un.org/intradoc/groups/public/.../unpan022443.p

Cirocco, M. (2007). How reflective practice improves nurses' critical thinking ability. *Gastroenterology Nursing, 30*, 407–413. Retrieved from http://dx.doi.org/10.1097/01.SGA.0000305221.78403.e9

Clancy, T. R. (2006). Decision-making skills. In D. L. Huber (Ed.), *Leadership and nursing care management* (3rd ed., pp. 149–178). Philadelphia, PA: Saunders Elsevier.

Effken, J. A., Verran, J. A., Logue, M. D., & Hsu, Y. (2010). Nurse managers decisions: Fast and favoring remediation. *Journal of Nursing Administration, 40*(4), 188–195.

Ennis, R. H., & Weir, E. (1985). *The Ennis-Weir critical thinking essay test.* Pacific Grove, CA: Midwest Publications.

Frank, B. (2006). Critical thinking skills. In D. L. Huber (Ed.), *Leadership and nursing care management* (3rd ed., pp. 131–147). Philadelphia, PA: Saunders Elsevier.

Goethals, S., Dierckx de Casterle, B., & Gastmans, C. (2013). Nurses' decision-making process in cases of physical restraint in acute elderly care: A qualitative study. *International Journal of Nursing Studies, 50*(5), 603–612.

Grahm-Dickerson, P., Houser, J., Thomas, E., Casper, C., ErkenBrack, L., Wenzel, M., & Siegrist, M. (2013). The value of staff nurse involvement in decision making. *Journal of Nursing Administration, 43*, 286–292. Retrieved from http://dx.doi.org/10.1097/NNA.0b013e31828eec15

Guo, K. L. (2008). DECIDE: A decision making model for more effective decision making by health care managers. *Health Care Manager, 27*(2), 1–8.

Halpern, E. R. (2007). *Halpern critical thinking assessment using everyday situations: Background and scoring standards.* Claremont, CA: Claremont McKenna College.

Hammond, K. R. (1988). Judgment and decision making in dynamic tasks. *Information and Decision Technologies, 14*, 3–14.

Hammond, K. R. (1996). *Human judgment and social policy: Irreducible uncertainty, inevitable error.* New York, NY: Oxford University Press.

Hammond, K. R. (2000). *Judgment under stress.* New York, NY: Oxford University Press.

Harbison, J. (2001). Clinical decision making in nursing: Theoretical perspectives and their relevance to practice. *Journal of Advanced Nursing, 35*(1), 126–133.

Pokorski, S., Moraes, M. A., Chirelli, R., Costanzi, A. P., & Rabelo, E. R. (2009). Nursing process: From literature to practice. What are we actually doing? *Revista Latino-Americana de Enfermagem, 17*(3), 302–307.

Porter-O'Grady, T., & Malloch, K. (2015). *Quantum leadership building better partnerships for sustainable health* (4th ed.). Burlington, MA: Jones & Bartlett.

Robbins, F. (2005). Provide information to support decision making. *Nursing Residential Care, 7*(11), 492–495. Retrieved from http://dx.doi.org/10.12968/nrec.2005.7.11.20007

Shearer, D. A. (2012). Management styles and motivation. *Radiology Management, 34*(5), 47–52.

Staib, S. (2003). Teaching and measuring critical thinking. *Journal of Nursing Education, 42*, 498–508.

Taylor, A.G. (1978). Decision making in nursing: An analytical approach. *Journal of Nursing Administration, 8*(11), 22–30.

Tversky, A., & Kahneman, D. (1982). Judgement under uncertainty: Heuristics and biases. In D. Kahneman, P. Slovic, & A. Tversky (Eds.), *Judgement under uncertainty: Heuristics and biases.* New York, NY: Cambridge University Press.

Watson, G., & Glaser, E. M. (1980). *Watson-Glaser critical thinking appraisal.* Cleveland, OH: Psychological Corporation.

EMOTIONAL INTELLIGENCE

Emotional intelligence (EI) is the ability to use emotions effectively. EI consists of five attributes: *self-awareness, self-regulation, motivation, empathy,* and *social skill* (Goleman, 2004). Individuals with strong EI skills perceive and regulate emotions that positively impact communication, motivation, and teamwork to achieve the best possible results from relationships (Mayer & Salovey, 1997). EI affects many different aspects of daily life, including the way people behave and the way they interact with others.

Salovey and Mayer (1990) introduced the term *emotional intelligence* into mainstream American psychology in their landmark article "Emotional Intelligence." In 1995, the concept of EI was popularized after publication of psychologist and *New York Times* science writer Goleman's book, *Emotional Intelligence: Why It Can Matter More than IQ*. Goleman argued that human intelligence was far too narrow and showed that people with high intelligence quotient (IQ) were not necessarily successful. He proposed that emotional factors such as self-awareness, self-discipline, and empathy contributed to a different way of being smart. According to Goleman, these factors are not fixed at birth; they are shaped by childhood experiences and can be nurtured and shaped throughout adulthood with immediate benefits to health, relationships, and work. In 1998, Goleman published a sequel, titled *Working with Emotional Intelligence*, which applied EI to leadership and success in organizations and corporate life.

Research clearly demonstrates a relationship between successful business leaders and high levels of EI. Akerjoret and Sevreinsson (2008) found that nurses who displayed high EI enhanced organizational, staff, and patient outcomes. If someone has a high EI, they perform better at work (O'Boyle, Humprhey, Pollack, Hawver, & Story, 2011) and in school (Petrides, 2004). Individuals with high EI also report more positive relationships (Mavroveli, Petrides, Rieffe, & Bakker, 2007) and better health (Costa, Petrides, & Tillmann, 2014).

Executive nurse leaders are well aware of how critical nurse managers and bedside nurses are to the success of any organization, as these individuals influence how hospital teams work together to consistently achieve high-quality, patient-centered care. Nurse managers who possess high levels of EI are more effective in leading teams to achieve efficient outcomes regarding quality, patient satisfaction, employee satisfaction and retention, and financial well-being.

DEFINING ATTRIBUTES

EI consists of five attributes: *self-awareness, self-regulation, motivation, empathy,* and *social skill* (Goleman, 2004).

The first attribute, self-awareness, is the ability to have insight into one's emotions, strengths, and weaknesses, and to see how one's feelings affect others. People with self-awareness have a rich understanding of emotions, strengths, weaknesses, needs, and drives (Goleman, 1995). They are very honest with themselves and others and avoid the extremes of being overly critical and unrealistically hopeful. Furthermore, these people know how their feelings affect them, others, and job performance (Goleman, 2004).

The second attribute, self-regulation, involves controlling one's impulses, and with holding judgment until enough information has been gathered. People with a high degree of self-regulation are more capable of facing change and the ambiguities of an advancing industry than those whose degree of self-regulation is low. Furthermore, people with a high level of self-regulation can help enhance the integrity of an organization by not making bad decisions through impulsive behaviors.

Motivation, the third attribute, can be described as passion, quest for challenges, a desire to learn, pride in one's work, high performance expectations, resilience, and/or stick-to-itiveness. People who are motivated actively search for solutions to problems and pursue goals with energy and commitment. Highly motivated people constantly raise their performance expectations for themselves, their team, and their organization. One of their greatest qualities is remaining optimistic even though they have experienced failure or a setback. This quality is beneficial because it means that a motivated person is committed to seeing the organization succeed in reaching its goals and objectives.

The fourth attribute is empathy, the ability to understand others' feelings and emotions when making decisions. People with empathy have acute organizational awareness, possess a service orientation, and are attentive to others (Goleman, 2004). When using teams, empathetic individuals can be extremely effective leaders because of their ability to recognize and understand other opinions. Empathetic leaders play a key role when globalization is a factor because they can understand the importance of others' cultural differences. These individuals are also effective in retaining talent because they are able to develop personal rapport with new employees during coaching and mentoring stages. An empathetic leader can provide the effective feedback and constructive criticism that is essential in employee retention and advancement.

The fifth attribute is social skill, which involves the ability to manage and forge relationships with others. Social leaders are able to build a rapport easily by finding some type of common ground with everyone, thus establishing a broad circle of acquaintances (Goleman, 1995). In addition, the social individual is an effective persuader and is able to effectively manage teams.

DEFINITION

EI is the ability to understand one's emotions (self-awareness), control those emotions (self-regulation), understand others' emotions (empathy), promote emotional and intellectual growth (motivation), and build effective relationships with others (social skill).

MODEL CASE

A model case example was provided by Richman in a 1994 *Fortune* article titled "How to Get Ahead in America." In this article, Michael Iem from Tandem Computers employed all of the attributes of EI to convince his company to adopt a new way of thinking about the business. Shortly after Iem joined the company as a junior analyst, he noticed the market trend away from mainframe computers to networks that linked workstations and personal computers (empathy). Iem realized that unless Tandem responded to this trend, its products would become obsolete (motivation). He had to convince Tandem's managers that their old "tried and true" emphasis on mainframes was no longer appropriate (social skill), and then develop a system using new technology. He was aware that as a junior analyst, he might have been resented or not taken seriously, so he moved slowly and respectfully, ensuring that he followed appropriate steps and political protocols of the company (self-awareness). Over the next 4 years, he presented his idea regarding the new system to customers and company sales personnel before the new network applications were fully accepted (self-regulation). In this example, Iem employed all five attributes of EI and in doing so achieved personal and organizational success.

RELATED CASE

Organizations have used the Myers-Briggs tool to assess certain personality variables such as introversion and extroversion, as well as other variables, to determine how groups of people in organizations and on teams relate to one another. Introverts hold back, are less spontaneous, more thoughtful, and will not be the first ones to speak; extroverts think out loud, will be the first to enter a conversation, and speak without thinking about consequences.

Bill Gates is an example of a business leader who is considered highly focused (motivation): an introvert who values privacy, needs quiet time alone to recharge, and feels more comfortable being alone than being with others.

These traits enable him to be thoughtful and display self-awareness and self-regulation. Yet, he has been known to end conversations by saying, "That's the stupidest thing I've ever heard" (failed social skill). One might say he lacked social awareness or that he was insensitive to and unaware of the feelings provoked by such a statement (failed empathy). Although personalities play a role in job performance and team dynamics and are related to the EI elements, personality variables are more limited, provide a much narrower view, and do not account for all of the attributes of EI.

BORDERLINE CASE

The U.S. Air Force used the EQ-I to select recruiters (the Air Force's front-line human resources personnel) and found that the most successful recruiters scored significantly higher in the EI competencies of assertiveness (self-regulation), social awareness (empathy), happiness (motivation), and emotional insight (self-awareness). The Air Force also found that by using EI to select recruiters, they increased their ability to predict successful recruiters by nearly threefold. The immediate gain was an annual savings of 3 million dollars. These gains resulted in the Government Accountability Office (GAO) submitting a report to Congress, which led to a request that the Secretary of Defense order all branches of the armed forces to adopt this procedure in recruitment and selection (Cherniss, 1999). The GAO report, titled *Military Recruiting: The Department of Defense Could Improve Its Recruiter Selection and Incentive Systems*, was submitted to Congress on January 30, 1998. This case study did not identify relationship management as an essential attribute (failed social skill).

CONTRARY CASE

Goleman (1998) described an excellent example of a contrary case. IQ or traditional intelligence (measured by academic knowledge, above-average grades, and IQ tests) is used to describe a computer programmer who has excellent skills in writing computer programs but who does not meet his client's needs because he does not have EI. The programmer describes the technical capabilities of the machine and does not consider the customer's request that the data be converted to a simple format that fits on one page. The programmer's inability to understand and address the customer's request (failed EI) resulted in an unsuccessful product. Thus, the programmer lacks the attributes of EI (failed self-awareness, self-regulation, motivation, empathy, and social skill).

ANTECEDENTS

The antecedents of EI are internal locus of control, thin mental boundaries, and self-determination. EI has been studied with variables such as motivation (Christie, Jordan, Troth, & Lawrence, 2007) and the big five personality construct

(Vakola, Tsaousis, & Nikolaou, 2004), leading one to hypothesize that locus of control might be correlated with EI. A study by Barbuto and Story examined the relationship between EI, internal locus of control, and mental boundaries. Using a cross-sectional survey design, the researchers found a positive correlation between internal locus of control, thin mental boundaries, and EI. Results indicated that internal locus of control and thin mental boundaries accounted for 18% of the variance in EI among 382 county employees (Barbuto & Story, 2010).

EI exists when a person possesses an internal locus of control and a thin mental boundary (Barbuto & Story, 2010). An internal locus of control is characterized by individuals who put forth more effort and perform better. Persons with an internal locus of control are reported to have higher work motivation, perform better, exert more effort, and have higher job satisfaction. A person with a thin mental boundary is less structured, spontaneous, and more likely to face challenges with motivation. People with a thin mental boundary relate to others' emotions and feel a sense of connectedness.

In a study published in 2014, researchers found that self-determination was considered an antecedent for EI (Perreault, Mask, Morgan, & Blanchard, 2014). At the core of the self-determination theory is the notion that the individual is motivated and geared toward the greater good. Data from two different samples of students and workers supported the hypothesis that self-determination may account for differences in EI.

CONSEQUENCES

The consequences of EI are workplace success, leadership effectiveness, happiness, and positive outcomes. According to Goleman (1998), emotionally intelligent individuals excel in human relationships, show marked leadership abilities, and perform well at work. Thus, it is not surprising that studies have demonstrated that persons with high EI are also happy (Casey, 2009). Nurses who display high EI enhance organizational, staff, and patient outcomes (Akerjordet & Sevreinsson, 2008).

EMPIRICAL REFERENTS

Empirical referents are ways to measure a concept. These referents provide observable phenomena by which to measure EI. Empirical referents for EI include self-confidence, emotional self-control, empathy, and leadership. Because EI is a measure of an individual's capability, it requires tools to assess this capability.

The most prominent measure of ability EI is the Multifactor EI Scale (MEIS; Mayer, Caruso, & Salovey, 1999) and its successor, the Mayer-Salovey-Caruso EI Test (MSCEIT; Mayer, Salovey, & Caruso, 2002). Critics of the ability EI tests cite the inherent subjectivity of the emotional experience (Watson, 2000). Unlike standard cognitive ability tests, tests of EI ability cannot be objectively scored because in most cases, there are no clear criteria for what constitutes a correct response. Researchers argue, however, that ability EI tests have improved considerably over the years (Matthews, Zeider, & Roberts, in press).

According to Mayer and Salovey (1997), the gold standard for measuring EI is an ability-based test known as the MSCEIT. This test measures one's ability by way of actual performance in solving emotional problems. The overall score on the MSCEIT indicates the ability of a respondent to perceive, use, understand, and manage emotion.

The MSCEIT measures the four branches of Mayer and Salovey's EI model. The tool consists of 141 items and takes 30 to 45 minutes to complete. The MSCEIT is reliable and valid. Mayer et al. (2003) found a correlation of R (705) = 0.908, the full-test split-half reliability was r (1985) = 0.93 for general and 0.91 for expert consensus scoring.

Two of the most common measures (and the most recent) of trait EI are the Trait Meta-Mood Scale (TMMS) and the emotional quotient inventory (EQ-i); however, there has been an explosion in the number of trait EI measures. Perez, Petrides, and Furnham maintain that few trait EI measures have been developed within a clear theoretical framework, and even fewer have sturdy empirical foundations. TMMS (Salovey et al., 1995)—the first measure of EI, in general, and of trait EI, in particular—is loosely based on the original model by Salovey and Mayer (1990). It comprises 30 items, which are responded to on a 5-point Likert scale. The TMMS produces scores on three factors namely: attention to emotion, emotional clarity, and emotional repair.

The Bar-On EQ-I (Bar-On, 1997) is one of the most widely used measures of trait EI in the literature. Its theoretical background is somewhat vague, having been converted from a well-being inventory to an EI questionnaire. The structure of the EQ-I is 133 items, 15 subscales, and 5 higher-order factors: intrapersonal, interpersonal, adaptation, stress management, and general mood. A concept map that illustrates all aspects of EI appears in Figure 22.1.

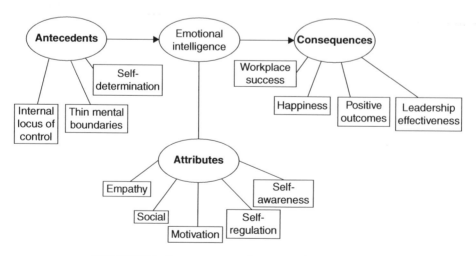

FIGURE 22.1 Concept map of emotional intelligence.

SUMMARY

This chapter included description of the characteristics of EI with attention to the attributes, antecedents, and consequences of EI.

REFERENCES

Akerjordet, K., & Severinsson, E. (2008). Emotionally intelligent nurse leadership: Literature review study. *Journal of Nursing Management, 16*(5), 65–77.

Barbuto, J. E., & Story, J. S. (2010). Antecedents of emotional intelligence: An empirical study. *Journal of Leadership Education, 9*(1), 144–154.

Casey, P. (2009). *The effects of emotional intelligence on happiness and well-being. Can EI predict significant life outcomes?* Edinburgh Research Archive.

Cherniss, C. (1999). The business case for emotional intelligence. Retrieved from www.eiconsortium.org

Christie, A., Jordan, P., Troth, A., & Lawrence, S. (2007). Testing the links between emotional intelligence and motivation. *Journal of Management and Organization, 13*, 212–226.

Costa, S., Petrides, K.V., Tillman, T. (2014). Trait emotional intelligence and inflammatory disease. *Psychology, Health*, and *Medicine, 19*(2), 180–189.

Goleman, D. (1995). *Emotional intelligence: Why it can matter more than IQ*. New York, NY: Bantam.

Goleman, D. (1998). *Working with emotional intelligence*. New York, NY: Bantam.

Goleman, D. (2004). What makes a leader? *Harvard Business Review, 82*(1), 82–91.

Matthews, G., Zeidner, M., & Roberts, R. D. (in press). Measuring emotional intelligence: Promises, pitfalls, solutions? In A. D. Ong & M. van Dulmen (Eds.), *Handbook of methods in positive psychology*. Oxford, UK: Oxford University Press.

Mavroveli, S., Petrides, K. V., Rieffe, C., & Bakker, F. (2007). Trait emotional intelligence, psychological well-being and peer–rated social competence in adolescence. *British Journal of Developmental Psychology, 25*(2), 263–275.

Mayer, J. D., Caruso, D. R., & Salovey, P., (1999). Mayer-Salovey-Caroso-Emotional Intelligence Test. (MEIS: Users Manual). Toronto, ON, Canada: MultiHealth Systems.

Mayer, J. D., Salovey, P., Goldman, S., Turvey, C., Palfai, T. (1995). Emotional attention, clarity, and repair: Exploring emotional intelligence using the Trait Meta Mood Scale. In J.W. Pennebaker (Ed.), *Emotion, disclosure and health* (pp. 125–154). Washington DC; American Psychological Association.

Mayer, J. D., & Salovey, P. (1997). What is emotional intelligence? In P. Salovey & D. J. Sluyter (Eds.), *Emotional development and emotional intelligence: Educational implications* (pp. 3–31). New York, NY: Basic Books.

Mayer, J. D., & Salovey, P., Caruso, D. R. (2002). Mayer-Salovey-Caroso-Emotional Intelligence Test. (MSCEIT: Users Manual).Toronto, Canada: MultiHealth Systems.

O'Boyle, E. H., Humphrey, R. H., Pollack, J. M., Hawver T. H., & Story, P. A. (2011). The relation between emotional intelligence and job performance: A meta-analysis. *Journal of Organizational Behavior, 32*(5), 788–818.

Perreault, D., Mask, L., Morgan, M., & Blanchard, C. (2014). Internalizing emotions; self–determination as an antecedent of emotional intelligence. *Personality and Individual Differences,* 641–646.

Petrides, K.V., Frederickson, N., & Furnham, A. (2004). The role of trait emotional intelligence in academic performance and deviant behavior at school. *Personality and Individual Differences, 36,* 277–293.

Richman, L. S. (1994, May 16). How to get ahead in America. *Fortune,* 46–54.

Salovey, P., Mayer, J.D., Goldman, S.L., Turvey, C., & Palfai, T.P. (1995). Emotional attention, clarity and repair: Exploring emotional intelligence using the Trait Meta-Mood Scale, In J.W. Pennebaker (Ed.). *Emotion, disclosure and health* (pp. 125–154). Washington, D. C: American Psychological Association.

Salovey, P., & Mayer, J. D. (1990). Emotional intelligence. *Imagination, Cognition and Personality, 9*(3), 185–211.

Vakola, M., Tsaousis, I., & Nikolaou, I. (2004). The role of emotional intelligence and personality variables on attitudes toward organizational change. *Journal of Managerial Psychology, 19*(2), 88–110.

Watson, D. (2000). *Mood and temperament.* New York, NY: Guilford.

23

EMPATHY

Empathy is a broad concept with varying definitions and views. Much like the concept of love, it is often intangible. Nonetheless, when present it seems apparent, and there is usually a positive effect. This concept analysis aims to examine the basic defining aspects of empathy in an effort to distinguish it from other concepts that may be similar to it, but are not the same.

American psychologist Carl Rogers further examined empathy as part of the core of interrelated conditions he asserted were required for successful patient psychotherapy. Rogers stated that empathy is when a therapist communicates his or her desire to understand and appreciate the client's perspective.

Empathy remains an elusive concept requiring added exploration, as several sources offer various definitions. According to Carl Rogers, empathy can be seen as the ability to communicate a sensing of the client's feelings as though they are the therapist's own, but without losing a sense of self (Pike, 1990). According to Williams and Stickley (2010), empathy may be described as the ability to supportively communicate affirmation of another person's feelings. Kalisch (1973) states that empathy is the ability to enter into the life of a patient and accurately perceive his or her current feelings and effectively communicate them to the patient (Kalisch, 1973, p. 1548). Furthermore, genuine empathy involves practitioners who are concerned with understanding the patient's perspective and are able to communicate their understanding back to their patients through acknowledgment of emotions and accurate reflections of patient statements (Bayne, Neukrug, Hays, & Britton, 2013, p. 213).

Some authors propose dividng empathy into two major components: affective empathy and cognitive empathy. Affective empathy involves listening to patients' words, gestures, and voice about their feelings and elic- iting an appropriate emotional response, whereas cognitive empathy is the capacity to understand the patient's perspective and/or mental state (Parvan et al., 2014).

Empathy has been the focus of a multitude of articles and research studies, all illustrating the diverse influences empathy has within health care practice. Various issues relative to empathy are described, such as the use of empathy in optimizing patient outcomes by way of alleviating patient stress and demonstrating care and concern. Conversely, researchers report how the lack of empathy in nurses can produce patient dissatisfaction. The article by Bayne et al. (2013) discusses the inherent qualities of an empathic practitioner; these qualities being interpersonal ease, active listening, and use of reflective communication. It seems that empathetic ability is also enhanced in caregivers who are honest and have greater self-awareness and genuineness. Topics such as practitioner perspectives of empathy, whether or not empathy can be taught, and structured empathy training in nursing school curriculum were also noted during publication review.

A predominant theme among the majority of the literature is that empathy serves as an integral part of the nurse–patient relationship. Bayne et al. (2013) states that the use of empathy can significantly strengthen the relationship between a caregiver and patient as it establishes greater trust. Consequently, with greater trust in their caregiver, patients seem to have increased rates of treatment compliance, lower malpractice claim tendencies, and higher patient satisfaction (Bayne et al., 2013). Patients cared for by empathic practitioners have also been linked to positive health outcomes measured in terms of reduced anxiety, improved pain management, easier emotional adjustment to chronic illness, and the ability to maintain hope (Williams & Stickley, 2010). Nurses must be able to understand the patient's perspective, thereby being empathetic, in order to meet the patient's individual needs (Pike, 1990). Furthermore, use of empathic understanding allows for increased communication by encouraging a more open dialogue between nurse and patient.

Several research studies conducted were qualitative in nature, scoring practitioner empathy levels using questionnaires, participant journals, and formulated empathy measurement tools. One study's design incorporated an interactive educational program called "Take a Walk in My Shoes" for health care employees at a long-term health care facility. Led by nursing students, the program consisted of an educational lecture, case studies, and simulation stations in order to provide employees an experience of physical ailments associated with the geriatric population. At the end of the program, nursing student and participant journals revealed increased empathy toward older adults (Eymard, Crawford, & Keller, 2010). Another study examined the effects of a structured empathy course taken by medical and nursing school students; the results demonstrated significantly higher student empathic skills and empathic tendency scores following their empathy course (Ozcan, Oflaz, & Bakir, 2012). Herbek and Yammarino (1990) assessed the effectiveness of an empathy training program for hospital staff nurses. Although the results of the pre- and postempathy scores among participants showed small practical significance, the nurses in the experimental group who received empathy training reported better teamwork, paid more attention to the emotional needs and concerns of their patients, and had greater job satisfaction.

DEFINING ATTRIBUTES

The defining attributes of empathy are *the ability to understand the perspective and feelings of another person's experience,* and *ability to effectively communicate this understanding to the person, both verbally and nonverbally.*

DEFINITION

Empathy is the ability to understand the perspective and feelings of another person's experience, and the ability to effectively communicate this understanding to the person, both verbally and nonverbally.

MODEL CASE

An obese woman is being counseled in a weight loss clinic. Faced with documents illustrating a strict diet food plan and exercise regimen, the woman begins to cry and shouts, "I can't do it. I just can't do it." A counselor gently places her hand on the woman's hand and states in a caring manner, "Losing weight is not easy; I was overweight most of my life, so I can understand your frustration [ability to understand the perspective and feelings of another person's experience]. It can seem really daunting at the beginning." The woman exclaims, "Yes, it's way too much." The counselor responds by saying, "It may help to try and take it one day at a time" (ability to effectively communicate this understanding to the person, both verbally and nonverbally).

This model case exemplifies the two defining characteristics of empathy. Based on the woman's verbal and physical cues, as well as having personal insight regarding weight issues, the counselor was able to gain understanding of the woman's frustrations with weight loss and then verbalize this understanding to the woman.

RELATED CASE

Related cases show similarity to the concept at hand, but do not contain all the defining characteristics required. An exemplary case related to empathy could involve a discussion between two patients sharing a hospital room.

In room 305, Patient A is being discharged and has begun packing up personal items. From behind the curtain separating the patient beds, Patient B begins to cry just after being seen by the medical team. Patient A inquires "What's wrong? What happened?" (ability to understand the perspective and feelings of another person's experience). Patient B states, "The doctor just told me I'll have to stay another week in the hospital." Patient A responds, "Oh, I'm sorry" (failed ability to effectively communicate this understanding to the person, both verbally and nonverbally).

In this case example, Patient A recognizes the other patient's despair and seems to show sympathy via the acknowledging statement made. The concept of sympathy may resemble empathy; however, it usually only relates to moments of suffering, whereas empathy can be utilized in almost all situations. Additionally, sympathy probably does not have the same emotional and intellectual depth of empathy. As seen in the scenario, Patient A acknowledged Patient B's sorrow, but more than likely did not fully comprehend Patient B's perspective, as there was no communicated recognition of this understanding.

BORDERLINE CASE

A man attends the funeral of his best friend's parent. The man notices that his friend is despondent and sitting apart from everyone else at the funeral home. Having lost his own parent the year before, the man goes over to his friend, gives the friend a hug, and states, "It'll be okay" (ability to understand the perspective and feelings of another person's experience; failed ability to effectively communicate this understanding to the person, both verbally and nonverbally).

This situation comes close to demonstrating empathy, though it probably leans more toward describing compassion. In this instance, the man acknowledges that his friend is experiencing some type of emotional turmoil. He probably has a good grasp on how his friend actually feels. He even hugs the friend in order to provide some comfort. Nevertheless, the man fails to specifically communicate his understanding of the friend's feelings to his friend, thus omitting an important attribute of empathy.

CONTRARY CASE

In contrary cases, none of the defining attributes of a concept are present. An example of a contrary case for empathy could be as follows.

A surgical patient, following abdominal surgery, slowly reaches for the call bell and presses the button. The patient is holding his stomach, has facial grimacing and groaning. A nurse enters the patient's room and announces, "We're right in the middle of report. Someone will attend to you afterward" and walks out of the room (failed ability to understand the perspective and feelings of another person's experience; failed ability to effectively communicate this understanding to the person, both verbally and nonverbally).

Evidently, the nurse in this case does not exhibit any of empathy's defining attributes. Even if the nurse did notice the patient's physical and verbal pain cues, it does not seem to have had any effect on the nurse. The nurse does not exhibit any sense of understanding the patient's experience and certainly does not convey any understanding of it to the patient.

ANTECEDENTS

Antecedents for empathy include a person's past experiences, the five senses (sight, hearing, smell, taste, and touch), and emotional intelligence. People's past experiences can definitely enhance their ability to better understand another person's perspective of a situation if they have also experienced it themselves. The five senses are also necessary for empathy to occur, as they allow someone to pick up on the visual and/or physical signals of how another person feels. Additionally, a person must have emotional intelligence in order to truly empathize with another person.

CONSEQUENCES

A consequence of empathy is enhanced communication between nurse and patient. Empathy facilitates the development of mutual trust between a nurse and patient; hence, a patient feels more comfortable to freely share with his or her nurse (Williams & Stickley, 2010, p. 752). The quality of patient care is improved, as empathy allows a nurse to be more attuned to treating the patient's specific needs. Use of empathy can also contribute to a practitioner's sense of personal accomplishment, which can increase clinical competency and better her patient management (Ozcan et al., 2012). Moreover, if a practitioner can employ empathy in his practice, he is likely to be more compassionate with patients.

EMPIRICAL REFERENTS

An empirical referent should be available for each defining attribute. Measuring the first defining attribute of empathy—a practitioner's ability to understand the patient's perspective and feelings of the patient's experience—could include observations for acknowledging gestures (e.g., eye-to-eye contact, head nodding). To measure the second defining attribute of empathy, which is the practitioner's ability to effectively communicate understanding of the patient's perspective/feelings, one could use interviewing as a way to gather data. Interviews could be performed one on one or with Likert-scale questionnaires specific to topics related to aspects of a nurse–patient interaction (e.g., the nurse effectively communicated that your feelings were understood by the nurse).

Likert-scale questionnaires such as the Empathic Tendency Scale and the Empathic Communication Skills Scale formalized by Dokmen (Ozcan et al., 2012) could be given to patients after nurse–patient interaction to gauge the nurse's empathy level; a high score indicates increased empathic tendency in the nurse. In addition, an observational tool could be created to score/record the number of acknowledging gestures (e.g., appropriate hand touching, maintenance of eye contact, and head nodding) during nurse–patient interactions. Again, a higher score would be demonstrative of a higher level of empathy (Figure 23.1).

SUMMARY

Empathy remains somewhat of an enigmatic concept even after conduct of this concept analysis. Nonetheless, the concept analysis did help to distinguish empathy from related concepts such as sympathy, compassion, and emotional intelligence. It also identified two defining attributes of empathy,

Concept Map

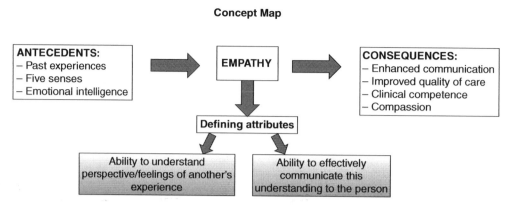

FIGURE 23.1 Empathy.

as well as the concept's antecedents, consequences, and empirical referents. Elements of the concept of empathy are provided in a diagram to facilitate understanding.

REFERENCES

Bayne, H., Neukrug, E., Hays, D., & Britton, B. (2013). A comprehensive model for optimizing empathy in person-centered care. *Patient Education and Counseling, 93,* 209–2015. doi:10.1016/j.pec.2013.05.016

Eymard, A. S., Crawford, B. D., & Keller, T. (2010). Take a walk in my shoes: Nursing students talk a walk in older adults' shoes to increase knowledge and empathy. *Geriatric Nursing, 31*(2), 137–141. doi:10.1016/j.gerinurse.2010.02.008

Herbek, T., & Yammarino, F. (1990). Empathy training for hospital staff nurses. *Group and Organizational Management, 15,* 279–295. doi:10.1177/105960119001500304

Kalisch, B. (1973). What is empathy? *American Journal of Nursing, 73*(9), 1548–1552.

Ozcan, C. T., Oflaz, F., & Bakir, B. (2012). The effect of a structured empathy course on the students of a medical and a nursing school. *International Nursing Review, 59,* 532–538. doi:10.1111/j.1466-7657.2012.01019.x

Parvan, K., Ebrahimi, H., Zamanzadeh, V., Seyedrasooly, A., Dadkhah, D., & Jabarzaddeh, F. (2014). Empathy from the nurses' viewpoint in teaching hospitals of Tabriz University of Medical Sciences, Iran. *Journal of Caring Sciences, 3*(1), 29–36. doi:10.5681/jcs.2014.004

Pike, A. W. (1990). On the nature and place of empathy in clinical nursing practice. *Journal of Professional Nursing, 6*(4): 235–240.

Williams, J., & Stickley, T. (2010). Empathy and nurse education. *Nurse Education Today, 30,* 752–755. doi:10.1016/j.nedt.2010.01.018

MIRIAM BELL *24*

INTERPROFESSIONAL COLLABORATION

For almost 40 years, interprofessional collaboration has been advocated as the means to achieve integration of increasingly fragmented health care services worldwide. In 1978, the World Health Organization (WHO), through the declaration of Alma Ata, declared collaborative practice as being essential for the effective and efficient delivery of primary care services. A decade later, WHO published *Learning Together to Work Together for Health* (WHO, 1988), advocating that health professionals be educated together to develop the competencies required for collaborative practice. In a macrosociological analysis of the trends in interprofessional research in the 40 years between 1970 and 2010, Paradis and Reeves (2013) identified more than 100,488 collaboration-related articles in the health care literature. International investigations into alleged poor care in the intervening years all refer, either explicitly or implicitly, to collaborative practice in health care as being essential for patient safety and quality of care (Francis, 2010; Government of Ireland, 2006; Health Information and Quality Authority [HIQA], 2011; Institute of Medicine, 2000; Sinclair, 1994). Yet, despite this drive for collaborative practice, 40 years on the empirical literature demonstrates little evidence of actual collaboration in practice (Klinar et al., 2013; Lundon et al., 2013; Martin et al., 2005; Onishi, Komi, & Kanda, 2013) and differing interpretations of the term *collaboration* (Nair, Fitzpatrick, McNulty, Click, & Glembocki, 2012). However, based on the review of current literature, the following four attributes are proposed.

DEFINING ATTRIBUTES

The defining attributes are *shared care goals*, *shared decision making*, *nonhierarchical relationships*, and *power sharing*.

The first attribute, shared care goals, places the patient at the center of care (D'Amour & Oandasan, 2005; Irvine, Kerridge, & McPhee, 2004; Irvine, Kerridge, McPhee, & Freeman, 2002; McNair, 2005; Miller et al., 2008; Nadolski et al., 2006; Orchard, Curran, & Kabene, 2005; Pullon, 2008). Working from this perspective, professional boundaries become less evident as the "work" of health care takes priority. The complexity of a patient's health care needs determines the number and variety of health care professionals on a team, and these professionals work interdependently toward patient-centered common goals.

Shared decision making (Gravel, Legare, & Graham, 2006; Orchard et al., 2005), the second attribute, becomes a natural consequence of patient-centered care goals. Planning a patient's care becomes a team activity in which all relevant expertise is considered and all team members are individually accountable for outcomes.

The third attribute, nonhierarchical relationships (D'Amour & Oandasan, 2005; Irvine et al., 2002, 2004; Orchard et al., 2005), involves all members of the health care team working in an egalitarian way, where all are considered full and equal members of the health care team. All contributions to care are treated with equal importance. This creates an environment where team members feel safe contributing their expertise and enables effective communication.

The final attribute of interprofessional collaboration is power sharing (D'Amour & Oandasan, 2005; Irvine et al., 2002, 2004; Orchard et al., 2005), where power is based on knowledge and expertise, rather than role or title (Henneman, Lee, & Cohen, 1995). Organizational culture plays a significant role in promoting and supporting power sharing.

DEFINITION

Interprofessional collaboration can be defined as occurring when two or more health care professionals from different disciplines work together in a respectful, egalitarian, nonhierarchical relationship where they have shared care goals and shared decision making and in which there is power sharing.

MODEL CASE

Susan is a geriatric liaison nurse specialist working in a large academic teaching hospital. The objective of her role is to prevent hospital readmissions in the over-65 patient population. To achieve this, she reviews patients as they are admitted to the emergency department. She is called to the emergency department to review a 90-year-old man who has presented after falling with no obvious injuries sustained. The man lives alone with no formal home supports. Susan undertakes a comprehensive assessment of this man, who appears unkempt and has significant orthostatic hypotension. He is unsteady when mobilizing and at risk of falling. He scores poorly on a brief cognitive assessment. Susan recommends admission under the care of a geriatrician for full multidisciplinary team input (power sharing and nonhierarchical working). This result in rationalization of his medications, provision of a walking aid, initiation of a home care package, and a new diagnosis of mild cognitive impairment (shared decision making and shared care goals). The man was discharged home after a short hospital stay, with planned follow-up review.

RELATED CASE

Concepts frequently used interchangeably with interprofessional collaboration are *multidisciplinary team working* and *interdisciplinary team working*. Both concepts can be explained using the ward round for context. Susan, the geriatric liaison nurse specialist, the admitting medical consultant, junior doctors, the ward manager, staff nurse, social worker, and occupational therapist are all in attendance, leading one to believe that interprofessional collaboration is evident (nonhierarchical relationships). The case of the elderly man is being reviewed. The consultant asks for a report of the man's recent blood tests; his junior doctors provide the information. The consultant says he is satisfied that the man can be discharged (failed shared decision making and hierarchical working). Susan and the social worker disagree and are supported by the occupational therapist (failed shared patient care goals). The consultant reiterates that the patient is medically fit for discharge and orders the "team" to arrange for this to occur (failed power sharing). This scenario is perhaps extreme, but it highlights the "silo" mentality of unidisciplinary working and professional boundaries that are at play under the guise of multidisciplinary or interdisciplinary team working.

BORDERLINE CASE

Using the same scenario as for the first model case, Susan is called to the emergency department to review a 90-year-old man who has presented after falling. She undertakes a comprehensive geriatric assessment and recommends admission, as the man is clearly off baseline; he is admitted under the care of the medical team on call (shared care goals and nonhierarchical working) but is discharged home soon afterward (failed power sharing and decision making). Some days later, he is found at home after having fallen and fractured his femur; he is admitted and after a prolonged stay and failed rehabilitation he is discharged to a long-term care facility.

CONTRARY CASE

Susan, a geriatric liaison nurse specialist whose job is to review patients over 65 years of age as they are admitted to the emergency department, hears from a nursing colleague that a 90-year-old man has been admitted to the emergency department. She queries why she has not been paged to review this patient. The emergency department consultant she speaks to tells her that the man is a straightforward admission and that he has ordered (failed nonhierarchical relationship) the emergency department nurse to arrange for his immediate transfer back home (failed shared care goals and decision making). This case highlights the complete absence of all attributes of interprofessional collaboration.

ANTECEDENTS

For the purposes of this concept analysis, the following are considered antecedents: a clear sense of professional identity (Bleakley, Boyden, Hobbs,

Walsh, & Allard, 2006; Irvine et al., 2004; McNair, 2005; Miller et al., 2008); an understanding of other disciplines' roles (Bleakley et al., 2006; Miller et al., 2008; Nadolski et al., 2006; Orchard et al., 2005); emotional intelligence (Atwal & Caldwell, 2006; Gaboury, Bujold, Boon, & Moher, 2009; Miller et al., 2008; O'Brien, Martin, Heyworth, & Meyer, 2009; Pullon, 2008; Tame, 2012); trust (Irvine et al., 2002, 2004; Miller et al., 2008; Orchard et al., 2005; Pullon, 2008); professional competence and confidence (Baxter & Brumfitt, 2008; Clancy, Gressnes, & Svensson, 2012; El Sayed & Sleem, 2011; Miller et al., 2008; Orchard et al., 2005; Pullon, 2008; Tame, 2012); tolerance of difference (Croker, Trede, & Higgs, 2012; D'Amour & Oandasan, 2005); a supportive organizational culture and leadership behaviors (D'Amour & Oandasan, 2005; Irvine et al., 2002; Kvarnstrom, 2008; Odegard & Strype, 2009; Orchard et al., 2005); mutual respect (Clancy et al., 2012; Makowsky et al., 2009; Piquette, Reeves, & Leblanc, 2009; Suter et al., 2009); and education and training around working collaboratively (Fouche, Butler, & Shaw, 2013; Makowsky et al., 2009; Pype et al., 2012; Wittenberg-Lyles, Parker Oliver, Demiris, & Regehr, 2010).

CONSEQUENCES

Consequences of interprofessional collaboration present in health care are improved patient outcomes and improved safety and quality of care (Bleakley et al., 2006; Braithwaite et al., 2013; Gravel et al., 2006; Nadolski et al., 2006; Orchard et al., 2005). When health care professionals collaborate, the patient is more likely to benefit from a holistic approach to care in which all needs are met and errors in care are minimized.

Improved staff morale and job satisfaction, with subsequent improvement in staff retention (Bleakley et al., 2006; D'Amour & Oandasan, 2005), is another outcome of true interprofessional collaboration.

Reduced length of patient stay can result from collaborative practice (D'Amour & Oandasan, 2005; Irvine et al., 2002; Nadolski et al., 2006; Orchard et al., 2005); a therapeutic context is created (Braithwaite et al., 2013; D'Amour & Oandasan, 2005; Orchard et al., 2005; Irvine et al., 2002); and a relaxation of professional boundaries leads to more integrated working.

EMPIRICAL REFERENTS

The four defining attributes of interprofessional collaboration are shared care goals, shared decision making, nonhierarchical relationships, and power sharing. Each attribute requires an empirical referent. *Empirical referents* are defined as "phenomena that by their existence or presence demonstrate the occurrence of the concept" (Walker & Avant, 2005, p. 73), in this case, inter-professional collaboration.

Ushiro's (2009) Nurse-Physician Collaboration Scale is a 3-factor, 51-item instrument that can be used to measure the four attributes of interprofessional collaboration. Power sharing and nonhierarchical relationships are measured through 6 items within the dimension cooperativeness; 9 items measure shared care goals, termed *sharing of patient information*; and 12 items are used to determine the degree of shared decision making within the dimension "joint participation in the cure/care decision-making process."

The Jefferson Scale of Attitudes Toward Physician-Nurse Collaboration (Hojat et al., 1999) utilizes four domains to study the degree of interprofessional collaboration. The four domains—shared education and teamwork, caring as opposed to curing, nurses' autonomy, and physician dominance—provide a means to measure the four defining attributes.

Interprofessional collaboration has a positive effect on staff engagement which can be effectively measured using the Utrecht Work Engagement Scale (Schaufeli & Bakker, 2003). Person centeredness can be measured using various instruments, for example, the Person-Centered Climate Questionnaire (Edvardsson et al., 2013).

SUMMARY

This concept analysis of interprofessional collaboration has identified four defining attributes and highlighted antecedents which must be in place for collaborative practice to occur. For almost four decades, interprofessional collaboration has been advocated as a means of addressing the increasing fragmentation of health care. It is seen as an essential component for the provision of safe, high-quality patient care. Yet despite this, and despite generally positive attitudes of health care professionals toward the ideal of collaboration, little empirical evidence exists of *actual* collaboration in practice. Differing conceptualizations of collaboration may contribute to this situation. Based on the four defining attributes, a definition of interprofessional collaboration has been proposed. The concept can be measured through several existing instruments that measure collaboration. The defining attributes, antecedents, consequences, and empirical referents of interprofessional collaboration can be seen in Figure 24.1.

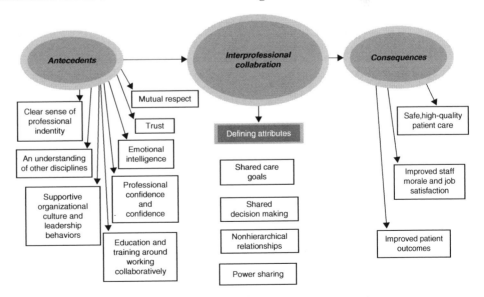

FIGURE 24.1 Interprofessinal collaboration.

REFERENCES

Atwal, A., & Caldwell, K. (2006). Nurses' perceptions of multidisciplinary team work in acute health-care. *International Journal of Nursing Practice, 12*, 359–365.

Baxter, S., & Brumfitt, S. M. (2008). Professional differences in interprofessional working. *Journal of Interprofessional Care, 22*(3), 239–251.

Bleakley, A., Boyden, J., Hobbs, A., Walsh, L., & Allard, J. (2006). Improving teamwork climate in operating theatres: The shift from multiprofessionalism to interprofessionalism. *Journal of Interprofessional Care, 20*(5), 461–470.

Braithwaite, J., Westbrook, M., Nugus, P., Greenfield, D., Travaglia, J., Runciman, W., ... Westbrook, J. (2013). Continuing differences between health professions' attitudes: The saga of accomplishing systems-wide interprofessionalism. *International Journal for Quality in Health Care, 25*(1), 8–15.

Clancy, A., Gressnes, T., & Svensson, T. (2012). Public health nursing and interprofessional collaboration in Norwegian municipalities: A questionnaire study. *Scandinavian Journal of Caring Sciences, 27*, 659–668.

Croker, A., Trede, F., & Higgs, J. (2012). Collaboration: What is it like?—Phenomenological interpretation of the experience of collaborating within rehabilitation teams. *Journal of Interprofessional Care, 26*, 13–20.

D'Amour, D., & Oandasan, I. (2005). Interprofessionality as the field of interprofessional practice and interprofessional education: An emerging concept. *Journal of Interprofessional Care, 19*(Suppl. 1), 8–20.

Edvardsson, D., Sjogren, K., Lindjvist, M., Taylor, M., Edvardsson, K., & Sandman, P. O. (2013). Person-centred climate questionnaire (PCQ-S): Establishing reliability and cut-off scores in residential aged care. *Journal of Nursing Management.* doi:10.1111/jonm.12132 [Epub ahead of print]

El Sayed, K. A., & Sleem, W. F. (2011). Nurse-physician collaboration: A comparative study of the attitudes of nurses and physicians at Mansoura University Hospital. *Life Science Journal, 8*(2), 140–146.

Fouche, C., Butler, R., & Shaw, J. (2013). Atypical alliances: The potential for social work and pharmacy collaborations in primary health care delivery. *Social Work in Health Care, 52*, 789–807.

Francis, R. (2010). *Investigation into Mid Staffordshire NHS Foundation Trust.* London, UK: The Stationery Office.

Gaboury, I., Bujold, M., Boon, H., & Moher, D. (2009). Interprofessional collaboration within Canadian integrative healthcare clinics: Key components. *Social Science and Medicine, 69*, 707–715.

Government of Ireland. (2006). *The Lourdes hospital inquiry: An inquiry into peripartum hysterectomy at our Lady of Lourdes Hospital, Drogheda: Report of Judge Maureen Harding Clark. S.C.* Dublin, Ireland: The Stationery Office.

Gravel, K., Legare, F., & Graham, I. D. (2006). Barriers and facilitators to implementing shared decision-making in clinical practice: A systematic review of health professionals' perceptions. *Implementation Science, 1*, 16. Retrieved from http://www.implementationscience.com/content/1/1/16

Health Information and Quality Authority. (2011). *Report of the investigation into the quality and safety of services and supporting arrangements provided by the Health Service Executive at Mallow General Hospital.* Dublin, Ireland: Author.

Henneman, E. A., Lee, J. L., & Cohen, J. I. (1995). Collaboration: A concept analysis. *Journal of Advanced Nursing, 21*, 103–109.

Hojat, M., Fields, S. K., Veloski, J. J., Griffiths, M., Cohen, M. J. M., & Plumb, J. D. (1999). Psychometric properties of an attitude scale measuring physician-nurse collaboration. *Evaluation and the Health Professions, 22*, 208–220.

Institute of Medicine. (2000). *To err is human: Building a safer health system.* Washington, DC: National Academy Press.

Irvine, R., Kerridge, I., & McPhee, J. (2004). Towards a dialogical ethics of interprofessionalism. *Journal of Postgraduate Medicine, 50*(4), 278–280.

Irvine, R., Kerridge, I., McPhee, J., & Freeman, S. (2002). Interprofessionalism and ethics: Consensus or clash of cultures? *Journal of Interprofessional Care, 16*(3), 199–210.

Klinar, I., Ferhatovic, L., Banozic, A., Raguz, M., Kostic, S., Sapunar, D., & Puljak, L. (2013). Physicians' attitudes about interprofessional treatment of chronic pain: Family physicians are considered the most important collaborators. *Scandinavian Journal of Caring Sciences, 27*, 303–310.

Kvarnstrom, S. (2008). Difficulties in collaboration: A critical incident study of interprofessional healthcare teamwork. *Journal of Interprofessional Care, 22*(2), 191–203.

Lundon, K., Kennedy, C., Rozmovits, L., Sinclair, L., Shupak, R., Warmington, K., ... & Soever, L. (2013). Evaluation of perceived collaborative behaviour amongst stakeholders and clinicians of a continuing education programme in arthritis care. *Journal of Interprofessional Care, 27*(5), 401–407.

Makowsky, M. J., Schindel, T. J., Rosenthal, M., Campbell, K., Tsuyuki, R. T., & Madill, H. M. (2009). Collaboration between pharmacists, physicians and nurse practitioners: A qualitative investigation of working relationships in the inpatient medical setting. *Journal of Interprofessional Care, 23*(2), 169–184.

Martin, J. J., Kulinna, P. H., McCaughtry, N., Cothran, D., Dake, J., & Fahoome, G. (2005). The theory of planned behavior: Predicting physical activity and cardiorespiratory fitness in African American children. *Journal of Sport & Exercise Psychology, 27*(4), 456–469.

McNair, R. P. (2005). The case for educating health care students in professionalism as the core content of interprofessional education. *Medical Education, 39*, 456–464.

Miller, K. L., Reeves, S., Zwarenstein, M., Beales, J. D., Kenaszchuk, C., & Gorlib Conn, L. (2008). Nursing emotion work and interprofessional collaboration in general internal medicine wards: A qualitative study. *Journal of Advanced Nursing, 64*(4), 332–343.

Nadolski, G. J., Bell, M. A., Brewer, B. B., Frankel, R. M., Cushing, H. E., & Brokaw, J. J. (2006). Evaluating the quality of interaction between medical students and nurses in a large teaching hospital. *BMC Medical Education, 6*(23). Retrieved from http://www.biomedcentral.com/1472-6920/6/23

Nair, D. M., Fitzpatrick, J. J., McNulty, R., Click, E. R., & Glembocki, M. M. (2012). Frequency of nurse-physician collaborative behaviours in an acute care hospital. *Journal of Interprofessional Care, 26*, 115–120.

O'Brien, J. L., Martin, D. R., Heyworth, J. A., & Meyer, N. R. (2009). A phenomenological perspective on advanced practice nurse-physician collaboration within an interdisciplinary healthcare team. *Journal of the American Academy of Nurse Practitioners, 21*, 444–453.

Odegard, A., & Strype, J. (2009). Perceptions of interprofessional collaboration within child mental health care in Norway. *Journal of Interprofessional Care, 23*(3), 286–296.

Onishi, M., Komi, K., & Kanda, K. (2013). Physicians' perceptions of physician-nurse collaboration in Japan: Effects of collaborative experience. *Journal of Interprofessional Care, 27,* 231–237.

Orchard, C. A., Curran, V., & Kabene, S. (2005). Creating a culture for interdisciplinary collaborative professional practice. *Medical Education Online, 10*(11). Retrieved from http://www.med-ed-online.org

Paradis, E., & Reeves, S. (2013). Key trends in interprofessional research: A macrosociological analysis from 1970 to 2010. *Journal of Interprofessional Care, 27,* 113–122.

Piquette, D., Reeves, S., & Leblanc, V.R. (2009). Interprofessional intensive care unit team interactions and medical crises: A qualitative study. *Journal of Interprofessional Care, 23*(3), 273–285.

Pullon, S. (2008). Competence, respect and trust: Key features of successful interprofessional nurse-doctor relationships. *Journal of Interprofessional Care, 22*(2), 133–147.

Pype, P., Symons, L., Wens, J., Van den Eynden, B., Stess, A., Cherry, G., & Deveugele, M. (2012). Healthcare professionals' perceptions toward interprofessional collaboration in palliative home care: A view from Belgium. *Journal of Interprofessional Care, 27,* 313–319.

Schaufeli, W., & Bakker, A. (2003). *UWES Utrecht Work Engagement Scale preliminary manual version 1, November 2003.* Sweden: Occupational Health Psychology Unit, Utrecht University.

Sinclair, M. (1994). *The report of the Manitoba pediatric cardiac surgery inquest: An inquiry into twelve deaths at the Winnipeg Health Sciences Centre in 1994.* Manitoba, Canada: Provincial Court of Manitoba.

Suter, E., Arndt, J., Arthur, N., Parboosingh, J., Taylor, E., & Deutschlander, S. (2009). Role understanding and effective communication as core competencies for collaborative practice. *Journal of Interprofessional Care, 23*(1), 41–51.

Tame, S. L. (2012). The effect of continuing professional education on perioperative nurses' relationships with medical staff: Findings from a qualitative study. *Journal of Advanced Nursing, 69*(4), 817–827.

Ushiro, R. (2009). Nurse–Physician Collaboration Scale: Development and psychometric testing. *Journal of Advanced Nursing, 65,* 1497–1508.

Walker, L. O., & Avant, K. C. (2005). *Strategies for theory construction in nursing* (4th ed.). Upper Saddle River, NJ: Pearson Prentice Hall.

Wittenberg-Lyles, E., Parker Oliver, D., Demiris, G., & Regehr, K. (2010). Interdisciplinary collaboration in hospice team meetings. *Journal of Interprofessional Care, 24*(3), 264–273.

25

MINDFULNESS

In today's fast-paced world, people are required to do more with less time; multitasking is valued and expected. Adults and children alike have a phone or electronic device at all times to keep them connected to the world. Everyday tasks are often done on autopilot while one's mind plans the day and wanders from thought to thought. Dr. Killingsworth, a professor at Harvard University, explains the results of his research, in which he tracked real-time thoughts five to six times a day from more than 15,000 people worldwide via a phone application. His findings showed that the more the mind is simultaneously thinking, wandering, and processing, the more a person's happiness decreases (Killingsworth & Gilbert, 2010). At a Technology Education and Design conference, Killingsworth explained in a video presentation that a person's happiness is increased if he or she is fully dedicated to the task, even if the person finds the task unenjoyable. That is, even if they do not like the task they are doing, they are happier as long as they are aware of doing it and fully present in the moment (Killingsworth, 2012). This focused behavior is referred to as *mindfulness*.

Mindfulness is gaining popularity among health professionals; however, it is not a new concept. Mindfulness has roots in Buddhist traditions dating back more than 2,500 years. The term *mindfulness* in Buddhist tradition is often associated with specific meditations, and refers to a mental quality, a self-regulation of attention (Shapiro, Oman, Thoresen, Plante, & Flinders, 2008). The introduction of mindfulness in health care is credited to Dr. Jon Kabat-Zinn. In 1979, he created a formalized education program called mindfulness-based stress reduction (MBSR) for patients with chronic illnesses (Bazarko, 2014).

Mindful meditation has shown the positive results of reducing stress. Overall well-being, decreased physical ailments, decreased pain, decreased anxiety, and depression are a few benefits of using mindful techniques (Brown & Ryan, 2003; Kemper et al., 2011; Shapiro et al., 2008). As one's stress decreases, the body can boost the immune system and inflammation is lowered (Davidson et al., 2003; Smith, 2014). Mindful meditation has the power to change the brain, even when done for short periods of time

(Davidson et al., 2003; Holzel et al., 2011). Holzel et al. (2011) found that with meditation, the fight-or-flight part of the brain known as the amygdala became smaller, while the parts of the cerebral cortex responsible for attention, memory, and emotional integration became thicker.

Patient safety is a concern of hospitals and practitioners. Safety is a top priority for nurses and it is not always an easy task. There are many challenges to stay focused in a busy environment, and when errors occur they are often linked to distractions, overconfidence, or not having all the information necessary before acting (Brady, Malone, & Fleming, 2009). The benefits of mindfulness, lower stress, increased empathy, and becoming aware of one's own thoughts and feelings has the potential to decrease errors and increase patient safety (Sibinga & Wu, 2010).

DEFINING ATTRIBUTES

The defining attributes of mindfulness are *noticing, nonjudgmental with self-acceptance*, and *awareness of present moment*.

Noticing is the first defining attribute. One needs to be able to notice and pay attention (Shapiro et al., 2008, p. 842). The act of noticing includes directing awareness to how a situation is making the body feel, or noticing the thoughts that are in the stream of consciousness. The act of noticing brings attention and focus back to the present moment. Ott (2004) explains that the practice of mindfulness allows individuals to observe what is happening without getting pulled away to other things, either in the past or thoughts about the future.

Nonjudgmental with acceptance is the second defining attribute. To obtain a state of mindfulness, it is imperative to be cognizant of your own thoughts and feelings in a nonjudgmental way. As thoughts intrude, simply acknowledge and dismiss them, then refocus on the task at hand. One needs to notice the thoughts and feelings from moment to moment, accept them, not judge them in any way; simply dismiss the thoughts and refocus. Offering loving kindness to one's self is crucial to the development of a state of mindfulness (Kabat-Zinn, 1990).

Awareness of present moment is the third defining attribute. Awareness in the context of mindfulness is different from that of normal functioning. It is an enhanced, acute awareness of the present moment and all experiences that the senses are feeling (Brown & Ryan, 2003; Kabat-Zinn, 1990). Being aware of the present moment is the opposite of multitasking. Multitasking while your brain is on autopilot diminishes the experience of the task. In contrast, being solely focused on your initial task allows you to fully experience the moment and have cognitive memory of it. Instead of trying to complete multiple items at once, on autopilot and therefore not experiencing any of them or doing any of them really well, is not being mindful. Awareness of the moment is taking each task as it comes and moving on to the next, having experienced the moment, with cognitive memory of it. When we complete tasks on autopilot, it becomes hard to remember having done them. Have you ever arrived at your destination only to wonder how you got there?

DEFINITION

Mindfulness is the ability to notice one's thoughts and feelings, to have an awareness of the present moment, and react nonjudgmentally with self-acceptance.

MODEL CASE

A nurse working on a busy acute care floor finds that the long hours, tending to sick patients and their families, and the politics of the floor are adversely affecting her (awareness of present moment). She notices that she constantly feels stressed, is short-tempered with her family, cannot sleep at night, and her stomach is in knots (noticing). A friend suggests mindfulness techniques and resources. She enrolls in a class and reads everything she can (nonjudgmental with self-acceptance). Now, at work she understands how she feels when she gets anxious or stressed (noticing). She is aware of the present moment and what she is doing, she does not judge the feeling or the constant stream of thoughts in her head. Instead, she dismisses them, takes a breath, and returns to the present moment.

RELATED CASE

A nursing instructor is aware that her students have increased anxiety before exams (noticing). The instructor plays relaxation music before the test and talks the students through breathing exercises (awareness of present moment). She helps them understand how the body feels before a test. Although the students are participating in relaxation, they are not fully aware of the present moment (failed nonjudgmental with self-acceptance).

BORDERLINE CASE

Let us continue with the example of the nurse on the busy acute care floor. She realizes that something has to change. Her stress from her job is affecting her health and her family (noticing). She educates herself on mindfulness techniques and uses them at work (awareness of present moment). She tries to take a breath to settle herself down. She gets frustrated with the constant stream of thoughts in her head. Instead of dismissing them, she gets annoyed and preoccupied with the list of things to do and gives up (failed nonjudgmental with self-acceptance).

CONTRARY CASE

In the case of the nurse working on the acute care unit, she is stressed and feeling the effects of her job on her professional and personal life (failed noticing). She does not make any changes for managing her stress (failed awareness of present moment); she feels this is just the way it is and she needs to accept it (failed nonjudgmental with self-acceptance).

ANTECEDENTS

Before mindfulness can exist, two antecedents must be present. A person must experience a moment of awakening and be open to change. Something must happen where the person realizes he or she is living life on autopilot. This could be a parent who realizes that a child is getting older and the parent is missing out on the child's youth. Or perhaps someone is having trouble remembering, or the stress of multitasking her life away is finally catching up with her. Most people go about the day not really aware of or present in their activities. Individuals often complete the morning routine without thinking: While showering, we are planning the day, rather than smelling the shampoo or feeling the warm water as it flows over the body. One pours a cup of coffee and moves on without smelling the coffee, feeling the cup, or tasting the liquid. Instead, the mind is off and planning, thinking, analyzing the past, or preparing for the future.

The individual must have an openness to change. It is one thing to say one wants to change, but it is another to be open to change and take action. The individual must want to better his life, value personal growth, and have the courage to change.

CONSEQUENCES

The consequences of mindfulness are increased overall well-being, decreased stress/anxiety, and increased coping skills. The goals of mindfulness meditation are to increase attention and empower individuals to respond to moments with intentional actions (Kabat-Zinn, 1990). Several studies on health care personnel have shown that MBSR increases coping skills, improves the immune system, and decreases stress and anxiety (Pipe et al., 2009).

Mindfulness can be practiced by everyone, and benefits have been linked to engagement in mindfulness techniques. Mindfulness helps one to disengage from automatic activities, thoughts, and habits, and helps to regulate behavior, which has long been associated with increased well-being (Brown & Ryan, 2003). Research has indicated that mindfulness practice decreases negative consequences (Robins, Kiken, & McCain, 2014). There is a large database of studies with results showing that mindfulness increases overall well-being (Eberth & Sedlmeier, 2012; Robins et al., 2014; Shapiro et al., 2008; Smith, 2014).

EMPIRICAL REFERENTS

Empirical referents are measurable ways to demonstrate the occurrence of the concept. Each defining attribute should have an empirical referent. Each element of the concept of mindfulness has been separated. Noticing is often used interchangeably with words like *attention*. It is the act of noticing the feelings in your body or thoughts in your head. There are currently no scales that solely measure noticing; however, when combined with awareness of the present moment, more measurement tools exist. In the literature, a scale often used to measure awareness is the Mindful Attention Awareness Scale (MAAS) created by Brown and Ryan (2003). The purpose of their research was creation of the scale to link mindfulness and well-being (Brown & Ryan, 2003). The tool is a 15-item scale that lends itself to participant completion in a timely manner.

The construction of the Freiburg Mindfulness Inventory (FMI) was particularly inspired by the Buddhist roots of mindful meditation, and measures mindful presence, nonjudgmental acceptance, openness to experiences, and insight. The scale contains 30 items and may be useful to measure the defining attributes of mindfulness (Bergomi, Tschacher, & Kupper, 2012; Figure 25.1).

SUMMARY

Nurses have a unique privilege to witness the human experience at its most vulnerable state. As a nurse, one can witness the healing of the mind, body, and spirit. A patient deserves a health care provider who is authentically present. Mindfulness allows for an inner calmness, decreased stress and anxiety, and increased awareness of each moment. By allowing the body and mind to relax and slow, one can make better decisions and be open to new opportunities. In this chapter, the concept of mindfulness has been explored with particular attention to cases in nursing practice.

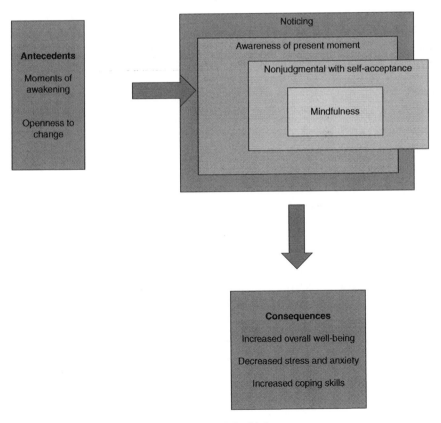

FIGURE 25.1 Mindfulness.

REFERENCES

Bazarko, D. (2014). *Mindfulness and you: Being present in nursing practice*. Silver Spring, MD: American Nurses Association.

Bergomi, C., Tschacher, W., & Kupper, Z. (2012). The assessment of mindfulness with self-report measures: Existing scales and open issues. *Mindfulness, 4,* 191–202.

Brady, A. M., Malone, A. M., & Fleming, S. (2009). A literature review of the individual and systems factors that contribute to medication errors in nursing practice. *Journal of Nursing Management, 17,* 679–697.

Brown, K. W., & Ryan, R. M. (2003). The benefits of being present: Mindfulness and its role in psychological well-being. *Journal of Personality and Social Psychology, 84*(4), 822–848. doi:10.1037/0022-3514.84.4.822

Davidson, R., Kabat-Zinn, J., Schumacher, J., Rosenkranz, M., Muller, D., Santorelli, S., & Sheridan, J. (2003). Alterations in brain and immune function produced by mindfulness meditation. *Psychosomatic Medicine, 65*(4), 564–570.

Eberth, J., & Sedlmeier, P. (2012). The effects of mindfulness meditation: A meta-analysis. *Mindfulness, 3,* 174–189. doi:10.1007/s12671-012-0101-x

Holzel, B., Carmody, J., Vangel, M., Congelton, C., Yerramsetti, S., Gard, T., & Lazar, S. (2011). Mindfulness practice leads to increases in regional brain gray matter density. *Psychiatry Research: Neuroimaging, 191*(1), 36–43.

Kabat-Zinn, J. (1990). *Full castastrophe living: Using the wisdom of your body and mind to face stress, pain, and illness*. New York, NY: Dell.

Kemper, K., Bulla, S., Krueger, D., Ott, M. J., McCool, J. A., & Gardiner, P. (2011). Nurses' experiences, expectations and preferences for mind-body practices to reduce stress. *Complementary and Alternative Medicine, 11,* 26. Retrieved from www.biomedcentral.com/1472-6882/11/26

Killingsworth, M. (2012, November 5). *Want to be happier? Stay in the moment*. [Video file]. Retrieved from https://www.ted.com/speakers/matt_killingsworth

Killingsworth, M., & Gilbert, D. (2010, November 12). A wandering mind is an unhappy mind. *Science, 330*(6006), 932. doi: 10.1126/science.1192439/

Ott, M. J. (2004). Mindfulness meditation a path of transformation and healing. *Journal of Psychosocial Nursing, 42*(7), 21–29.

Pipe, T., Bortz, J. J., Dueck, A., Pendergast, D., Buchda, V., & Summers, J. (2009). Nurse leader mindfulness meditation program for stress managment. *Journal of Nursing Administration, 39*(3), 130–137.

Robins, J. L., Kiken, L., & McCain, N. L. (2014). Mindfulness: An effective coaching tool for improved physical and mental health. *Journal of the American Association of Nurse Practitioners, 26,* 511–518.

Shapiro, S. L., Oman, D., Thoresen, C. E., Plante, T. G., & Flinders, T. (2008). Cultivating mindfulness: Effects on well-being. *Journal of Clinical Psychology, 64*(7), 840–862. doi:10.1002/jclp.20491

Sibinga, E., & Wu, A. (2010). Clinician mindfulness and patient safety. *Journal of the American Medical Association, 304,* 3532–3533.

Smith, S. A. (2014). Mindfulness-based stress reduction: An intervention to enhance the effectiveness of nurses' coping with work-related stress. *NANDA International, 25,* 119–130.

MARY E. QUINN AND MARY T. QUINN GRIFFIN

26

NURSE MANAGER ACCOUNTABILITY

The concept of accountability has been defined in various ways in the literature. A search of the literature indicates that the concept of accountability has only been used since 1980s. In social sciences, *accountability* is defined as the implicit or explicit expectation that one may be called on to justify one's beliefs, feeling, and actions to others (Lerner & Tetlock, 1999). Wood and Winston (2007) noted that leader accountability requires a level of ownership that includes making, keeping, and proactively answering for personal commitments. Other disciplines, such as business administration and leadership (Ferris et al., 1997), define *accountability* as the "extent to which one's actions are evaluated by some external constituency who has salient reward or sanctions that are made contingent on the evaluation" (p. 163). Connors, Smith, and Hickman (1994), developers of "The Oz Principle,®" define *accountability* as the guiding principle that defines how we make commitments to one another, how we measure and report our progress, how we interact when things go wrong, and how much ownership we take to get things done. Wakeman (2013) defines *personal accountability* as the "belief that you are fully responsible for your own actions and their consequences and comprised of four factors: commitment, resilience, ownership, and continuous learning" (pp. 79, 83).

Accountability as a term used in nursing literature was noted as early as 1978, in articles related to accountability as a requirement for the independent practice of nursing (Jordan, 1978). Krautscheid (2014) noted the level of variation in how accountability is defined in medical and allied health literature, citing the inconsistent terminology used within nursing. However, within the literature there are linkages between the terms *responsibility*, *commitment*, and *accountability*. Krautscheid cites numerous definitions and distinctions between these terms and highlights Dohmann's (2009) differentiation of responsibility and accountability as follows: "responsibility equates to having the authority to accomplish an activity, whereas accountability arises out of one's free choice and strong personal commitment to ensuring that a result is achieved" (p. 45). *Professional nursing practice* is defined as "taking responsibility for one's nursing judgments, actions, and omissions as they relate to life-long learning, maintaining competency, and upholding both quality patient care outcomes and standards of the profession while being answerable to those who are influenced by one's nursing practice" (Krautscheid, 2014, p. 46).

The American Nurses Association (ANA) *Code of Ethics* (2015, Provision 4, Section: 4.2, pp. 15–16) specifies that "nurses in all roles are accountable for decisions made and actions taken in the course of nursing practice." In other nursing references, *accountability* is defined as "an ethical duty status that one should be answerable legally, morally, ethically, or socially for one's activities" (Cherry & Jacob, 2002, p. 198). Maas (1989) highlighted nurse accountability as being answerable to the patient, peer, and organization for the outcomes of her or his actions. The nurse manager role has been identified as critical in the retention and organizational commitment of staff nurses and provision of high-performing, highly reliable, effective, and efficient patient care at the unit level (Laschinger, Finegan, & Wilk, 2009). The nurse manager is responsible for ensuring that the appropriate systems and processes are in place to support the staff in the delivery of quality and safe patient care in accordance with regulatory standards of care. In addition, the nurse manager is accountable for continually evaluating staff performance, the patient's level of satisfaction with the care delivered, balancing financial management of resources, and facilitating performance improvement for improved outcomes. The manager's role has expanded in both scope and accountability. However, there is no clear succinct definition for the concept of nurse manger accountability. With the concept of nurse manager accountability, the first step is to get a clear definition of what is meant by the term that describes what it is and what it looks like.

DEFINING ATTRIBUTES

The defining attributes of nurse manager accountability are *organizational commitment, openness, answerability*, and *resilience*. These defining attributes of nurse manager accountability were identified from a review of the literature for common themes or characteristics of the concept.

Organizational commitment has been defined in several ways in the literature. It is associated with terms such as *loyalty, pledging*, or *dedication of oneself*. Mowday, Steers, and Porter (1979) summarize organizational commitment as an attitude that transcends loyalty to an organization; it is the active relationship between an individual and the organization in which "individuals are willing to give something of themselves in order to contribute to the organization's well-being" (p. 226). Connors et al. (1994) emphasize that accountability is the foundation and guiding principle that defines how we make commitments to one another. A search of the term *nurse manager commitment* produces articles that highlight the role of the nurse manager related to nurse manager motivation, staff nurse job satisfaction, staff nurse turnover, and organizational commitment. According to the Wakeman personal accountability model, commitment is one of the four factors of personal accountability and is described as "the willingness to do what it takes to get results" (Wakeman, 2013, p. 83). Avolio, Zhu, Kho, and Bhatia (2004) conducted a study to explore the relationship between transformational leadership and organizational commitment. Avolio et al. (2004) referenced prior research suggesting that transformational leadership is "positively associated with organizational commitment." Leach (2005) conducted a study of 101 chief nursing officers, 148 nurse managers, and 651 staff nurses to identify how transformational leadership style influences organizational commitment. The study results showed that when transformational leadership was practiced by the chief nursing officers and nurse managers, staff members reported being less alienated and more strongly committed to the organization. Wood and Winston (2005) surmised within their construct of leader accountability that one of the critical prepositions is that "accountable leaders are more effective, both from a transactional and transformational perspective, than non-accountable leaders" (p. 92).

Openness is defined as being open to new ideas and to change one's behavior or work pattern based on these new ideas. Wood and Winston (2005) cite several references that note how scholars in the past have described accountability using terms such as *openness* and *transparency* (Bavly, 1999) and others (Mondale, 1975) cite "openness" and "candor" as key virtues of accountability (p. 89). The ANA's *Nursing Administration: Scope and Standards of Practice* (2009) states that one of the key elements of the nurse administrator role is to promote "open communication between staff and administration" (p. 11).

Answerability is defined as being responsible to someone for one's actions, responsible to a supervisor for your decisions, or responsible for an assigned activity. The terms *accountability, responsibility*, and *answerability* are frequently found to be used synonymously in the literature. The prior version of the ANA (2001) *Code of Ethics for Nurses* linked accountability and answerability: "accountability means to be answerable to oneself and others for one's own actions" (Provision 4.2). However, the newly released version of the ANA (2015) *Code of Ethics for Nurses*, Provision 4, now highlights the role of the nurse as related to "authority, accountability, and responsibility" (p. 15). As nurse manager, one core skill for success is the ability to fully understand the role and being answerable for all aspects of that role. Nurse managers who understand, and are answerable, lead from a place of grounded integrity and are highly regarded, trusted, and followed by their staff. They take full responsibility for their actions and overall unit performance and take measures to fix any problems and address issues related to the work environment, staff satisfaction, and quality of patient care.

Resilience is defined as the a dynamic attribute that is identified as "the relative resistance to environmental risks or overcoming stress or adversity"

(Rutter, 2006, p. 10). Wakeman (2013, p. 84) places resilience as the second factor in her personal accountability conceptual model and defines it as the "ability to stay beyond the course in the face of obstacles and setbacks." According to Fletcher and Sarkar (2013), Polk described the nursing model of resilience as an ability to turn disastrous situations into meaningful growth experiences and to learn and gain new insight from those experiences. A nurse manager is responsible for leading his or her staff in performance improvement activities and needs to demonstrate resilience in continually evaluating unit performance, identifying process improvements needed, implementing process change, and re-evaluating effectiveness of those outcomes. This is a cyclical process that must occur until desired outcomes are met. Also integral to the nurse manager role is consistent and sustained effort in maintaining a healthy work environment and work force.

DEFINITION

Nurse manager accountability is characterized by the nurse manager's organizational commitment to take whatever measures are necessary for goal attainment and outcomes, openness in communication with staff and receptiveness to feedback, answerability for the process and outcomes, and resilience in managing whatever barriers or obstacles that present to obtaining the goal and desired outcomes.

MODEL CASE

Mary is a nurse manager of a 32-bed medical/surgical unit and supervises 40 nurses and 10 ancillary support staff. A review of unit performance indicated an increase in patient fall events. Mary understands that in order to reduce falls, a concerted effort is needed on the part of both unit leadership and staff. She calls a unit staff meeting during both shifts to share the data and facilitates an open discussion among staff as to the potential causes and elicits their feedback and ideas for improvement (openness). The nurse manager shares with staff the organizational goal for falls reduction and that she is committed (organizational commitment) to achieving their unit targets and determined to support all efforts to reduce falls to improve patient safety on their unit (resilience). She highlights that this is a team effort and that it will require not only her commitment, but also the full support of and dedicated effort by all unit staff to achieve this goal, and that they are all accountable for their unit performance (answerability). Staff nurses volunteer as project leaders and present a plan that outlines leadership and staff roles and responsibilities and a target goal to reduce falls by 10% within 4 months (answerability). Mary reports to her supervisor that she is responsible for the unit performance (answerability) and is committed (organizational commitment) to reducing fall events and shares the action plan to reduce falls and asks for feedback (openness). Daily huddles (resilience) are held with staff to discuss patients at risk for falls and interventions needed to reduce the risk of a fall event; Mary validates implementation of fall precautions and works with staff as needed (answerability, resilience). A reduction of fall events during the month was celebrated by staff, and their efforts continue (resilience).

RELATED CASE

Beth is a nurse manager of a 24-bed pediatric unit and supervises a staff of 24 staff nurses and 8 ancillary staff. She receives compensation for managing the budget and other administrative functions to ensure that adequate resources are available to deliver patient care. She reports to her supervisor that she takes responsibility for and is committed (organizational commitment) to achieving unit performance targets with regard to operational and outcome measures, but lists several reasons why she is not meeting targets. Her supervisor provides feedback on her performance as nurse manager and highlights a need for consistency and follow-through with staff in order to improve. Mary acknowledges the need to improve (openness) and states that she understands her responsibility and what she needs to do as the nurse leader (answerability). She subsequently gathers her staff and asks for feedback, posts the unit's performance with regard to outcome measures related to central line associated bloodstream infection (CLABSI) rates, and reviews the CLABSI bundle for catheter line maintenance. She asks senior nurses to work with novice staff nurses to validate competencies with regard to CLABSI bundle implementation. This is a related case in that it describes the role and function of a nurse manager related to the job and tasks but does not include many of the defining attributes (failed answerability and failed resilience).

BORDERLINE CASE

John is a nurse manager of a 36-bed surgical intensive care unit and manages 75 staff members. Employee engagement scores show low staff satisfaction with regard to staff decision making. Increasing staff nurse autonomy is a key priority of the organization. John is perplexed by these scores and reports to his manager that he understands the goal and is committed (organizational commitment) to improving scores. John informs staff that they need to improve on decision making; staff listen, but no ideas are presented. John indicates to staff that it is a joint responsibility of unit leadership and staff (answerability) to develop a plan on how to improve these scores. He develops a plan (answerability), reviews it with staff, and posts it on the unit; there is no plan on how updates will be provided. John reports to his manager that he has implemented a plan for the unit. Next quarter's performance shows a decline in performance; John is perplexed, because he thought his plan was being implemented and followed by staff and expected improved scores. In this scenario, only two of the defining attributes are present. John indicates that he is committed (organizational commitment) to improve scores and develops a plan to improve staff decision making (answerability). However, staff were not provided any specific data or information on their unit performance with regard to decision making, nor were they asked to provide input on what they think is needed (failed openness). There was no organized approach for periodic updates from staff on how they think the plan is working and there was a lack of leadership in performing any type of ongoing validation of the effectiveness of the interventions (failed resilience).

CONTRARY CASE

Paul is a nurse manager on an oncology unit and notes that his unit's fall with injury rate is the highest in the hospital. When reviewing the data with his supervisor, he lists reasons for the increased fall events: the acuity of the oncology patient population, overall lack of patient compliance in use of the call bell to request assistance, and inadequate ancillary support on the unit for patient care. He summarizes that he will "do his best" to decrease falls, but says that these factors are just "out of his control" (failed answerability). His supervisor outlines some strategies that have worked for them in the past, but Paul states that until the resource issues are addressed he cannot effect change (failed openness and failed organizational commitment). Paul meets with staff and states that they must improve and that he does not want to hear any comments from staff (failed openness). Staff verbalize that they feel unsupported by their manager and disillusioned about trying anything new. No other meetings are held with staff related to the unit's performance related to falls reduction (failed resilience). Unit performance related to fall events further declines.

ANTECEDENTS

The antecedents of nurse manager accountability are *rules*, *self-awareness*, *motivation*, and *engagement*.

Rules refer to having expectations and goals that are clear and specific. Nurse managers must understand the key responsibilities of their role, the level of importance of these responsibilities, and expectations in carrying out their responsibilities. The nurse manager's job description typically provides a high-level listing of responsibilities, but does not provide the specific metrics that the manager is held accountable for. Annual performance metrics and targets are generally set at the organizational level and nurse managers are expected to achieve those targets. Rachel (2012) notes a difference between responsibility and accountability in that responsibility overarches accountability. She further streses the need for clarity in setting goals and expectations. Otherwise, how can nurse managers be expected to be accountable for meeting these requirements?

In their landmark study, Duval and Wicklund (1972) described self-awareness as "the system comparing self against standards only operates in as much as attention is directed inward on the self" (Duval & Silvia,

2002, p. 51). They further note that "when self-awareness is low, the relationship between self and any given standard is indistinct and obscure to the person" (Duval & Silvia, 2002, p. 51). Self-awareness consists of being conscious of your strengths and weaknesses and acknowledging what you still have yet to learn. To be successful, nurse managers must be able to continually self-assess to determine their need for additional knowledge and skills.

Burns (1978) highlights motivation as one of the characteristics of transformational leadership: instilling pride and motivation, sharing vision for the organization, providing staff direction in attaining organizational goals, and demonstrating openness to staff input and ideas.

Kerfoot (2007) describes the importance of engagement in fostering a work environment in which staff are loyal, highly productive, and excited about their work. Critical to creating this work environment is the role of the nurse manager/leader in being engaged, because staff tend to replicate behaviors of their leader (engagement or disengagement) (Kerfoot, 2007).

Nurse managers must have an understanding of the rules with in which they work, have a self-awareness of their skills and competencies, be motivated to excel in performance, and be able to work with their staff in the delivery of patient care.

CONSEQUENCES

The consequences of nurse manager accountability are *empowerment*, *teamwork*, *goal attainment*, and *job satisfaction*.

Regan and Rodriguez (2011) studied the role of middle management (nurse managers and assistant nurse managers) in creating an empowering work environment for their staff in acute care hospital setting. They cited the definition of *empowerment* from Greco, Laschinger, and Wong (2006) as the "ability to get things done and includes a capacity to mobilize resources and to provide support, opportunity, and information" (p. 101).

As the leader of a unit, a nurse manager must foster a work environment that promotes teamwork in order to achieve unit goals and improved outcomes.

Goal attainment is described in the Theory of Goal Attainment as developed by Imogene King in the early 1960s (King, 1960). The model has three interacting systems: personal, interpersonal, and social. Each of these systems has its own set of concepts. The concepts for the personal system are perception, self, growth and development, body image, space, and time. The concepts for the interpersonal system are interaction, communication, transaction, role, and stress. The concepts for the social system are organization, authority, power, status, and decision making. In 2006, King expanded use of the Theory of Goal Attainment in providing the foundational structure and process for nurses, health care professionals, and administrators in the formation of partnerships to achieve organizational goals. Within this structure, and central to the process, is the nurse administrator. King emphasizes the role of the nurse administrator as:

> one of the central individuals who interacts with human beings as individuals, with two, three, or more individuals as interpersonal systems, and with large groups, such as the board of directors, in making decisions. The perceptions, communications, interactions, and transactions with individuals in the three interacting systems are crucial in establishing mutual goals in a health care system on the basis of differentiated roles and responsibilities that lead to outcomes and cost-effectiveness (King, 2006, p 104).

The nurse manager is accountable for understanding organizational goals and facilitating a leading staff in goal attainment at the unit level.

The relationship between nursing leadership and job satisfaction can be found in the literature (Kleinman, 2004). Shader, Broome, Broome, West, and Nash (2001) conducted a study and found that effective nursing leadership is associated with greater work satisfaction among staff nurses. An accountable nurse manager has the confidence to drive staff empowerment, foster teamwork, and meet and exceed performance goals, all of which leads to a positive work environment and satisfaction among staff.

EMPIRICAL REFERENTS

To measure the defining attributes of accountability, a search of the literature provides various tools utilized in past studies. Organizational commitment can be measured using Mowday, Steers, and Porter's Organizational Commitment Questionnaire (OCQ; Mowday et al., 1979). The OCQ contains 15 items that measure 3 factors of organizational commitment: "(1) a strong belief in and acceptance of the organization's goals and values; (2) a willingness to exert considerable effort on behalf of the organization; and (3) a strong desire to maintain membership in the organization" using a 7-point Likert scale ranging from strongly disagree to strongly agree (Mowday et al., 1979, p. 226).

One method to measure openness is through use of the Authentic Leadership Questionnaire (ALQ) authored by Walumbwa, Avolio, Gardner, Wernsing, and Peterson (2008). The ALQ contains 16 questions that measure the dimensions of self-awareness, transparency, ethical/moral, and balanced processing (Walumbwa et al., 2008). Transparency measures the level of leadership openness with others using a 5-point Likert scale ranging from strongly disagree to strongly agree.

Both openness and answerability can be measured using Wood and Winston's (2007) tool that was developed to measure three dimensions of accountability: responsibility, openness, and answerability. Both scales, openness and answerability, contain 10 items and use a 10-point response range from zero to 10, with zero paired with "never" and 10 with "always."

Resilience can be measured using the Wakeman Reality Check Accountability Scale, which is a 12-item instrument. This scale measures the

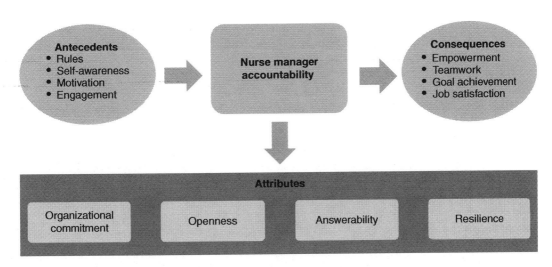

FIGURE 26.1 Nurse manager accountability.

four primary characteristics of accountability: commitment, resilience, ownership, and continuous learning (Wakeman, 2010).

SUMMARY

As noted throughout this concept analysis, the work of the nurse manager is complex, multifaceted, and guided by various leadership and management behaviors. The purpose of this concept analysis was to examine and identify the attributes, antecedents, and consequences of nurse manager accountability. A succinct definition of the concept was provided, listing four attributes which support the potential empirical referents that may measure nurse manager accountability. Each of the concept's attributes is highlighted in case examples related to the nurse manager role. Antecedents and consequences were provided and described, focusing on the role and responsibilities of the nurse manager. To facilitate understanding of the concept of nurse manager accountability, a schematic representation is provided (Figure 26.1).

REFERENCES

American Nurses Association. (2001). *Code of ethics for nurses with interpretive statements*. Retrieved from http://www.nursingworld.org/provision-4

American Nurses Association. (2009). *Nursing Administration: Scope and standards of practice*. Silver Spring, MD: Nursingbooks.org

American Nurses Association. (2015). *Code of ethics for nurses with interpretive statements*. Retrieved from http://www.nursingworld.org/MainMenuCategories/EthicsStandards/CodeofEthicsforNurses/Code-of-Ethics-For-Nurses.html

Avolio, B. J., Zhu, W., Koh, W., & Bhatia, P. (2004). Transformational leadership and organizational commitment: Mediating role of psychological empowerment and moderating role of structural distance. *Journal of Organizational Behavior, 25,* 951–968. doi:10.1002/job.283

Bavly, D. A. (1999). *Corporate accountability and governance: What role for the regulator, director, and auditor?* Westport, CT: Quorum.

Burns, J. (1978). *Leadership.* New York, NY: Harper & Row.

Cherry, B., & Jacob, S. R. (2002). *Contemporary nursing: Issues, trends, & management* (2nd ed.). St. Louis, MO: Mosby.

Connors, R., Smith, T., & Hickman, C. (1994). *The Oz principle: Getting results through individual and organizational accountability.* New York, NY: Portfolio.

Dohmann, E. (2009). *Accountability in nursing. Six strategies to build and maintain a culture of commitment.* Marblehead, MA: HCPro, Inc.

Duval, T. S., & Silvia, P. J. (2002). Self-awareness, probability of improvement, and the self-serving bias. *Journal of Personality and Social Psychology, 82*(1), 49–61. Retrieved from http://psycnet.apa.org/journals/psp/82/1/49.pdf

Duval, T. S., & Wicklund, R. A. (1972). *A theory of objective self-awareness.* New York, NY: Academic Press.

Ferris, G. R., Dulebohn, J. H., Frink, D. D., George-Falvy, J., Mitchell, T. R., & Matthews, L. M. (1997). Job and organizational characteristics, accountability, and employee influence. *Journal of Managerial Issues, 9*(2), 162–175.

Fletcher, D., & Sarkar, M. (2013). Psychological resilience: A review and critique of definitions, concepts, and theory. *European Psychologist, 18*(1), 12–23. doi:10.1027/1016-9040/a000124

Greco, P., Laschinger, H. K., & Wong, C. (2006). Leader empowering behaviours, staff nurse empowerment and work/engagement burnout. *Nursing Leadership, 19*(4), 41–56.

Jordan, C. A. (1978). Accountability for nursing practice. *AORN Journal, 27*(6), 1076–1080.

Kerfoot, K. (2007). Staff engagement: It starts with the leader. *Nursing Economics, 25*(1), 47–48. Retrieved from http://web.b.ebscohost.com/ehost/pdfviewer/pdfviewer?sid=057c31e9-17e5-4cc4-8592-daccc4aa7eb%40sessionmgr198&vid=1&hid=110

King, I. M. (1960). *Theory of goal attainment.* Retrieved from http://nursing-theory.org/theories-and-models/king-theory-of-goal-attainment.php

King, I. M. (2006). A systems approach in nursing administration: Structure, process, and outcome. *Nursing Administration Quarterly, 30*(2), 100–104.

Kleinman, C. (2004). The relationship between managerial leadership behaviors and staff nurse retention. *Hospital Topics, 82*(4), 2–9.

Krautscheid, L. C. (2014). Defining professional nursing accountability: A literature review. *Journal of Professional Nursing, 30*(1), 43–47. doi:10.1016/j.profnurs.2013.06.008

Laschinger, H. K., Finegan, J., & Wilk, P. (2009). Context matters: The impact of unit leadership and empowerment on nurses' organizational commitment. *Journal of Nursing Administration, 39*(5), 228–235. doi:10.1097/NNA.0b013e3181a23d2b

Leach, L. S. (2005). Nurse executive transformational leadership and organizational commitment. *Journal of Nursing Administration, 35*(5), 228–237.

Lerner, J. S., & Tetlock, P. E. (1999). Accounting for the effects of accountability. *Psychological Bulletin, 125*, 255–275.

Maas, M. L. (1989). Professional practice for the extended care environment: Learning from one model and its implementation. *Journal of Professional Nursing, 5*(2), 66–76. Retrieved from http://dx.doi.org/10.1016/S8755-7223(89)80009-2

Mondale, W. F. (1975). *The accountability of power: Toward a responsible presidency.* New York, NY: David McKay Company.

Mowday, R. T., Steers, R. M., & Porter, L. W. (1979). The measurement of organizational commitment. *Journal of Vocational Behavior, 14*(2), 224–247.

Rachel, M. (2012). Accountability: A concept worth revisiting. *American Nurse Today, 7*(3), 36–40.

Regan, L. C., & Rodriguez, L. (2011). Nurse empowerment from a middle-management perspective: Nurse managers' and assistant nurse managers' workplace empowerment views. *Permanente Journal, 15*(1), 101–107.

Rutter M. (2006). Implications of resilience concepts for scientific understanding. *Annals of the New York Academy of Sciences, 1094*, 1–12.

Shader, K., Broome, M., Broome, C., West, M., & Nash, M. (2001). Factors influencing satisfaction and anticipated turnover for nurses in an academic medical center. *Journal of Nursing Administration, 31*(4), 210–216.

Walumbwa, F. O., Avolio, B. J., Gardner, W. L., Wernsing, T. S., & Peterson, S. J. (2008). Authentic leadership: Development and validation of a theory-based measure. *Journal of Management, 34*(1), 89–126.

Wakeman, C. (2010). *Reality-based leadership: Ditch the drama, restore sanity to the workplace, & turn excuses into results.* San Francisco, CA: Jossey-Bass.

Wakeman, C. (2013). *The reality-based rules of the workplace: Know what boosts your value, kills your chances, and will make you happier.* San Francisco, CA: Jossey-Bass.

Wood, J. A., & Winston, B. E. (2005). Towards a new understanding of leader accountability: Defining a critical construct. *Journal of Leadership and Organizational Studies, 11*(3), 84–94. doi:10.1177/107179190501100307

Wood, A., & Winston, B. E. (2007). Development of three scales to measure leader accountability. *Leadership and Organizational Development Journal, 28*(2), 167–185. doi:10.1108/01437730710726859

27

SOCIAL SUPPORT FOR NEW MOTHERS

Social support in health and chronic illness has been one of the most frequently researched concepts in the past decades, both as a coping resource (Cohen, Underwood, & Gottlieb, 2000) and as a protective factor related to stress and coping (Lazarus & Folkman, 1984). Becoming a mother is a major developmental transition and new mothers are faced with learning new skills relating to infant care practices (Forster et al., 2008; Leahy-Warren, 2007), as well as recovering physically and emotionally from childbirth (Forster et al., 2008). There are health implications for babies and mothers affected by parental capacity issues, as well as being a serious public health concern. The World Health Organization (WHO) recommends that expectant mothers be supported throughout the perinatal period and that they receive not only medical support but also comfort and reassurance. The term *support* also frequently appears in the international and national strategy and policy documents (Child and Family Agency, 2013; Child and Family Agency Commissioning Strategy, 2013; Department of Health & Children [DOH&C], 2001; WHO, 2005), particularly those relating to supporting new mothers in the community. Furthermore, the term *social support* is habitually used in the context of the perinatal period in facilitating adaptation to motherhood (Corrigan, Kwasky, & Groh, 2015; Emmanuel, Creedy, St. John, Gamble, & Brown, 2008; Mercer, 2006), but frequently without a clear definition.

Social support is frequently proposed as the panacea for all issues regarding maternal and child health. However, there is lack of consensus on the conceptualization and definition of social support (Hupcey, 1998), which leads to health care professionals, particularly midwives and public health nurses (PHNs) being at a loss as to their required contribution to maternal and child health and well-being. The purpose of this concept analysis is to create clarify around the understanding of the concept of social support in early parenting. This is necessary to enable midwives and PHNs to accurately assess, plan, and implement strategies that promote maternal and child health and well-being.

SOCIAL SUPPORT

A review of the literature showed that the concept of social support has been examined by multidisciplinary researchers such as sociologists, psychologists, nurses, and midwives. This has resulted in a multiplicity of understandings and meanings of the concept. For example, it has been described in terms of a process, interaction, or relationship (Veiel & Baumann, 1992); social integration; and interactive processes and supportive interactions (Hupcey, 2001). The commonality of terms indicates that social support is a positive concept of acting as a buffer or cushioning in preventing or relieving stress (Leahy-Warren, 2014). Support for new mothers has been described as the availability of individuals, either health care professionals in the hospital (Tarkka, Paunonen, & Laippala, 1999) or family and friends in the home (Ugarriza, 2002). Social support has also been operationalized as telephone follow-up calls, home visits, peer support groups, professional support groups, and/or the inclusion of written or video material (Corrigan et al., 2015; Leahy-Warren, 2007). Therefore, there is a lack of clarity as to what constitutes social support for new mothers; hence, the importance of making the meaning of the concept more explicit for research and practice.

DEFINING ATTRIBUTES

Defining attributes of social support are *structural social support* (formal and informal), and *functional social support* (informational, instrumental, emotional, and appraisal).

Structural Social Support

Social supportive behaviors cannot occur without a structure of social networks, which include formal and informal structural social supports. Therefore, availability of a social network is a necessary attribute of social support. This social network can be made up of informal social support sources such as family or friends, or formal social support sources which are health care professionals, for example, PHNs/ midwives/general practitioners (GPs). While it is important to identify the sources of social support within an individual's social network, it is also necessary to identify the interactions that occur within the process (Leahy-Warren, 2014).

Functional Social Support

From the literature reviewed, four functional social support attributes were identified: informational, instrumental, emotional, and appraisal support (Barrera, 1986; Cronenwett, 1985; House, 1981; Khan & Antonucci, 1980; Power & Parke, 1984; Tilden & Weinert, 1987).

Informational support means that a new mother receives pertinent relevant information about her child's health and well-being from a knowledgeable source, either a health care professional (Leahy-Warren, McCarthy, & Corcoran, 2011; Leahy-Warren et al., 2012; Shorey, Chan, Chong, & He, 2014;

Tarkka et al., 1999) or her own mother (Leahy-Warren, 2005, 2007). These sources provide the new mother with information, advice, and directives, which the individual can use in coping with personal and environmental problems.

Emotional support is delineated as those acts that provide empathy, concern, caring, love, and trust. It would thus appear that emotional support is the transfer of some form of caring attributes to an individual. This could be in the guise of providing comfort either of a physical or a psychological nature. Findings from a qualitative study of new mothers ($n = 10$) indicated that emotional support, particularly from the baby's father, was very important (Podkolinski, 1998), as was that provided within a breastfeeding support group (Dennis, Hodnett, Gallop, & Chalmers, 2002). Mothers felt it was important to have someone with whom to share their feelings at this time when everything was so new.

Instrumental support is characterized as access to behaviors that directly help the person in need, such as aid in money, time, or labor. New mothers have also indicated the importance of having someone to help them with caring for the baby and with household chores (Häggman Laitila, 2003; Shaw, Levitt, Kaczorowsk, & Wong, 2007).

Appraisal support is identified as the transmission of information relevant to self-evaluation, which may be derived from affirmation, feedback, and social comparison opportunities. Appraisal support or comparison support means some type of communication of expectations, evaluation, and shared worldview with individuals in a similar position. This attribute is crucial in the development or enhancement of a new mother's belief in her ability to parent her infant, which is known as *maternal parental self-efficacy* (Leahy-Warren, McCarthy, & Corcoran, 2012). Maternal parental self-efficacy enables new mothers to cope with the stress of learning the skills of parenting and adapting to new motherhood (Leahy-Warren et al., 2011, 2012; Shorey, Chan, Chong, & He, 2015) and reduces the risk of postnatal depression.

DEFINITION

Social support is defined as the process through which social relationships promote health and well-being through structural and functional elements that are inextricably linked. Structural social support comprises both formal (from health care professionals) and informal (from family/friends) support. Functional social support comprises informational (knowledge), instrumental (practical support), emotional (love, care, and empathy to new mothers) and appraisal (constructive feedback and affirmation to enable self-evaluation by mothers) elements.

MODEL CASE

Aoife is a new first-time breastfeeding mother who receives a first visit from the PHN. On arrival, the PHN is greeted by Aoife's partner (John), who is new baby David's dad. Aoife is feeling tired and tearful, and her nipples are sore from David's frequent feeding. John sits beside Aoife and puts his arm on her shoulder (emotional support) while listening to the PHN. The PHN asks if she can observe Aoife latching David onto the breast and shows her (instrumental support) how to use the football position so that David latches onto the nipple from the noncracked side, thus reducing the pain on initiation (informational support). Immediately, the baby settles on the breast and the relief on Aoife's face is evident as the pain subsides. The PHN tells Aoife what a great job she is doing, as her baby is thriving on her breast milk (appraisal support). John and Aoife express their concern to the PHN that once John is back at work in a few days, Aoife will not be able to cope alone. The PHN recommends that Aoife attends the PHN mother/infant support group (formal support) the following Thursday and asks that John also attend so he can be assured that Aoife will have peer support (informal support) when he is back at work. They both thank the PHN and assure her that they will attend the mother/infant support group. It is clear that this case includes all attributes of social support.

RELATED CASE

A related case is an instance that is closely related to the concept, but does not show all the attributes. Aoife is a first-time mother who receives a first home visit from the PHN. On arrival, Aoife is alone and tearful, and her nipples are sore from her infant David's continuous feeding. Aoife's nipples are bleeding, but she refuses the PHN's request to examine them or to observe her breastfeeding. She lives alone and has no family and friends close by, as she is new to the area (failed availability of informal social support). In the course of conversation, she expresses concern about the PHN visit, as she had previously negative experience with the health services. She allows the PHN to weigh the baby and the PHN praises Aoife for the way she is parenting her son (appraisal social support), as he is relaxed and content and has gained weight since discharge from the hospital. Aoife accepts the invitation to attend the drop-in weight clinics at the health center and will consider attending the PHN mother/infant support group (informal social support). She has failed availability of informal informational, instrumental, emotional, and appraisal social support, but formal social support, is being facilitated and mobilized by the PHN.

BORDERLINE CASE

Aoife is a first-time mother who receives a first postnatal visit from the PHN. On arrival, Aoife is alone and tearful, and her nipples are sore from her infant David's continuous feeding. The PHN asks to observe Aoife feeding David, but Aoife feels too embarrassed and says she thinks she will give David a bottle of formula, as she thinks he is too hungry and she does not have enough milk for him. Aoife is lacking in her self-belief as a new mother. The PHN praises Aoife for the way she is parenting her son (appraisal social support), as he is relaxed and content and has gained weight since discharge from the hospital. The PHN talks to Aoife (formal social support) about infant feeding and shows her how to make a bottle of formula. The PHN asks Aoife about her family and friends and Aoife says that she can call her mom if she needs information with regard to David (informational social support), but as she lives 100 miles away and cares for her own mother, she will make only a short visit on the weekend. Aoife and David's dad are no longer in a relationship and he will not be helping her to care for David (failed emotional social support). The PHN invites Aoife to the PHN mother/infant support group (appraisal social support) on Thursdays to meet with other new mothers who live in her neighborhood. Aoife agrees to attend the mother/infant support group (informal social support) to meet with other new mothers. Aoife's case is described as borderline because she has low availability of informal social support, especially informal emotional support, but the PHN can facilitate and mobilize potential informal peer social support.

CONTRARY CASE

Aoife is a first-time mother who receives a first home visit from the PHN. Aoife answers the door but refuses to allow the PHN to enter. Aoife has poor English-language skills, but the PHN establishes that she has recently arrived in Ireland and has no family or friends (failed availability of informal social support). She does not trust the PHN or the health care professionals because she had a bad experience in her home country with the health services. She refuses to take the contact details of the PHN and the offer of a translator to come for another visit. Aoife also refuses to consider attending the mother/infant clinic to meet with other new mothers (failed availability of formal social support).

ANTECEDENTS

The identification of antecedents is helpful in identifying underlying assumptions about the concept. In order for social support to be initiated, a new mother must *perceive a need* for assistance and be a *willing recipient* in accepting support (Barclay, Everett, Rogan, Schmied, & Wyllie, 1997; Hupcey, 2001). These factors are influenced by new mothers' perceptions of their coping abilities and their expectations of others (Lackner, Goldenberg, Arrizza, & Tjosvold, 1994). Supportive interactions are objective transactions of social support, whereas the perceptions of being supported are very much subjective. Perceiving certain interactions as being supportive is based on the "needs" of the recipient as well as her expectations with respect to that "need." In turn, a potential provider of social support must identify the need for support and be a *willing provider* (Scott, Brady, & Glynn, 2001). Social support cannot occur unless there is some form of social competence, where the recipient and the provider are both in a position of a *positive social climate* of assistance and protection (Langford, Bowsher, Maloney, & Lillis, 1997). Social supportive behaviors cannot occur unless there is a structure of social networks with the quality of connectedness in a favorable environment of assistance and safety. Thus, it is this favorable environment, which is regarded as a social climate, that is a necessary antecedent of social support (Figure 27.1).

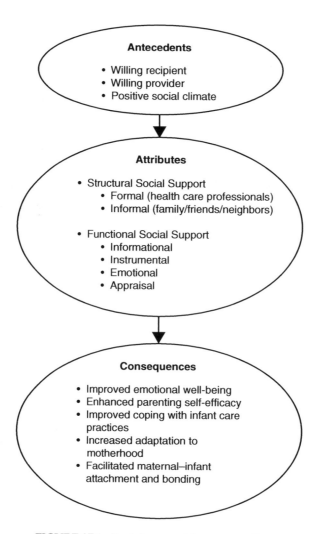

FIGURE 27.1 Social support for new mothers.

CONSEQUENCES

There are a number of consequences for new mothers of receiving social support. Social support for new mothers is associated with increase in confidence and improved coping with infant care (Leahy-Warren, 2007), enhanced maternal parental self-efficacy (Leahy-Warren et al., 2011; Shorey et al., 2015), increased adaptation to motherhood (Hui Choi et al., 2012), facilitation of infant bonding (Kinsey & Hupcey, 2013) and infant attachment (Condon & Corkindale, 1998), and improved emotional well-being (Leahy-Warren et al., 2012). A significant correlation was found between total social support, in addition to the informational, instrumental, and appraisal subscales of functional support, and the risk of postnatal depression (PND; Shorey et al., 2014). Furthermore, Leahy-Warren et al. (2011) found that formal structural support and emotional functional support were independently predictive of PND at 12 weeks. A Cochrane systematic review on psychosocial and psychological interventions (Dennis & Dowswell, 2013) of 28 trials in

Europe and South America with 16,912 women concluded that women who received a psychosocial intervention were significantly less likely to develop postpartum depression compared with those receiving standard care (20 trials, 14,727 women). In Norway, Glavin, Smith, Sørum, and Ellefsen (2010), with a sample of postnatal women (*n* = 228), found significant decreased depression scores in the intervention group where the intervention was the provision of intensive, individualized postpartum home visits provided by PHNs. A recent randomized controlled trial with first-time mothers (*n* = 122) by Shorey et al. (2015) in Singapore found that a midwife home visit intervention enhanced maternal parental self-efficacy, yielded higher social support scores on the Perinatal Infant Care Social Support Scale (PICSS), and reduced the risk of postnatal depression (Shorey et al., 2015).

EMPIRICAL REFERENTS

Establishing availability of social support in the perinatal period from a research perspective has required the use of a variety of methods and instruments. Some of these include the modified Kendler Social Support Interview (Schuster, Kessler, Aseltine, 1990); birth scenarios (Ford & Ayers, 2009); the Interpersonal Support Evaluation List (ISEL; Lau, 2011); the Norbeck social support questionnaire (McClennan-Reece, 1993); Cohen's Dimensions of Social Support Scale (Gjerdingen & Chaloner, 1994); daily logs (Pridham & Zavoral, 1988); daily diary (Maloni, 1994); and formal structural support networks such as midwives only (Haggerty Davis, Brucker, & MacMullen, 1988; Beger & Cook, 1998) or PHNs only (Tarkka & Paunonen, 1996). Some or most of these scales omit items that are important to women in the context of infant care practices. Only one instrument, the Support Behaviors Inventory (SBI; Browne, 1986), is specific to pregnancy, but it is conceptualized in terms of functional social support only and does not include structural social support as in social networks. The Postpartum Social Support Questionnaire (PSSQ; Hopkins & Campbell, 2008) was developed in the context of postpartum adaptation only and is not underpinned by theory. The only available social support instrument that has been developed with a strong theoretical underpinning in the context of the postnatal period is the PICSS (Leahy-Warren et al., 2011, 2012; Shorey et al., 2014). The PICSS is comprised of 22 items of a 4-point Likert scale in the Social Support Functional Scale. It includes four functional elements: informational support (7 items), instrumental support (7 items), appraisal support (4 items), and emotional support (4 items). The subscales within the Social Support Functional Scale are scored by the sum score of each subscale. For both the informational and the instrumental support subscales, the scores ranged from the lowest at 7 to the highest at 28. For the appraisal and emotional subscales, the scores ranged from 4 to 16. Structural social support is measured by asking participants to identify the persons available to provide the four types of functional social support (36 items). The persons from the participants' social network include both formal (health care professionals) and informal sources. The number of persons who provide at least one type of functional social support is taken as the total informal structural support score.

SUMMARY

As a result of this concept analysis, social support was defined as containing structural and functional components that are inextricably linked. The concept was defined, and antecedents, attributes, and consequences identified in the context of new mothers. A schematic representation was provided to facilitate understanding of the concept.

REFERENCES

Barclay, L., Everett, L., Rogan, F., Schmied, V., & Wyllie, A. (1997). Becoming a mother—An analysis of women's experience of early motherhood. *Journal of Advanced Nursing, 25,* 719–728.

Barrera, M. (1986). Distinctions between social support concepts, measures, and models. *American Journal of Community Psychology, 14*(4), 413–445.

Beger, D., & Cook, C. (1998). Postpartum teaching priorities: The viewpoints of nurses and mothers. *Journal of Obstetric, Gynaecologic, and Neonatal Nursing, 27*(2), 161–168.

Browne, M. (1986). Social support during pregnancy: A unidimensional or multidimensional construct? *Nursing Research, 35*(1), 4–9.

Child and Family Agency. (2013). *Investing in families: Supporting parents to improve outcomes for children.* Retrieved from http://www.childandfamilyresearch.ie/sites/www.childandfamilyresearch.ie/files/cfa_parenting_support_strategy_0.pdf

Child and Family Agency Commissioning Strategy. (2013). Retrieved from http://www.childandfamilyresearch.ie/sites/www.childandfamilyresearch.ie/files/cfa_commissioning_strategy_0.pdf

Cronenwett, L. (1985). Parental network structure and perceived support after birth of first child. *Nursing Research, 34*(6), 347–352.

Cohen, S., Underwood, L., & Gottlieb, B. (2000). *Social support measurement and intervention.* London, UK: Oxford University Press.

Condon, J. T., & Corkindale, C. J. (1998). The assessment of parent-to-infant attachment: Development of a self-report questionnaire instrument. *Journal of Reproductive and Infant Psychology, 16*(1), 57–76.

Corrigan, C., Kwasky, A., & Groh, C. (2015). Social support, postpartum depression, and professional assistance: A survey of mothers in the Midwestern United States. *Journal of Perinatal Education, 24*(1):48–60.

Dennis, C. -L., & Dowswell, T. (2013). Psychosocial and psychological interventions for preventing postpartum depression. *Cochrane Database Systematic Review, 2,* CD0001134.

Dennis, C. -L, Hodnett, E., Gallop, R., & Chalmers, B. (2002). The effect of peer support on breastfeeding duration among primiparous women: A randomized controlled trial. *Canadian Medical Association Journal, 166,* 21–28.

Department of Health & Children. (2001). *Quality and fairness: A health system for you.* Dublin, Ireland: Stationary Office.

Emmanuel, E., Creedy, D., St. John, W., Gamble, J., & Brown, C. (2008). Maternal role development following childbirth among Australian women. *Journal of Advanced Nursing, 64*(1), 18–26.

Ford, E., & Ayers, S. (2009). Stressful events and support during birth: The effect on anxiety, mood and perceived control. *Journal of Anxiety Disorders, 23*(2), 260–268.

Forster, D. A., McLachlan, H. L., Rayner, J., Yelland, J., Gold, L., & Rayner, S. (2008). The early postnatal period: Exploring women's views, expectations and experiences of care using focus groups in Victoria, Australia. *BMC Pregnancy & Childbirth, 8*(1), 27–29.

Gjerdingen, D., & Chaloner, K. (1994). Mothers' experience with household roles and social support during the first postpartum year. *Women and Health, 21*(4), 57–74.

Glavin, K., Smith, L., Sørum, R., & Ellefsen, B. (2010). Redesigned community postpartum care to prevent and treat postpartum depression in women—A one year follow up study. *Journal of Clinical Nursing, 19*, 3051–3062.

Haggerty Davis, J., Brucker, M., & MacMullen, M. (1988). A study of mothers' postpartum teaching priorities. *Maternal-Child Nursing, 17*(1), 41–50.

Häggman-Laitila, A. (2003). Early support needs of Finnish families with small children. *Journal of Advanced Nursing, 41*(6), 595–606.

Hopkins, J., & Campbell, S. (2008). Development and validation of a scale to assess social support in the postpartum period. *Archives of Womens Mental Health, 11*(1), 57–65.

House, J. (1981). *Work, stress and social support.* Reading, MA: Addison-Wesley.

Hui Choi, W., Lee, G., Chan, C., Cheung, R., Lee, I., & Chan, C. (2012). The relationships of social support, uncertainty, self-efficacy, and commitment to prenatal psychosocial adaptation. *Journal of Advanced Nursing, 68*(12), 2633–2645.

Hupcey, J. (1998). Social support: Assessing conceptual coherence. *Qualitative Health Research, 8*(3), 304–318.

Hupcey, J. (2001). The meaning of social support for the critically ill. *Intensive and Critical Care Nursing, 17*(4), 206–213.

Khan, R., & Antonucci, T. (1980). Convoys over the life course: Attachment, roles and social support. In P. Baltes & O. Brim (Eds.), *Life span development and behaviour* (pp. 253–268). New York, NY: Academic Press.

Kinsey, C. B., & Hupcey, J. E. (2013). State of the science of maternal–infant bonding: A principle-based concept analysis. *Midwifery, 29*(12), 1314–1320.

Lackner, S., Goldenberg, S., Arrizza, G., & Tjosvold, I. (1994). The contingency of social support. *Qualitative Health Research, 4*, 224–243.

Langford, C., Bowsher, J., Maloney, J., & Lillis, P. (1997). Social support: A conceptual analysis. *Journal of Advanced Nursing, 25*(1), 95–100.

Lau, Y. (2011). A longitudinal study of family conflicts, social support, and antenatal depressive symptoms among Chinese women. *Archives of Psychiatric Nursing, 25*(3), 206–219.

Lazarus, R. S., & Folkman, S. (1984). Coping and adaptation. In W. D. Gentry (Ed.), *The handbook of behavioral medicine* (pp. 282–325). New York, NY: Guilford.

Leahy-Warren, P. (2005). First-time mothers: Social support and confidence in infant care. *Journal of Advanced Nursing, 50*(5), 479–488.

Leahy-Warren, P. (2007). Social support for first-time mothers: An Irish study. *MCN American Journal of Maternal Child Nursing, 32*(6), 368–374.

Leahy-Warren, P. (2014). Social support theory. In G. McCarthy & J. Fitzpatrick (Eds.), *Theories guiding nursing research* (ch. 6). New York, NY: Springer.

Leahy-Warren, P., McCarthy, G., & Corcoran, P. (2011). Postnatal depression in first-time mothers: Prevalence and relationships between functional and social support. *Archives of Psychiatric Nursing, 25*(3), 174–184.

Leahy-Warren, P., McCarthy, G., & Corcoran, P. (2012). First time mothers: Social support, maternal parental self-efficacy and postnatal depression. *Journal of Clinical Nursing, 21*(3–4), 388–397.

Maloni, J. (1994). The content and sources of maternal knowledge about the infant. *Maternal-Child Nursing Journal, 22*(4), 111–119.

McClennan-Reece, S. (1993). Social support and the early maternal experience of primiparas over 35. *Maternal and Child Journal, 21*(3), 91–98.

Mercer, R. (2006). Nursing support of the process of becoming a mother. *Journal of Obstetric, Gynecologic, and Neonatal Nursing, 35*(5), 649–651.

Podkolinski, J. (1998). Women's experiences of postnatal care. In S. Clement & L. Page (Eds.), *Psychological perspectives on pregnancy and childbirth* (pp. 205–225). London, UK: Churchill Livingstone.

Power, T., & Parke, R. (1984). Social network factors and the transition to parenthood. *Sex Roles, 10*(11/12), 949–973.

Pridham, K., & Zavoral, J. (1988). Help for mothers with infant care and household tasks: Perceptions of support and stress. *Public Health Nursing, 5*(4), 201–208.

Schuster, T. L., Kessler, R. C., & Aseltine, R. H. (1990). Supportive interactions, negative interactions, and depressed mood. *American Journal of Community Psychology, 18*, 423–438.

Scott, D., Brady, S., & Glynn, P. (2001). New mother groups as a social network intervention: Consumer and maternal and child health nurse perspectives. *Australian Journal of Advanced Nursing, 18*(4), 23–29.

Shaw, E., Levitt, C., Kaczorowsk, I., & Wong, S. (2007). Effectiveness of postpartum support. *Birth, 34*(2), 188–189.

Shorey, S., Chan, S. W. C., Chong, Y. S., & He, H. G. (2014). Maternal parental self-efficacy in newborn care and social support needs in Singapore: A correlational study. *Journal of Clinical Nursing, 23*(15–16), 2272–2283.

Shorey, S., Chan, S. W. C., Chong, Y. S., & He, H. G. (2015). A randomized controlled trial of the effectiveness of a postnatal psychoeducation programme on self-efficacy, social support and postnatal depression among primiparas. *Journal of Advanced Nursing, 71*(6), 1260–1273.

Tarkka, M., & Paunonen, M. (1996). Social support provided by nurses to recent mothers on a maternity ward. *Journal of Advanced Nursing, 23*, 1202–1206.

Tarkka, M., Paunonen, M., & Laippala, P. (1999). Social support provided by public health nurses and the coping of first time mothers with childcare. *Public Health Nursing, 16*(2), 114–119.

Tilden, V., & Weinert, C. (1987). Social support and the chronically ill individual. *Nursing Clinics of North America, 22*(3), 613–620.

Ugarriza, D. (2002). Postpartum depressed women's explanation of depression. *Journal of Nursing Scholarship, 34*(3), 227–233.

Veiel, H., & Baumann, U. (1992). The many meanings of social support. In H. Viel & U. Baumann (Eds.), *The meaning and measurement of social support* (pp. 1–9). New York, NY: Hemisphere.

World Health Organization. (2005). *Make every mother and child count. The World Health Report 2005.* Geneva, Switzerland: Author.

MARY JOY GARCIA-DIA and DEIRDRE O'FLAHERTY *28*

RESILIENCE

Many disciplines and fields of science, ranging from ecology, business, sociology, psychology, engineering, medicine, nursing, and even the military, have studied the phenomenon of resilience. Historically, the origin of resilience in the literature reaches back to World War I and the extraordinary journey of the explorer Ernest Shackleton and his crew's expedition to Antarctica in 1914. After 2 years of being shipwrecked and stranded in the adverse conditions of the Antarctic, the entire crew survived. Sir Shackleton is recognized for his legendary courage and heroism in leading his crew to safety (Lansing, 2001), and his leadership behavior became a role model for successful managers (Harland, Harrison, Jones, & Reiter-Palmon, 2005).

The theory of cumulative factors contributing to outcomes was established by Garmezy and Rodnick (1959) in their study of children in poverty. They proposed that a personality trait of the individual is not the sole source of an outcome, but a product of both internal and external factors. This combination of psychosocial elements and biological predispositions, acting as both risk and "protective factors," helped define what is now known as resilience. Garmezy's early focus in the 1960s on the competence of children at risk for psychopathology laid the groundwork for the Project Competence Longitudinal Study in 1970, which aimed to understand children's ability to overcome adversity, identify protective processes, and measure key aspects of competence. His interest in studying disease states led him to investigate why some patients could "bounce back" by demonstrating positive behavioral adaptation and do well in life and others could not. The first epidemiologic studies published in 1973 addressed major issues; Garmezy suggested that the availability of psychosocial resources might contribute to counteracting the negative influence of an adversity such as schizophrenia, and promote positive behavioral adaptation (Garmezy, 1973; Garmezy & Rodnick, 1959). Subsequent researchers proposed integrating the concept of protective processes within the framework of resilience (Kumpfer, 1999; Luthar, 1999; Masten, 1994; Rutter, 1987), which eventually helped determine which individuals are at risk for maladaptation, apply points of intervention, and change the course to positive behavioral adaptation. Individuals possess personality traits, protective factors, and experiences accumulated through life, all of which precipitate resilience to surface from within as a process, and/or develop as an outcome (Garcia-Dia, Dinapoli, Garcia-Ona, Jakubowski, & O'Flaherty, 2013).

Resilience is complex, diverse, and dynamic in nature and has been linked to economics, research, and professional practice, making it applicable to many populations. Elder and Liker (1982) did a systematic comparison of the psychological health and coping resources of women who suffered hardships in the 1930s. The research examined the economic impact of the Great Depression and its influence on the women's coping mechanism, finding that it resulted in varying outcomes: enhanced efficacy, sense of control, and resilience as opposed to social withdrawal, sense of victimization, and somatic symptoms. Similarly, Werner and Smith (1992) conducted a longitudinal study of children born in 1955 in Hawaii who grew up in poverty and examined the long-term impact of adverse events (divorce, alcoholism, mental illness) on their adaptation to life.

There has also been an attempt to address the biologic and physiologic aspects of resilience and to integrate this research into the earlier research on protective factors. The phenomenon that Southwick and Charney (2012) defined as "neuroplasticity" refers to the ability of the human brain to change as a result of one's experiences. They have suggested that although neuroplasticity is exhibited throughout an individual's life, its greatest effectiveness is subject to a limited window of time, and thus it is recommended that interventions be started early on. By practice and training, stress protective factors can be increased, thus improving adaptation and decreasing chances of developing stress-related depression or a decline in mood, health, and general well-being (Garcia-Dia et al., 2013).

According to Dunkel Schetter and Dolbier (2011), the majority of individuals are able to withstand trauma and continue to function reasonably. Traumatic events that happened in New York (World Trade Center attack in 2001; Hurricane Sandy in 2012), as well as other states like Connecticut (Sandy Hook shooting) and Louisiana (Hurricane Katrina), demonstrate how individuals and families remain resilient despite their traumatic experience (Garcia-Dia et al., 2013). Although some may experience posttraumatic stress symptoms, positive outcomes leading to posttraumatic growth may occur for other individuals.

Shakespeare-Finch, Gow, and Smith (2005) described characteristics that support resilience in the workplace, such as include extroversion, openness, agreeableness, conscientiousness, humor, altruism, adeptness at facing fears, and optimism. In a study examining the relationship between resilience and work engagement of Malaysian staff nurses, resilience was shown to have a positive and significant effect, thus making resilient nurses an essential element in an ever-changing health care system (Jackson, Firtko, & Edenborough, 2007; Othman, Ghazali, & Ahmad, 2013).

Mallak (1998) found critical understanding and effective use of information to be key factors in resilience. He believes that nurses' understanding of work situations or chaotic work environments, navigating the system confidently to access resources, and browsing through multiple sources of information can be major strategy for building resilience in nursing. McAlister and McKinnon (2009) advocate that resilience theory should be included in the curriculum for nursing education and in orientation programs, to encourage individuals to explore and develop their professional identity and build their coping capacity. The emphasis on the use of role models, storytelling, and narrative reflection reflects that these strategies are a valuable resource for students and a way to sustain and empower new graduates in the work environment.

DEFINING ATTRIBUTES

Self-efficacy, *coping*, and *hope* have been identified as defining attributes of resilience (Gillespie, Chaboyer, & Wallis, 2007; Hart, Brannan, & deChesnay, 2012).

Self-Efficacy

Defined as the belief in one's ability to achieve a goal or overcome an event, *self-efficacy* is related to many stages, forms, and levels of resilience. Self-efficacy refers to beliefs about having the capabilities to organize and perform tasks successfully within a specific domain, thereby influencing the outcome of circumstances (Bandura, 1997). Bandura also indicated that self-efficacy convictions influence resilience to adversity. It is often the reason "why some people snap and others snap back" (Earvolino-Ramirez, 2007, p. 77; Rutter, 1993). Research by Richardson (2002) indicates that resilient individuals have the potential not only to return to previous levels of functioning after experiencing adversity, but also to manifest gains in self-esteem, self-efficacy, autonomy, and a change in life perspective that serve to make them stronger than they were before. Such gains in adaptive behavior have been termed *thriving* or *flourishing* (Carver, 1998; Keyes, 2006; Ryff & Singer, 2003).

Coping

Coping refers to efforts to deal with something difficult, and these efforts may include cognitive, behavioral, or psychosocial strategies that an individual uses to alleviate stress when events challenge the routine predictions of the world (Kleinke, 1998). Constructive coping is seen as a characteristic of resilient people when making the effort to manage situations that they appraise as potentially stressful or harmful (Kleinke, 1998; Lazarus & Folkman, 1984; Zeidner & Endler, 1996). Chesney, Neilands, Chambers, Taylor, and Folkman (2006) combined the coping and self-efficacy concepts and introduced the coping self-efficacy construct (and measuring instrument). *Coping self-efficacy* refers to a person's perceived ability to cope effectively with life challenges or threats. Once an adverse event occurs or is present, it must be interpreted as being physically and/or psychologically traumatic. Like Bandura, Chesney et al. (2006) indicate that beliefs about one's ability to perform specific coping behaviors or coping self-efficacy would influence the outcomes of adverse situations. In the current study, *coping self-efficacy* refers to the belief of the professional nurses that through developing coping behavior or strategies, they will be successful in dealing with the work stresses they encounter (Koen, van Eden, & Wissing, 2011).

Hope

Hope is the ability to plan pathways to reach desired goals despite obstacles, and the motivation to use these pathways. Hope is closely related to optimism and was conceptualized by Snyder (2000) as involving two main components: pathway thoughts that formulate positive goal outcomes and agency thoughts that create efficacy expectations to reach the goals. Resilient individuals, especially nurses, can apply hope to adapt to change, accept challenges, and cope with adversity. For professional nurses, hope allows individuals to set realistic goals in the nursing profession and find the ways and will to achieve these despite difficulties they may encounter.

DEFINITION

Resilience is defined as the possession of hope that is characterized by self-efficacy and coping.

MODEL CASE

Mary Ann completed her bachelor of science in nursing 10 years ago. She started her career in a medical–surgical unit as a staff nurse caring for a diverse population of patients suffering from either acute or chronic illnesses. During her second year working as a nurse, her own mother was diagnosed with colon cancer. She took a leave of absence and took care of her mom, who underwent surgery and chemotherapy. However, due to the late diagnosis, the prognosis was poor and eventually, her mother transitioned to hospice care and passed away. As a result of this experience, Mary Ann requested to transfer to the adult oncology unit, where she found satisfaction in taking care of patients who were undergoing an experience similar to that of her mom. Mary Ann feels that the most important part of her practice is actually taking care of the patient as a whole person. She is comfortable in assessing their emotional state or their spiritual distress and to ask questions: "Would you like me to just be here and hold your hand?" "Can I give you a hug?" "Would you like me to pray for you?" "Can I call the pastoral care for you?" She considers treating the whole person as the best part of her job. Through the process of intense personal reflection, Mary Ann began to resolve the dilemmas and personal turmoil associated with discerning her fit in the reality of professional practice, demonstrating self-efficacy. Satisfaction derived from patient care, knowing that one can make a difference, and a strong spiritual belief appeared to be the driving forces facilitating her own coping and her hope for her patients. As Mary Ann began to confirm her professional identity, she became more self-directed and performed with greater confidence and self-determination.

Based on this case study, Mary Ann demonstrated positive outcomes and was able to have a successful professional career despite the impact of her mother's death coinciding with her entry into the nursing workforce. The interpersonal relationship, the challenges, and hardship associated with taking care of oncology patients who face constant pain and death did not dissuade Mary Ann in her nursing career, but rather helped her find meaning in her personal and professional life.

RELATED CASE

One of Mary Ann's classmates in high school, Ed, was an accountant. Due to the company's downsizing, Ed lost his job during the time that Mary Ann was taking care of her mother. Observing Mary Ann while she was caring for her mom, Ed came to realize and appreciate the significant role of nurses. Mary Ann encouraged Ed to consider nursing. He went back to school and completed an Associate Degree in Nursing. After passing the board exam, Ed was immediately hired as an operating room (OR) nurse, thus rebounding back into the professional workforce. The fast-paced, highly stressful environment took Ed by surprise. Due to his limited clinical experience, Ed had a hard time dealing effectively with the clinical demands by the surgeons and his other colleagues (failed coping). He found himself arguing with his co-workers most of the time and he dreaded the thought of coming to work. Despite his daily struggle, Ed continued to work in the OR. Although he could request a transfer to a less stressful workplace environment, Ed did not want to make any effort, feeling that wherever he goes, he will still encounter the same type of individuals (failed hope and self-efficacy).

BORDERLINE CASE

Mary Ann reaches out to Ed, who works in the same hospital, to check how he is adjusting in his new role in nursing. Ed shares his frustrations about his current position and mentions that he feels trapped and not challenged, but is unable to leave due to the current economic climate. Mary Ann asks if he has ever thought of combining his finance background with his OR skills and knowledge of instrumentation. She was recently appointed to serve on the Materials Management and Supply Committee and the team is looking for someone with a finance background. Although not initially interested, Ed joins the committee, as he has some hope that this might provide a key opportunity for his success in work. The team finds Ed's knowledge and financial acumen tremendously helpful and through his input they are able to get approval for a procurement management system. Ed is offered the manager's role in implementing the application. He is reluctant to take this on, but with Mary Ann's encouragement and leadership support from the committee, Ed accepts the challenge. Without admitting it to Mary Ann, he finds this new position to be as much of a struggle as his staff position in the OR was (failed self-efficacy and hope).

CONTRARY CASE

Amber had a substance-abuse problem prior to becoming a nurse. She had not used drugs or alcohol since high school and had been seeing a therapist for treatment. The daily stress of dealing with critically ill patients and their loved ones in the intensive care unit mentally weighs on her, and she considers leaving nursing. Every day it is a challenge to cope and she struggles with the temptation to resort to drugs or alcohol to combat the stress. After one particularly stressful day, Amber did not waste one of her patient's narcotics, but took it herself. Amber realized that diverting narcotics was an option and too great a temptation, so she continued to use drugs. Eventually, Amber was caught diverting Oxycontin and was immediately suspended, and referred for counseling. Amber drifted in and out of her addiction and was not able to re-enter the nursing workforce. This demonstrates the lack of adaptation and lack of conscious determination to "rise" above adversities (failed self-efficacy, hope, coping).

ANTECEDENTS

The primary antecedent of resilience is an adverse event, such as, trauma, stress, or illness. Any adverse or traumatic event can place an individual at risk for a compromised ability to cope. The individual has to have a realistic understanding of the circumstances, accept his or her situation, learn to cope, and become resilient (Garcia-Dia et al., 2013). Depending on their responses to these stressors, individuals might develop protective factors, which can decrease both the effects of and negative reactions to risk (Rutter, 1987).

Authors like Huber and Mathy (2002) and Rutter (2007) find that children who have suffered abuse and neglect undergo controlled exposure to cumulative risks rather than avoidance, making them liable to develop resilience as a protective factor. Despite the development of serious problems as adolescents, the majority of the children were able to turn their lives around, thus developing into caring, functional, and competent adults. The authors found that both external factors (family and community) and internal factors (one's personality, self-help skills, advanced motor and language skills) serve as protective factors or buffers and have a greater impact on one's life course than specific risk factors or stressful events. Solomon's (2007) study on rescue workers in Israel posited that resilience develops in response to stress and increased exposure to violent incidents in particular (in the case of these study subjects, working with recovering victims of terrorist attacks). This divergence from the traditional field helped theorists address day-to-day stressors (unexpected death of a spouse) as well as potentially acute traumatic events (terrorist attack or natural disaster) occurring at least once in one's lifetime (Bonanno, 2004; Kessler, Somega, Bromet, Hughes, & Nelson, 1995). Bonanno (2004) suggested that the variable responses could be described by four prototypical trajectories: chronic dysfunction, recovery, delayed reactions, and resilience.

CONSEQUENCES

The consequences of resilience are personal control, psychological adjustment, and personal growth. Effective coping can best be described as successfully dealing with an adverse event and still being able to live life to the fullest. In Holaday and McPhearson's (1997) research, individuals who experienced the horrific physical effects of burns were able to set and redefine goals, and were able to psychologically and physically recover from the effects of their severe burns. Nurses dealing with burn patients over time are able to develop and master coping skills and/or strategies enabling them to deal with the devastating psychological and physical injury that their patients endure through social support of the team, positive team dynamics, and humor (Kornhaber & Wilson, 2011). The length of employment enables staff to develop more coping skills. Hinsch (1982) reported that nurses in burn units stayed working for extended periods of time despite the stress experienced, thus highlighting the findings of Gillespie et al. (2007) and Waller (2007) that resilience is a dynamic process developing over time rather than a trait or characteristic.

EMPIRICAL REFERENTS

Shackleton, the exemplar of resilience was viewed as so stalwart that Connor and Davidson (2003), both researchers and the developers of the resilience scale, included two of Shackleton's personal characteristics—optimism and having faith—as factors used to measure resilience. The conceptual definitions of resilience from multiple disciplines (nursing, psychology, and psychiatry), age of a potential study population, and the context or framework of the study have to be considered when choosing the survey instrument (Gillespie et al., 2007). Due to the relevance of resilience to many different fields of study (business, education, medicine, mental health, social, welfare), locating and selecting a particular and appropriate scale to measure resilience is a daunting task; one must make an informed judgment about suitability before choosing an instrument for a particular purpose or population (O'Neal, 1999). For purposes of this chapter, the empirical referent discussion will focus on instruments used in measuring resilience in nursing population.

Windle, Bennett, and Noye's (2011) review of 19 resilience scales noted that four were refinements of the original measure. In their review, they found that the Connor–Davidson Resilience Scale (CD-RISC), the Resilience Scale for Adults, and the Brief Resilience Scale received the best psychometric ratings (Garcia-Dia et al., 2013). For a schematic representation of resilience, see Figure 28.1.

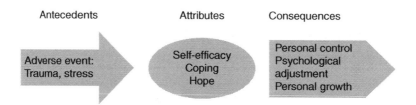

FIGURE 28.1 Schematic representation of resilience: concept, attributes, antecedents, and consequences.

1. CD-RISC has been used with clinical and nonclinical populations to measure resilience or capacity to change and cope with adversity using a 25-item scale.
2. The Resilience Scale for Adults measures five factors: personal competence, social competence, family coherence, social support, and personal structure.
3. The Brief Resilience Scale is a four-item scale on a point rating designed to measure coping tendencies and adaptation: personal coping resources, pain coping behavior, and psychological well-being (Gillespie et al., 2007).

Among these three, the Resilience Scale for Adults developed by Wagnild and Young in 1993 is the most frequently used measurement scale, with reliability and validity supported by several small studies since 1990: Cronbach's alpha coefficient was consistently acceptable and moderately high, ranging from 0.73 to 0.91 (Wagnild, 2009); and test-retest reliabilities range from 0.67 to 0.84 (O'Neal, 1999). The scale correlates with other instruments measuring morale, life satisfaction, health, perceived stress, symptoms of stress, depression, and self-esteem (O'Neal, 1999).

CD-RISC has been used in many nursing specialty studies (intensive care nurses, OR nurses) measuring and/or identifying resilient characteristics: these range from hardiness, challenge, and commitment in Kobasa's construct to Rutter's work that includes adaptability when coping with change, problem-solving skills, and experiences with success and achievements (Gillespie, Chaboyer, Wallis, & Grimbeek, 2007). The CD-RISC also measures valuable coping skills in highly stressful and tension-charged work environment: spirituality, supportive social network, optimism, resilient role model, exercising, and cognitive flexibility. Other professionals who are exposed to extremely stressful environments may benefit from and apply the CD-RISC to provide insights for leaders and management on how to create preventive resilience training programs and reduce posttraumatic stress disorder (PTSD) in the workplace (Mealer, Jones, & Moss, 2012).

SUMMARY

Nurse leaders and managers can use resilience as a theoretical framework in creating and planning staff development programs as the profession addresses nurses' satisfaction, adverse workplace environment, and challenges with retention and recruitment. Resilience building encompasses both seasoned and novice nurses; both can address the real and perceived adversities in the workplace, support each other as a team, and continuously cope with the daily challenges of known and unknown risks typical of the health care delivery system. Resilience offers hope to nurses in their daily lives as they continuously increase their protective factors, adjust to daily adversities, and find success and meaning in their own personal and professional journey with their patients.

REFERENCES

Bandura, A. (1997). *Self-efficacy: The exercise of control.* New York, NY: Freeman.

Bonanno, G. A. (2004). Loss, trauma, and human resilience: Have we underestimated the human capacity to thrive after extremely aversive events? *American Psychologist, 59*, 20–28.

Carver, C. S. (1998). Resilience and thriving: Issues, models and linkages. *Journal of Social Issues, 54*(2), 245–266.

Chesney, M. A., Neilands, T., Chambers, D., Taylor, J., & Folkman, S. (2006). A validity and reliability study of the coping self-efficacy scale. *British Journal of Health Psychology, 11*, 421–437. doi:10.1348/135910705X53155

Connor, K., & Davidson, J. (2003). Development of a new resilience scale: The Connor Davidson Resilience Scale (CD-RISC). *Depression and Anxiety, 18*, 76–82.

Dunkel Schetter, C., & Dolbier, C. (2011). Resilience in the context of chronic stress and health. *Social and Personality Psychology Compass, 5*(9), 634–652.

Earvolino-Ramirez, M. E. (2007). Resilience: A concept analysis. *Nursing Forum, 42*(2), 73–82.

Elder, G. H., Jr., & Liker, J. K. (1982). Hard-times in women's lives: Historical influences across forty years. *American Journal of Sociology, 88*(2), 241–269.

Garcia-Dia, M. J., Dinapoli-Reisman, J. M., Garcia-Ona, L., Jakubowski, R., & O'Flaherty, D. (2013). Concept analysis: Resilience. *Archives of Psychiatric Nursing, 27*, 264–270.

Garmezy, N. (1973). Competence and adaptation in adult schizophrenic patients and children at risk. In S. R. Dean (Ed.), *Schizophrenia: The first ten dean award lectures* (pp. 163–204). New York, NY: MSS Information.

Garmezy, N., & Rodnick, E. H. (1959). Promorbid adjustment and performance in schizophrenia: Implications for interpreting heterogeneity in schizophrenia. *Journal of Nervous and Mental Diseases, 129*(5), 450–466.

Gillespie, B. M., Chaboyer, W., & Wallis, M. (2007). Development of a theoretically derived model of resilience through concept analysis. *Contemporary Nurse: Journal for the Australian Nursing Profession, 25*, 124–135.

Gillespie, B. M., Chaboyer, W., Wallis, M., & Grimbeek, P. (2007). Resilience in the operating room: Developing and testing resilience model. *Journal of Advanced Nursing, 59*(4), 427–438. doi:10.1111/j.1365-2648.2007.04340.x

Harland, L., Harrison, W., Jones, J. R., & Reiter-Palmon, R. (2005). Leadership behaviors and subordinate resilience. *Journal of Leadership & Organizational Studies, 11*(2), 2–14.

Hart, P., Brannan, J., & deChesnay, M. (2012). Resilience in nurses: An integrative review. *Journal of Nursing Management, 21*(4), 1–15 doi:10.1111/j.1365-2834.01485x

Hinsch, A. (1982). The psychological effects on nursing staff working in a burns unit. *Australian Nurses Journal*, *11*, 25–26.

Holaday, M., & McPhearson, R. W. (1997). Resilience and severe burns. *Journal of Counseling and Development*, *75*(5), 246–357.

Huber, C. H., & Mathy, R. M. (2002). Focusing on what goes right: An interview with Robin Mathy. *Journal of Individual Psychology*, *58*(3), 214–224.

Jackson, D., Firtko, A., & Edenborough, M. (2007). Personal resilience as a strategy for surviving and thriving in the face of workplace adversity: A literature review. *Journal of Advanced Nursing*, *60*, 1–9.

Kessler, R., Somega, A., Bromet, E., Hughes, M., & Nelson, C. (1995). Posttraumatic stress disorder in the national comorbidity survey. *Archives of General Psychiatry*, *52*(12), 1048–1060.

Keyes, C. L. M. (2006). Subjective well-being in mental health and human development research worldwide: An introduction. *Social Indicators Research*, *77*(1), 1–10.

Kleinke, C. L. (1998). *Coping with the challenges* (2nd ed.). Pacific Grove, CA: Brooks Cole.

Koen, M. P., van Eden, C., & Wissing, M. P. (2011). The prevalence of resilience in a group of professional nurses. *Journal of Interdisciplinary Health Sciences*, *16*(1), 1–11.

Kornhaber, R., & Wilson, A. (2011). Building resilience in burns nurses: A descriptive phenomenological inquiry. *Journal of Burn Care & Research*, *32*(4), 481–488.

Kumpfer, K. L. (1999). Factors and processes contributing to resilience: The resilience framework. In M. D. Glantz & J. L. Johnson (Eds.), *Resilience and development: Positive life adaptations* (pp. 179–224). New York, NY: Academic/Plenum Publishers.

Lansing, A. (2001). *Endurance: Shackleton's incredible voyage*. London, UK: Weidenfeld & Nicolson.

Lazarus, R., & Folkman, S. (1984). *Stress, appraisal and coping*. New York, NY: Springer.

Luthar, S. (1999). *Poverty and children's adjustment. Developmental clinical psychology and psychiatry*. Thousand Oaks, CA: Sage Publications.

Mallak, L. (1998). Measuring resilience in health care provider organizations. *Health Manpower Management*, *24*(4), 148–152.

Masten, A. (1994). Resilience in individual development: Successful adaptation despite risk and adversity. In M. Wang & E. Gordon (Eds.), *Educational resilience in inner city America: Challenge and prospects* (pp. 3–25). Hillsdale, NJ: Erlbaum.

McAlister, M., & McKinnon, J. (2009). The importance of teaching and learning resilience in the health disciplines: A critical review of the literature. *Nurse Education Today*, *29*, 371–379.

Mealer, M., Jones, J., & Moss, M. (2012). A qualitative study of resilience and posttraumatic stress disorder in the United States ICU nurses. *Intensive Care Medicine*, *38*, 1445–1451. doi:10.1007/s00134-012-2600-6

O'Neal, M. R. (1999). *Measuring resilience*. Paper presented at the Annual Meeting of the Mid-South Educational Research Association, Point Clear, AL.

Othman, N., Ghazali, Z., & Ahmad, S. (2013). Resilience and work engagement: A stitch to nursing care quality. *Journal of Global Management*, *6*(1), 40–48.

Richardson, G. E. (2002). The metatheory of resilience and resiliency. *Journal of Clinical Psychology*, *58*(3), 307–321.

Rutter, M. (1987). Psychosocial resilience and protective mechanisms. *American Journal of Orthopsychiatry*, *57*(3), 316–331.

Rutter, M. (1993). Resilience: Some conceptual considerations. *Journal of Adolescent Health*, *14*, 598–611.

Rutter, M. (2007). Resilience, competence and coping. *Child Abuse and Neglect, 31*(3), 205–209.

Ryff, V. L., & Singer, B., (2003). Thriving in the face of challenge: The integrative science of human resilience. In F. Kessel & P. L. Rosenfield (Eds.), *Expanding the boundaries of health and social science: Case studies in interdisciplinary innovation* (pp. 181–205). Oxford, UK: Oxford University Press.

Shakespeare-Finch, J., Gow, K., & Smith, S. (2005). Personality, coping and posttraumatic growth in emergency ambulance personnel. *Traumatology, 11*(4), 325–334.

Solomon, Z. (2007). Posttraumatic stress disorder and posttraumatic growth among Israeli ex-POWs. *Journal of Traumatic Stress, 20*(3), 303.

Southwick, S. M., & Charney, D. S. (2012). The science of resilience: Implications for the prevention and treatment of depression. *Science, 338*, 79–82. doi:10.1126/science.1222942

Snyder, C. R. (2000). *Handbook of hope.* San Diego, CA: Academic Press.

Wagnild, G. (2009). A review of the resilience scale. *Journal of Nursing Measurement, 17*, 105–113.

Waller, M. A. (2007). Resilience in the ecosystemic context: Evolution of the concept. *American Journal of Orthopsychiatry, 71*, 290–297.

Werner, E. E., & Smith, R. S. (1992). *Overcoming the odds: High risk children from birth to adulthood.* Ithaca, NY: Cornell University Sage Press.

Windle, G. (2011). What is resilience? A review and concept analysis. *Reviews in Clinical Gerontology, 21*(2), 152–169.

Zeidner, M., & Endler, N. S. (Eds.). (1996). *Handbook of coping: Theory, research, applications.* New York, NY: Wiley.

TRIAGE NURSE EXPERTISE

The concept of triage nurse expertise has been widely examined and holds a particularly important role in the domain of nursing practice. Christensen and Hewitt-Taylor (2006) explore the concept of expertise in intensive care nursing practice, while Reimer and Moore (2010) present a discussion paper on flight nursing expertise which unveils a middle-range theory on the subject. More recently, Jelinek, Fahje, Immermann, and Elsbernd (2014) introduced an improvement strategy aimed at trauma triage accuracy, creating a trauma report nurse role which became the trauma nurse expert.

Jasper (1994) has defined *expert nurse* as a nurse who has developed the capacity for pattern recognition through high-level knowledge and skill and extensive experience in a specialist field, and who is identified as such by his or her peers. Benner (1982) notes that competent nurses are consciously aware that their actions are part of a plan and know what is most important and what can be ignored. This analysis of expertise focuses specifically on the role of the triage nurse in the emergency department. Positive patient outcomes and operational efficiency in the presence of high volume in the emergency department environment are dependent on the expertise of the triage nurse. Correlating positive outcomes with triage nurse "expertise" is a common theme in the literature. In the world of emergency nursing, the triage nurse must be highly competent and proficient in order to recognize illness and understand how to navigate within a fast-paced environment to rapidly move patients through the system. According to McNally (1996), novice emergency nurses are challenged to develop knowledge and skills to ensure that they can perform in dual roles as competent emergency and triage nurses. The Emergency Nurses Association (ENA) *Position Statement on Triage Qualifications* (2011) notes that emergency nurses need a standardized triage education course and ongoing education to further improve their triage knowledge, skills, and attitudes.

DEFINING ATTRIBUTES

The attributes for triage nurse expertise are *triage skill* and *triage knowledge*.

Triage skill is the first defining attribute of triage nurse expertise. Triage is an essential clinical skill in emergency nursing. Understanding the best way to facilitate this skill is vital when educating new nurses or providing continuing education to practicing nurses (Smith, 2013). In the world of emergency nursing, the triage nurse must be highly skilled and knowledgeable in order to recognize illness. Additionally, the triage nurse must understand how to navigate within a fast-paced environment to rapidly move patients through the system. The triage nurse must have advanced decision-making skills to ensure that patients are appropriately allocated to clinical areas for care (Fry & Stainton, 2005). Triage has been identified as a unique, specialized skill that allows the triage nurse to identify patient problems and prioritize these patients for care in a very different way than that used in other patient care areas (Zimmerman, 2002). Zimmerman (2002) notes that the skill involved in triaging is not limited to recognizing the severely ill patient but also includes the ability to recognize patients who might be seriously ill. Hohenhaus, Travers, and Mecham (2008) state that triage nurses caring for pediatric patients must have strong pediatric assessment skills to accurately triage children, as often child patients present with subtle signs and symptoms of illnesses and injuries.

Triage knowledge is the second attribute of triage nurse expertise because it is essential for the registered nurse to possess advanced education regarding clinical presentations and triage tools necessary to perform appropriate triage. Cone and Murray (2002) have stated that formal education is indicated as being necessary for an effective triage nurse, and that triage nurses should continue with education significant in triage and emergency situations. For expertise to be present, there must be a strong knowledge foundation starting with formal education and followed by continuing education coupled with clinical practice (Cleaver, 2003). Although triage decision-making skills mature as novice nurses gain clinical experience, the addition of multiple teaching strategies and methodologies such as simulation gives new nurses the needed advantage of recognizing patient problems early (Smith et al., 2013). The ENA position paper (2011) indicates that basic general nurse education is not sufficient to prepare the emergency nurse for the range of complexities inherent in the triage nurse role. The authors of this paper recommended that a nurse undergo a standardized triage education course with didactic and clinical components, coupled with a preceptorship experience, before working in a triage role (ENA, 2011).

DEFINITION

Triage nurse expertise is defined as the combination of triage skill and triage knowledge that results in appropriate assessment and nursing care interventions in any triage situations.

MODEL CASE

The model case contains all the defining attributes. A patient arrives at the emergency department at the same time as several other patients. The triage registered nurse (RN) is busy but notes the patient's arrival, taking in the patient's overall appearance. The triage RN notes a slow gait with facial grimace and the patient's hand clutching his chest. His color is pale and the patient is clearly diaphoretic (triage knowledge). The triage RN stops his or her current task and calls for a wheelchair as she begins a rapid screening interview while obtaining vital signs (triage skill). The patient is transferred back to a critical care bed within minutes of arrival, appropriately triaged so that care can begin immediately. This triage RN is skillful and knowledgeable, understands the situation, and has a sense of capability and an ease in addressing a very time-sensitive and life-threatening situation.

RELATED CASE

Expertise is often associated and used interchangeably with registered nurse *competency* and/or *capability*, as is evident in this case. In this scenario, a registered nurse is attending a dinner at a hotel. She is a very capable certified labor and delivery nurse. A woman at a nearby table "faints" and falls forward onto her table. The dinner attendees respond immediately, asking for medical assistance. The registered nurse acts competently as she responds and asks for 911 notification as she completes a quick assessment for airway, breathing, and circulation (triage skill). She waits with the patient for the emergency team. She fails to ask any questions regarding the woman's medical history. A quick question would have revealed that the woman is an insulin-dependent diabetic (failed triage knowledge). Without this information, the nurse was unable to provide skilled nursing interventions such as treating the patient quickly and appropriately by getting the woman to drink some orange juice, which would have improved the woman's mental status quickly. The labor and delivery RN, though competent and experienced, does not hold triage nurse expertise in this scenario.

BORDERLINE CASE

A borderline case has most of the defining attributes. A patient arrives at the emergency department along with several other patients. The triage RN is busy but notes this particular patient. He is clutching his chest and looks anxious (triage skill). The triage RN asks the patient to sign in and tells him he will be treated next as soon as she finishes with the current patient (failed triage knowledge). After a few minutes, the triage RN calls for a wheelchair and asks a technician to take vital signs on the patient. Once the technician completes the vital signs, the patient is transferred back to a critical care bed to await further care.

This triage RN understands the situation but is not skillful in handling the patient flow. Additionally, the decision making was inadequate and the action did not match the situation. Emergency department triage efforts, although founded in the patient urgency, also seek to accomplish a second goal, patient streaming: getting the right patient to the right resources at the right place and at the right time. This clinician lacks the facility to handle multiple patients, which is a frequent occurrence in triage.

CONTRARY CASE

A patient arrives at the emergency department along with several other patients. The triage RN is busy and notes many patients arriving. The triage RN becomes anxious and asks the registration clerk to take the names of the patients and have them take a seat and await their turn at triage. The triage RN fails to notice the man who is clearly in distress and clutching his chest. After 15 minutes the patient yells out that he is in excruciating pain and falls to the floor from his chair. The code team is called to the waiting room where the patient is in full cardiac arrest (failed triage knowledge and failed triage skill).

In this scenario, the triage RN lacks the knowledge and skill to recognize the severity and to handle multiple patients. Thus, the wrong decision and lack of action resulted in a poor outcome.

ANTECEDENTS

The antecedents to triage nurse expertise are *education*, *training*, and *experience*. In order for triage nurse expertise to be present, an individual nurse must have the education, training, and experience to adequately assess and prioritize patients for care. It is commonly accepted that it is through education, training, and experience that nurses acquire a knowledge base specific to their specialty. At first this can be general in nature, but subsequently the registered nurse needs to specialize in emergency department nursing as an antecedent to triage nurse expertise. Professional expertise requires extensive specialized skill and knowledge. This is important to understand in order to provide the appropriate training for the new triage nurse. An orientation specific for the triage area is essential. Often the triage nurse is triaging patients in practice areas away from the rest of the emergency room nursing team. Therefore, triage nurses need to be prepared for this changing context of practice if they are to adjust, enjoy, and succeed in the role (Fry & Stainton, 2005). In addition to training, knowledge and skill are dependent upon experience. It is common practice to have orientation to triage follow a specified time of working in the emergency department in order to understand the basic determinations between sick/not sick. Cioffi (2001) found that 63% of the nurses voiced that they used past experiences in their decision-making processes. Although discussion in the literature is ongoing regarding years of experience, Cone and Murray (2002) note that a minimum of one year emergency department experience and formal education is indicated as being necessary for an effective triage nurse. Unlike the expert nurse, the beginner nurse has little clinical experience and needs to follow specific procedures and protocols when making decisions about appropriate nursing interventions. Triage education programs must provide nurses with adequate practical experience in order to develop advanced decision-making skills (Fry & Stainton, 2005).

CONSEQUENCES

Appropriate action and *decision making* are the consequences of triage nurse expertise. According to Reimer and Moore (2010), good decision making is critical to function as an expert in flight nursing (a type of triage nursing) if optimal patient outcomes are to occur. Rapid and accurate decision making, along with appropriate action taken, are the desired outcomes of triage assessment. The expert triage nurse has the skill and knowledge to make the appropriate decision regarding the acuity level of the patient. The triage nurse is tasked with the responsibility of deciding which patients can wait for care and which need immediate medical attention (Gerdtz & Bucknall, 2001).

EMPIRICAL REFERENTS

A review of the literature does not reveal an explicit instrument to measure triage nurse expertise. Considering the antecedents, along with the attributes of triage skill and triage knowledge leading to appropriate decision making and action, there are a number of ways these attributes can be measured. Emergency department quality efforts are focused on rapid and timely patient care. The time from triage until the first intervention is an indicator of the skill and knowledge of the triage nurse. Similarly, the time taken to triage the patient is another indicator of the triage nurse's level of expertise. Retrospective chart reviews would reveal specific time stamps reflecting these quality measures.

Appropriate triage is reflected in the emergency severity index (ESI) level assigned to the patient. The ESI is a simple five-level triage tool that categorizes emergency department patients by evaluating both patient clinical presentation and resources (Agency for Healthcare Research and Quality, 2005). Retrospective chart review of ESI gives credible insight into triage nurse expertise.

The attributes—triage skills and triage knowledge—can also be measured using patient simulation scenarios. The advantage of using a simulated environment is that each triage nurse can be assessed using the same scenario and their performances can be compared to each other. Gaps in skills and knowledge can be identified easily and, if needed, continuing education modules can be developed and implemented to increase the nurses' knowledge and skills (Figure 29.1).

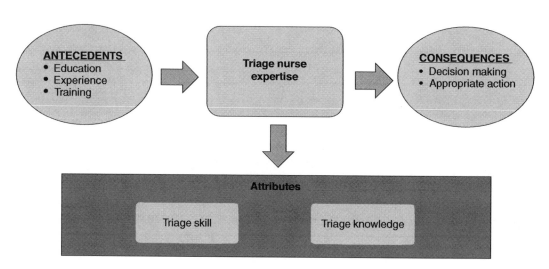

FIGURE 29.1 Triage nurse expertise.

SUMMARY

In this chapter, triage nurse expertise is defined. The attributes, antecedents, and consequences of this concept are identified. Case studies demonstrating the presence and absence of the attributes are provided. These provide clarity and understanding of the concept of triage nurse expertise. Empirical referents for the concept are proposed. These possible ways to measure the attributes can be incorporated into educational and evaluation programs to ensure that triage nurses have the key attributes of triage nurse expertise to make the appropriate decisions and take the necessary actions in every patient encounter.

REFERENCES

Agency for Healthcare Research and Quality. (2005). *Emergency severity index, version 4: Implementation handbook.* Rockville, MD: U.S. Department of Health and Human Services, AHRQ.

Benner, P. (1982). From novice to expert. *American Journal of Nursing, 82,* 402–407.

Christensen, M., & Hewitt-Taylor, J. (2006). Defining the expert ICU nurse. *Intensive and Critical Care Nursing, 22*(5), 301–307. doi:10.1016/j.iccn.2005.07.003

Cioffi, J. (2001). A study of the use of past experiences in clinical decision making in emergency situations. *International Journal of Nursing Studies, 38,* 591–599.

Cleaver, K. (2003). Developing expertise—The contribution of paediatric accident and emergency nurses to the care of children, and the implications for their continued professional development. *Accident and Emergency Nursing, 11*(2), 96–102. doi:10.1016/SO965-2302(02)00211-4

Cone, K., & Murray, R. (2002). Characteristics, insights, decision making, and preparation of ED triage nurses. *Journal of Emergency Nursing, 28*(5), 401–406. doi:10.1067/men.2002.127513

Emergency Nurses Association [ENA]. (2011). *Triage qualifications position statement.* Approved by ENA Board of Directors. Des Plaines, IL: Author.

Fry, M., & Stainton, C. (2005). An educational framework for triage nursing based on gatekeeping, timekeeping and decision-making processes. *Accident and Emergency Nursing, 13*(4), 214–219. doi:10.1016/j.aaen.2005.09.004

Gerdtz, M. F., & Bucknall, T. K. (2001). Triage nurses' clinical decision making: An observational study of urgency assessment. *Journal of Advanced Nursing, 35*(4), 550–561. doi:10.1046/j.1365-2648.2001.01871.x

Hohenhaus, S. M., Travers, D., & Mecham, N. (2008). Pediatric triage: A review of emergency education literature. *Journal of Emergency Nursing, 34*(4), 308–313. doi:10.1016/j.jen.2007.06.022

Jasper, M. A. (1994). Expert: A discussion of the implications of the concept as used in nursing. *Journal of Advanced Nursing, 20,* 769–776.

Jelinek, L., Fahje, C., Immermann, C., & Elsbernd, T. (2014). The trauma report nurse: A trauma triage process improvement project. *Journal of Emergency Nursing, 40*(5), 111–117. doi:10.1016/j.jen.2013.12.018

McNally, S. (1996). The triage role in emergency nursing: Development of an educational programme. *International Journal of Nursing Practice, 2*(3), 122–128.

Reimer, A., & Moore, S. (2010). Flight nursing expertise: Towards a middle-range theory. *Journal of Advanced Nursing, 66*(5), 1183–1192. doi:10.1111/j.1365-2648.2010.05269

Smith, A. (2013). Using a theory to understand triage decision making. *International Emergency Nursing, 21,* 113–117. doi:10.1016/j.ienj.2012.03.003

Smith, A., Lollar, J., Menhenhall, J., Brown, H., Johnson, P., & Roberts, S. (2013). Use of multiple pedagogies to promote confidence in triage decision making: A pilot study. *Journal of Emergency Nursing, 39*(6), 660–666. doi:10.1016/j.jen.2011.12.007

Zimmerman, P. G. (2002). Guiding principles at triage: Advice for new triage nurses. *Journal of Emergency Nursing, 28*(1), 24–33. doi:10.1067/men.2002.120058

PART III ORGANIZATION-FOCUSED CONCEPTS

MARGARET A. HARRIS

30

NURSE WORKAROUNDS

Although not specifically named as such, nurse workarounds were alluded to in the literature as early as 2002 (Patterson, Cook, & Render, 2002; Tucker & Edmondson, 2002). Their appearance followed the Institute of Medicine (IOM) report of significant errors with patients in the U.S. health care system (IOM, 1999). A *workaround* is a method used to overcome a technical problem without eliminating it, especially a problem that could prevent success.

Nurse workarounds have been described in the literature as nurses devising an alternative work procedure to address a block in the workflow (Rathert, Williams, Lawrence, & Halbesleben, 2012). With a somewhat negative connotation, nurse workarounds have also been described as finding ways to skirt the known and formal patient care process (Healthcare IT, 2013). Most recently, nurse workarounds were simply described as deviations from established policies, procedures, or work processes (Westphal, Lancaster, & Park, 2014).

Nurse workarounds start when the nurse is faced with a block or hurdle to expected processes. Standard procedures do not alleviate the block and unconventional means, *nurse workarounds*, are employed to proceed with patient care. With escalating integration of technology in health care systems, the need for nurse workarounds has surged. This is an anticipated phase of technology integration and eventual evolution. All too often, the end user of technology, in this case the nurse, is not included in the system design team. Upon implementation, this naturally leads to some gaps in the human–technology interface. Nurses may expect the technology to work in ways for which it was not designed. Likewise, nurses may not know all of the ways in which the technology can function, because of a lack of education or training. Nurses employ their experience and creativity to proceed outside of the system's protocol to complete their work. These maneuvers, called nurse workarounds, are detected by system surveillance and must be addressed. System modification, nurse reeducation, or both should occur to permanently resolve the impasse in workflow and evolve the system to a higher and more user-friendly level.

DEFINING ATTRIBUTES

The defining attributes of nurse workarounds are the *modification or circumvention of standard care or protocol, patient care directed to increase efficiency*, and the *issue temporarily addressed but not resolved*.

Nurses use their knowledge to create and execute modifications to achieve the desired goal of patient care (Ash, Berg, & Coiera, 2004; Koopman & Hoffman, 2003). Ash et al. (2004) simply described nurse workarounds as methods for achieving what the system does not let the nurse accomplish easily. A workaround has also been described as improvisation in one or more aspects of an existing work system with an emphasis on circumvention of standard protocol (Alter, 2014; Healthcare IT, 2013; Patterson et al., 2002). In a seminal research report, nurse workarounds were described as actions that deviate from the protocol of system designers and are nonstandard procedures (Koppel, Wetterneck, Telles, & Karshl, 2008).

When looking at consequences of introducing bar code medication administration (BCMA) systems, Patterson et al. (2002) described nurse workarounds as strategies that circumvent the intended use of the BCMA system to increase efficiency. Generally, workarounds are goal-driven adaptations (Alter, 2014). For nurses, who care for patients, nurse workarounds are patient care directed adaptations aimed at increasing efficiency in patient care (Ash et al., 2004; Koopman & Hoffman, 2003). This attribute rules out those actions taken by nurses for their own convenience without regard to patient needs.

The temporary nature of nurse workarounds is a primary attribute, in that any workaround that is adopted as standard practice ceases to be a workaround (Kobayashi, Fussell, Xiao, & Seagull, 2005). Nurse workarounds are informal, temporary, and many times spontaneous in origin. When successful, nurse workarounds may be repeated until the system changes and the workaround is no longer necessary (because it has become the system). Throughout the literature, the nature of workarounds has been a temporary address of a challenging issue, not a resolution of the issue (Alter, 2014; Ash et al., 2004). This defining attribute is intrinsically related to the temporal nature of nurse workarounds. Once a nurse workaround is adopted as a permanent resolution to standard protocol, it loses its identity as a nurse workaround.

DEFINITION

The definition of *nurse workarounds* is temporary, nonstandard modifications or circumventions of patient care processes to more efficiently meet the goals of patient care, by which the issue is temporarily addressed but not resolved.

MODEL CASE

The BCMA system presents many opportunities for nurse workarounds. The model case is a nurse who does not scan the patient's arm band prior to administering an intravenous (IV) medication. It is 2:00 a.m. and the identification (ID) band is on the patient's arm that is crossed under the other with a blanket tucked around it. The nurse has cared for this patient since 7:00 p.m. the previous evening and makes a visual ID in the dim lighting from the bathroom light. The nurse scans the medications and overrides the patient scan feature (modification or circumvention of standard patient care processes to more efficiently meet the goals of patient care). She proceeds to administer the IV medication without disturbing the patient's sleep.

The nurse perceived an obstacle in the accessibility of the patient's ID band for medication administration. With regard to the time of night and the mode of administration, the nurse intended to administer the medication without disturbing the patient's sleep (patient care directed). She did this by circumventing the patient scan feature of the system. This is a temporary measure to address the situation and does not resolve the issue.

RELATED CASE

A related case pertains to hand hygiene. The nurse cares for both patients in a double-occupancy room. Upon entering the room, she washes her hands and begins care for the patient in bed A. When finished, she begins to care for the patient in bed B without performing hand hygiene (modification or circumvention of standard care or protocol). When the nurse completes care for the patient in bed B, she washes her hands and departs from the room.

The action, or in this case inaction, is not patient care directed and does not address an issue (failed patient care directed). The nurse's omission of handwashing does not truly circumvent standard patient care, but ignores it (failed circumvent standard patient care). The lack of intention toward patient care categorizes this case as a mistake or error and not a nurse workaround.

BORDERLINE CASE

A borderline case pertains to BCMA. The nurse is caring for a patient who is transferring to another unit. The patient has medication due at the time of the transfer. The nurse brings the computer, scanner, and medication to the bedside for administration. The nurse scans the medication but not the patient's ID band (modification or circumvention of standard care or protocol). She then gives the patient the oral medication with water to drink. When asked why she did not scan the patient, the nurse responds that she had cared for this patient for several days, the arm band was on the opposite side to her, and the transport person was waiting to take the patient to the other unit.

In terms of attributes of nurse workarounds, a few are represented here. This was a temporary inaction probably related to a time constraint that the nurse perceived. It was a modification that circumvented standard protocol and increased efficiency for medication administration. However, it failed patient care directed. There was no benefit to the patient. The only benefit was to the nurse and transporter waiting to move the patient.

CONTRARY CASE

A contrary case pertains to an invasive procedure. The nurse prepares to start an IV access. He deliberately rips off the tip of the index finger of his glove to palpate for an appropriate vein (modification or circumvention of standard care or protocol). The nurse then cleanses the site and touches the intended access point with the ungloved fingertip. When asked about this, the nurse claims that he always immerses his ungloved finger in cleanser before touching the cleansed IV site.

This is purely unsafe nursing practice. There appears to be a regularity of this action, shown the nurse's response to why he touches his bare finger to the insertion site when he claims to "always" immerse his finger in cleanser. Therefore, there is failed temporary address in this action. This situation represents a lack of proper training and practice of initiating IV access. This action failed patient care directed as it poses a significant threat to the patient.

ANTECEDENTS

The antecedents to nurse workarounds include *nurse's perceived obstacle or dysfunction*; *system introduction or design*; *policy, procedure and work flow*; and *workload and time*.

The nurse perceives an obstacle or dysfunctional limitation (Koopman & Hoffman, 2003; Rathert et al., 2012) in the system. Regardless of reality, the nurse perceives an obstacle when a path to a goal is blocked or dysfunctional. These are typically structural constraints that the nurse perceives as preventing a desired level of achievement or efficiency in patient care (Alter, 2014).

Nurse workarounds are usually related to poorly designed systems or the introduction of new technology (Rathert et al., 2012). Unintended consequences of organizational or technological implementations create gaps in the human–technology interface which necessitate nurse workarounds, at least from the nurse's perspective (Cook, Render, & Woods, 2000). This frequently occurs when nurses are not part of the team that selects and develops technologies to be integrated in patient care processes. Training and implementation strategies can also contribute to these gaps. Health care technology must be user-friendly for nurses to adopt it fully (Voshall, Piscotty, Lawrence, & Targosz, 2013). Several approaches are recommended to facilitate nurses' adoption of new patient care technologies: test each system component for performance, adequacy, integration, and durability; encourage open communication with staff regarding quality improvement; and provide trained super users to support staff in the initial integration process (Halbesleben, Rathert, & Williams, 2013; Heinen, Geraldine, & Hamilton, 2003).

Institutional and unit policy and procedure can create blocks for the nurse's workflow. Sometimes these blocks are intentional (Halbesleben, Savage, Wakefield, & Wakefield, 2010; Halbesleben, Wakefield, & Wakefield, 2008). This is the case with safeguards like BCMA blocks that will not allow the nurse to proceed with standard processes if a particular medication is not currently ordered for the patient. The intention of this workflow block is patient safety. The nurse can, and sometimes needs to, employ workarounds to administer the medication outside of the system design. Sometimes workflow blocks are created unintentionally. An example of an unintentional workflow block is having only one supply cart of personal protective equipment to be employed with patients in isolation. When there are several isolation patients who are spread throughout the unit, nurses are challenged with the source of supplies and the physical location of patients for whom they care (Westphal et al., 2014).

Workload is directly related to time. When sufficient staffing allowed nurses to spend adequate amounts of time with each patient to deliver complete care, procedures were more likely to be followed without exception (Halbesleben et al., 2008). Likewise, during shifts where workload was heavy, nurses perceived that they did not have enough time to follow routine procedures (Westphal et al., 2014). Some reports referred to this phenomenon in terms of task-related causes of nurse workarounds (Koppel et al., 2008). Without regard to the designed safety mechanism of a particular task, if nurses perceived the task as inefficient, they felt authorized to execute a time-saving nurse workaround.

CONSEQUENCES

The consequences of nurse workarounds include destabilization of the system, error, and evolution of the system. Which consequence occurs depends upon a variety of factors.

One of the first consequences of nurse workarounds is destabilization of the system as the temporary and unreliable actions accumulate. Nurse workarounds, even the safe and successful ones, cannot continue over long periods of time because they degrade the stability of the system (Kobayashi et al., 2005). The conventional view is that the technology system is safe by design but can be degraded by the failure of its human interface (Seibert, Maddox, Flynn, & Williams, 2014). Therefore, bolstering the system can be achieved by decreasing the opportunities for human interface and increasing the automation through guidelines and regulations. However, the automation is only successful if it is logical to the human interface or user, namely the nurse.

Another consequence of nurse workarounds is error. Any time a system designed with safety features is circumvented, the chance for error increases (Seibert et al., 2014). Depending upon the area and extent of the nurse workaround, the chances that the error will reach the patient can be significant (Halbesleben et al., 2013). Invasive procedures and medication administration are two areas in which nurse workarounds carry high risk for deleterious patient outcomes (Westphal et al., 2014). A seemingly minor nurse workaround can result in serious consequences to the patient.

Optimally, nurse workarounds can contribute to the refinement and evolution of the system. Researchers have reported that an organizational culture that has (a) a learning orientation, (b) decentralization, (c) flexible implementation, (d) training, and (e) physician participation is better poised for successful implementation of quality programs (Tucker & Edmondson, 2002). These characteristics decrease the total number and types of nurse workarounds that lead to system destabilization and serious error. Within this type of culture, useful nurse workarounds can be identified, addressed, and, if appropriate, integrated into the system for improved patient care and safety.

Nurse workarounds can help coordinate work, especially under conditions of time restriction (Kobayashi et al., 2005). They are not inherently bad; nurse workarounds can be temporarily safe and successful. These types of nurse workarounds should be recognized, analyzed, and, when indicated, incorporated into the system; thereafter they are no longer nurse workarounds. This is the nature of a dynamic system that health care must embody: moving from a static culture of blame to a dynamic culture of safety (Pronovost & Wachter, 2014).

EMPIRICAL REFERENTS

Measurement of nurse workarounds has proven to be challenging. Part of the challenge is the individual nature of nurse workarounds. Measurement of nurse workarounds has to be specific to the practice area under examination. Nurses' perception, patient care focus, modification of expected actions, and bypass of standard patient care must be examined in the context of the nursing practice studied. Successful measurement of these attributes necessitates various methods of data collection. Koppel et al. (2008) employed five different modes to measure nurse workarounds in five hospitals where they identified 15 different nurse workarounds to BCMA. These kinds of studies are laborious, yet necessary to capture and measure the nuances of nurse workarounds.

Specific nurse workarounds can be identified in the electronic medication administration record as administration time changed to earlier times than scanned, changed doses, and lack of scanning either the patient or the medications. Nurse workarounds can be identified in hand hygiene by direct observation or by technology that scans nurses' (and other health care providers') ID badges upon entering the patient's room as well as when hand-washing equipment is activated. In the area of direct patient care (e.g., dressing changes, IV initiation, and other invasive procedures), direct observation of procedure adherence is necessary to determine the employment of nurse workarounds. The laborious process of direct observation proves to be a marked challenge in the measurement and the further understanding of relationships surrounding nurse workarounds (Figure 30.1).

Antecedents	Attributes	Consequences
Nurse's perceived obstacle/dysfunction	Modify or circumvent standard care or protocol	Destabilization of the system
System introduction or design	Patient care directed to increase efficiency	Error
Policy, procedure, workflow		Evolution of the system
Workload, time	Issue temporarily addressed but not resolved	

FIGURE 30.1 Nurse workarounds.

SUMMARY

From a variety of disciplines, workarounds have been reported as an anticipated component of the human–technology interface. Technology is increasingly being integrated into patient care processes. Therefore, nurse workarounds are anticipated as a natural component of this process. The use of, detection of, and response to nurse workarounds should be capitalized upon to maximize the safety and efficiency of patient care. The challenge of nurse workarounds is to capture their positive aspects—frontline resiliency and creativity—while simultaneously avoiding the consequences of relying too heavily on temporary fixes to long-standing problems (Tucker, 2009). Health care systems must look earnestly at nurse workarounds to incorporate the positive contributions while removing the threats to patient outcomes in order to deliver patient care with the highest levels of safety and efficiency. In an important way, nurse workarounds will play a significant role in the safe and efficient evolution of technology-rich patient care modalities across health care systems.

REFERENCES

Alter, S. (2014). Theory of workarounds. *Communications of the Association for Information Systems, 34*(55), 1041–1056. Retrieved from http://aisel.aisnet.org/cais/vol34/iss1/55

Ash, J. S., Berg, M., & Coiera, E. (2004). Some unintended consequences of information technology in health care: The nature of patient care information system-related errors. *Journal of the American Medical Informatics Association, 11*(2), 104–112. doi:10.1197/jamia.M1471

Cook, R. I., Render, M., & Woods, D. D. (2000). Gaps in the continuity of care and progress on patient safety. *British Medical Journal, 320*(7237), 791–794.

Halbesleben, J., Rathert, C., & Williams, E. S. (2013). Emotional exhaustion and medication administration work-arounds: The moderating role of nurse satisfaction with medication administration. *Health Care Management Review, 38*(2), 95–104. doi:10.1097/HMR.Ob013e3182452c7f

Halbesleben, J., Savage, G., Wakefield, D., & Wakefield, B. (2010). Rework and workarounds in nurse medication administration process: Implications for work processes and patient safety. *Health Care Management Review*, 35(2), 124–133. doi:10.1097/HMR.0b013e3181d116c2

Halbesleben, J., Wakefield, D., & Wakefield, B. (2008). Work-arounds in health care settings: Literature review and research agenda. *Health Care Management Review*, 33, 2–12. doi:10.1097/01.HMR.0000304495.95522.ca

Healthcare IT on the frontlines: Avoid workaround: Why they happen and how to avoid them. (2013). *Patient Safety Monitor Journal*, 14(11), 2–6.

Heinen, M. G., Geraldine, A. C., & Hamilton, A. V. (2003). Barcoding makes its mark on daily practice. *Nursing Management*, 34(10), 18–20.

Institute of Medicine. (1999). *To err is human: Building a safer health system*. Washington, DC: National Academy Press.

Kobayashi, M., Fussell, S. R., Xiao, Y., & Seagull, J. (2005). Work coordination, workflow, and workarounds in a medical context. In *CHI proceedings: Extended abstracts on human factors* (pp. 1561–1564). New York, NY: ACM Press.

Koopman, P., & Hoffman, R. R. (2003). Work-arounds, make-work, and kludges. *IEEE Intelligent Systems*, 18(6), 70–75. doi:10.1109/MIS.2003.1249172

Koppel, R., Wetterneck, T., Telles, J., & Karsh, B. (2008). Workarounds to barcode medication systems: Their occurrences, causes, and threats to patient safety. *Journal of the American Medical Informatics Association*, 15, 408–423. doi:10.1197/jamia.M2616

Patterson, E. S., Cook, R. I., & Render, M. L. (2002). Improving patient safety by identifying side effects from introducing bar coding in medication administration. *Journal of American Medical Informatics Association*, 9(5), 540–553. doi:10.1197/jamia.M1061

Pronovost, P. J., & Wachter, R. M. (2014). Progress in patient safety: A glass fuller than it seems. *American Journal of Medical Quality*, 29(2), 165–169. doi:10.1177/1062860613495554

Rathert, C., Williams, E. S., Lawrence, E. R., & Halbesleben, J. R. B. (2010). Emotional exhaustion and workarounds in acute care: Cross sectional tests of a theoretical framework. *International Journal of Nursing Studies*, 49, 969–977. doi:10.1016/j.ijnurstu.2012.02.11

Seibert, H., Maddox, R., Flynn, E., & Williams, C. (2014). Effect of barcode technology with electronic medication administration record on medication accuracy rates. *American Journal of Health-System Pharmacy*, 71, 209–218. doi:10.2146/ajhp130332

Tucker, A. (2009). *Workarounds and resiliency on the front lines of health care*. AHRQ Morbidity and Mortality Rounds on the Web. Retrieved from http://www.webmm.ahrq.gov/printviewperspective.aspx?perspectiveID=78

Tucker, A. L., & Edmondson, A. C. (2002). Managing routine exceptions: A model of nurse problem solving behavior. *Advances in Health Care Management*, 3, 87–113.

Voshall, B., Piscotty, R., Lawrence, J., & Targosz, M. (2013). Barcode medication administration work-arounds: A systematic review and implications for nurse executives. *Journal of Nursing Administration*, 43, 530–535. doi:10.1097/NNA.0b013e3182a3e8ad

Westphal, J., Lancaster, R., & Park, D. (2014). Work-arounds observed by fourth-year nursing students. *Western Journal of Nursing Research*, 36(8), 1002–1018. doi:10.1177/0193945913511707

31

ORGANIZATIONAL COMMITMENT

Organizations are goal-directed entities that can be created in society, business, health care, and family units. An organization has a deliberate structure that coordinates activities. Organizations do not stand alone, but affect and are affected by the outside environment (Daft, 2009). *Commitment* is broadly defined as a multidimensional theory that guides a course of action toward one or more goals (Meyer, Stanley, Herscovitch, & Topolnytsky, 2002). Commitment is viewed as a major variable in developing positive employee relations and can influence the quality of health care service. When nurses are highly committed, they feel greater responsibility for the care they deliver to their patients (Brooks & Swailes, 2002).

Organizational commitment (OC) consists of three behaviors: identification, loyalty, and involvement (Porter, Steers, Mowday, & Boulian, 1974). OC represents an employee's active relationship with an organization he or she works for. Individuals exhibit commitment-related behaviors by abandoning an alternative course of action and instead linking themselves to an organization and contributing to the well-being of that organization. A person's identity is associated with the organization because of a belief in similar goal or mission of the organization. The goals of the individual and the organization become interrelated as the person wants to continue to be part of this affiliation. An individual takes pride in association with the organization. The employee demonstrates a willingness to perform for the organization. She works to maintain that relationship. Commitment attitudes appear slowly but consistently over time as the employee contemplates the relationship between himself and the employer. OC is an acceptance of an organization's goals and values (identification), motivation to work for the organization (involvement), and willingness to stay with the organization (loyalty; Mowday, Porter, & Steer, 1979). It is a measure of an employee's global attitude toward an organization.

Another widely used definition of OC is Meyer, Allen, and Smith's (1993) three-component model of commitment. This model refers to the three forms of OC as affective, continuance, and normative. *Affective commitment* is explained as an emotional attachment to, identification with, and involvement with the organization. *Continuance* is a commitment because of the alleged costs associated with leaving the organization. *Normative commitment* refers to the perceived obligation to stay within the organization (Meyers et al., 1993). With this model, individuals continue with an organization because they want to, need to, or ought to.

DEFINING ATTRIBUTES

The defining attributes of OC in nursing practice are *multidimensional, continuous, collective goal seeking*, and *involvement*.

DEFINITION

Organizational commitment is defined as an individual's feeling and/or belief toward the institution he or she works for that is multidimensional and continuous, reflected in a sense of loyalty, collective goal seeking, and involvement within the organization.

OC is multidimensional in nature. It is a broader concept than just the particular task or role. OC includes all aspects of the work environment, such as job role, job satisfaction, financial benefits, job security, opportunity, and relationships with leadership/management and fellow colleagues (Mowday Porter, & Steers, 1979).

OC is a continuous dynamic process. When first entering into an organization, individuals may be uncertain of how to or to what degree they should commit. One may go through stages or degrees of developing commitment. It may start tentatively and develop into a passionate stage (Manion, 2004). This is an interactive process between the individual and the organization. Both contribute to this process.

Loyalty is a willingness to stay and identify with an organization. The individual may feel an obligation, desire, and need to remain a member (Meyer et al., 1993). One feels a sense of pride in being associated with the organization. The extent of commitment depends on the amount of positive feelings for the organization and ability to emotionally bond to that organization. This type of bonding occurs when affirmed by policies, actions, and events orchestrated by the organization that create an emotional connection (Manion, 2004; Meyer et al., 2002).

In collective goal seeking, there is a strong belief in a common mission. There is an acceptance of not only the organization, but also its goals and values. An individual actively assists the organization in pursuit of these goals (Liou, 2008).

Involvement is a motivation to work for the organization. Purposeful action is taken to contribute to the success of the organization. As more involvement occurs, the strength of the commitment increases (Zangaro, 2001).

MODEL CASE

Mary has been working at the hospital for 10 years. She started as a staff nurse in the intensive care unit. As part of the employee benefits, the hospital pays for continued education, which enabled Mary to return to school and attain her masters in nursing education. For the past 3 years (continuous), she has worked as the nurse educator for that unit. Mary enjoys her relationships with the intensive care unit (ICU) staff nurses and the ability to influence quality patient care (collective goal seeking). Mary participates in several of the hospital committees (involvement): documentation, infection control, and research, and works on carrying out the recommendations of these committees. She teaches a basic EKG course to new cardiac nurses. Here, she gets to interact with new employees, sharing her positive feelings about the hospital (loyalty) and enlightening them as to the opportunities that are available to them. She is a chairperson for the hospital's annual community health fair (multidimensional). For Mary, this is the best place to work. Mary's example encompasses all of the attributes of OC.

RELATED CASES

Related cases contain elements that are similar to the concept of OC but are not the same because they do not possess all the defining attributes. They are connected to the concept and may help us understand the meaning or purpose of a concept. The concept of job satisfaction is a related case. This refers to the degree to which an individual likes her or his job, simply defined as a pleasurable or positive emotional state resulting from one's job experience (Locke, 1976).

Sue works on the telemetry floor. She started orientation there 4 years ago with five other nurses. They studied together when they took their electrocardiogram (EKG) and advanced cardiac life support (ACLS) courses, and now they all are planning on getting their certification as cardiovascular (CV) nurses. The unit is very busy, but they work as a team (involvement) and have obtained high patient satisfaction scores over the past 6 months (continuous). Sue frequently goes out socially with a group of nurse from her floor, where they review their busy day and congratulate each other for making it through another shift. Sue loves working on the "tele" floor except when they have to take an admission from another unit (failed multidimensional). Administration does not understand that she needs to take care of "her" patients first (failed common goal) before accepting another assignment, and Sue has been spoken to about her delaying taking report. She thinks that if only her nurse manager would see things her way (failed loyalty), it would a perfect job.

OC is more global, reflecting a general affective response to the organization as a whole. Job satisfaction reflects one's response either to one's job or to a certain aspect of one's job. OC emphasizes attachment to the employing organization as evidenced by the employee's identification, loyalty, and involvement with the organization as a whole. One can have job satisfaction but not OC.

BORDERLINE CASE

Jill likes working at the hospital. This hospital has a good reputation for excellent patient care and she has suggested to several relatives that they come to this hospital for their care (collective goal seeking). She was able to start on day shift, and she has a good relationship with the other staff nurses and her nursing director (loyalty), who is fair in scheduling time off. She will occasionally be assigned to be charge nurse, but prefers not to because she really does not want to get involved with managing the unit (failed involvement). She instead wants to focus on providing quality care for her patients. When there is a unit meeting to discuss new policies or procedures, many of her colleagues speak up with ideas of how to implement them. Jill generally prefers not to offer suggestions because she does not want to "make waves." She will just follow the rules (failed multidimensional). Jill's goal is to work at this job for at least for 5 years and then look for a position in a doctor's office (failed continuous). This way she will not have to work weekends and holidays. Jill's case shows an example of the multidimensional nature of OC. She is loyal to her patients, and believes in the institution's values. She is proud to work there, but does not have long-term commitment plans. She is not willing to be involved or make contribution to the success or goals of specific hospital or unit projects.

CONTRARY CASE

John has been working on a surgery floor for 6 months. He hates it there (failed loyalty). He believes the patient load is too heavy, the medical residents do not answer their pages when he has questions about his patients' care, and the other nurses do not help him. He even got into an argument with one of the nurse's aides. He has reported these issues several times to his nursing director and nursing supervisor, but nothing changes. He feels that they really do not care. He thinks that all the hospital cares about is money, not quality of patient care (failed collective goal seeking). He decides that if he was sick, he would not come here. He was asked to be on the Skin Care committee, but declined (failed involvement); he knows that no one would listen to his ideas anyway. John just wants to collect his weekly paycheck and go home (failed multidimensional). He has applied to several other places and is just waiting to hear back when a position becomes available so he can leave (failed continuous). John demonstrates unshared perceived goals and lack of loyalty to his hospital. There is no continuance in his work plans and he is unwilling to become involved. This example did not display any defining attributes.

ANTECEDENTS

Antecedents are those events or incidents that must occur or be in place prior to the occurrence of a concept. Through the review of literature, there appear to be three broad categories of antecedents for OC: personal characteristic, work experience, and organizational environment.

The need for an individual to achieve is an antecedent that promotes OC. High-performing employees need a challenging environment. When organizations recognize this, behaviors can be fostered and OC can improve (Ingersoll, Olsan, Drew-Cates, DeVinney, & Davies, 2002).

Work experience antecedents include opportunities and job security. OC develops as a result of experiences that satisfy an employee's needs (professional, financial, or personal). Providing opportunities for growth within the organization can promote OC. Caykoylu, Egri, Havlovic, and Bradley (2011) developed a model that explains the antecedents and mediating factors predicting the OC of health care employees in different work roles. This study highlighted that the opportunity to obtain career advancement had a direct impact on OC. Employee's job-motivating potential and effective leadership were also important determinants of OC.

Employees do not favor risk taking. Individuals will be more committed to the organization if they feel secure in their positions (McNeese-Smith, 2001). They will be uncertain about making a commitment if their position or role is ambiguous, such as during times of layoff, changes in management or leadership, or mergers.

Organizational environment antecedents to OC are trust of the organization and leadership style. Leadership style, such as evidence based, perceptions of fairness, and transformational leadership, can strengthen OC (English & Chalon, 2011; McNeese-Smith, 1995; Yurumezoglu & Gulseren, 2012). Positive supervisor relationships can influence nurses' OC. This emphasizes the importance of leadership creating conditions that result in a committed nursing workforce (Laschinger, Finegan, & Wilk, 2009). The organization's dependability will set an early stage for an individual to trust. The development and implementation of policies and interventions aimed at creating more supportive work environments and greater trust in employers have influenced nurses' OC (Gregory, Way, LeFort, Barrett, & Parfey, 2007).

CONSEQUENCES

Consequences are the outcomes or the results that develop when a concept has occurred. One of the important consequences of OC is that once it exists, it empowers individuals and stabilizes behavior as circumstances change (Mowday et al., 1979). Yang, Liu, Chen, and Pan (2014) concluded that there was a strong relationship between empowerment, professional practice, and OC. By empowering the nursing staff, a positive practice environment is created, and this enhances OC. Strategic interventions that have improved OC can result in improved job retention, job satisfaction, productivity, and quality care (Idel et al., 2003; Porter et al., 1974). High correlation has been shown between OC and job satisfaction (Kim & Lee, 2001; Yang et al., 2014) and OC and job retention rates among nurses (Laschinger et al., 2009; Lee, Kim, & Yoom, 2011). OC directly affects employees' performance and therefore should be treated as an issue of great importance (Meyer et al., 2002).

EMPIRICAL REFERENTS

Empirical referents are ways to measure the defined attributes. Two widely known quantitative instruments have been utilized to measure OC. These instruments are the Organizational Commitment Questionnaire (OCQ) developed by Mowday et al. (1979) and the Affective, Continuance, and Normative Commitment Scale developed by Meyer et al. (1993).

The OCQ is a 15-item questionnaire that measures the three behaviors of OC: loyalty, identification, and involvement. It was intended that the scale items, when taken together, would provide a fairly consistent indicator of an employee's commitment level for most working populations. Meyer et al. (1993) developed their Three Component Model of Commitment Scale that consists of 18 questions (six for each of the three measures of Affective, Continuance, and Normative Commitment). This model explains that commitment to an organization is a psychological state. It consists of three distinct components that affect how employees feel about the organization that they work for. The three components are: (a) affection for the job (affective commitment), (b) fear of loss (continuance commitment), and (c) sense of obligation to stay (normative commitment; Figure 31.1).

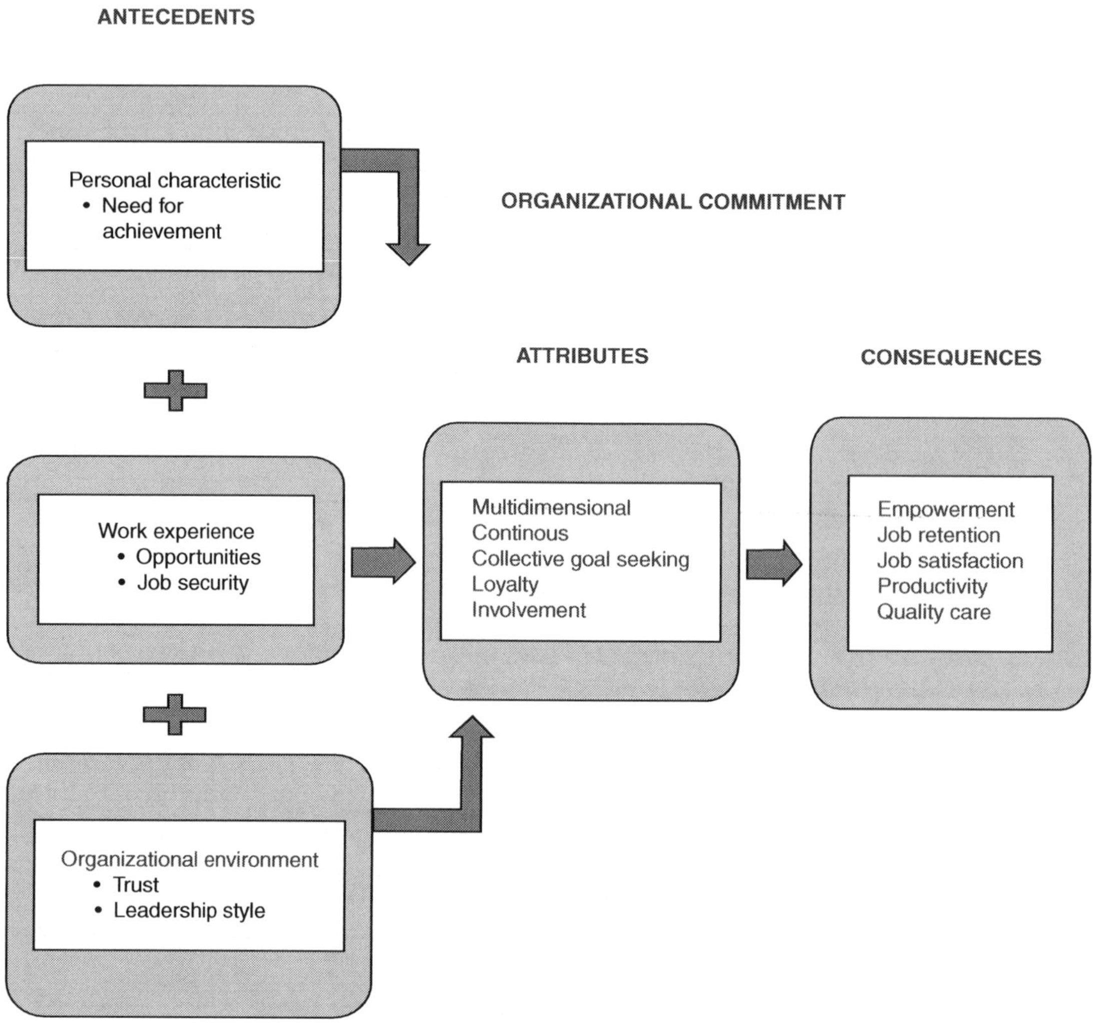

ANTECEDENTS

ORGANIZATIONAL COMMITMENT

Personal characteristic
• Need for achievement

ATTRIBUTES

CONSEQUENCES

Work experience
• Opportunities
• Job security

Multidimensional
Continous
Collective goal seeking
Loyalty
Involvement

Empowerment
Job retention
Job satisfaction
Productivity
Quality care

Organizational environment
• Trust
• Leadership style

FIGURE 31.1 Organization commitment.

SUMMARY

OC has a strong relationship with the employee behavior. In today's health care environment, it is imperative that hospital and nursing management have a clear understanding of the positive effects of this concept. Administration should take measures to develop OC from the initial point of contact with a new employee. The nurse should have a clear idea of what the institution's mission and goals are. The hospital should then provide work opportunities that foster these OC behaviors. Re-evaluation of OC is necessary, as it is an ongoing and dynamic process. Every nurse may not be at the same stage, so it is important that there be an open communication line between management and staff. The end results are employees who contribute to the financial success of the institution and improved quality of patient care.

REFERENCES

Brooks, I., & Swailes, S. (2002). Analysis of relationships between nurse influences over flexible working and commitment to nursing. *Journal of Advanced Nursing*, *38*, 117–126.

Caykoylu, S., Egri, C. P., Havlovic, S., & Bradley, C. (2011). Key organizational commitment antecedents for nurses, paramedical professionals and non-clinical staff. *Journal of Health Organization Management*, *25*(1), 7–33.

Daft, R. L. (2009). Organization and organization theory. In R. L. Daft (Ed.), *Organization theory and design* (10th ed., pp. 2–46). Mason, OH: South-Western Cengage Learning.

English, B., & Chalon, C. (2011). Strengthening affective organizational commitment: The influence of fairness perceptions of management practices and underlying employee cynicism. *Journal of Health Care Management*, *30*(1), 29–35. doi:10.1097/HCM.0b013e3182078ae2

Gregory, D. M., Way, C., LeFort, S., Barrett, B., & Parfey, P. (2007). Predictors of registered nurses' organizational commitment and intent to stay. *Health Care Manager Review*, *32*(2), 119–127.

Idel, M., Melamed, S., Merlob, P., Yahav, J., Hendel, T., & Kaplan, B. (2003). Influence of a merger on nurses' emotional well-being: The importance of self-efficacy and emotional reactivity. *Journal of Nursing Management*, *11*, 59–63.

Ingersoll, G. L., Olsan, T., Drew-Cates, J., DeVinney, B. C., & Davies, J. (2002). Nurses' job satisfaction, organizational commitment, and career intent. *Journal Nursing Administration*, *32*(5), 250–263.

Kim, H. O., & Lee, B. S. (2001). The influence of nursing organizational commitment and job satisfaction on intention of resignation of clinical nurses. *Journal of Korean Academy of Nursing Administration*, *7*, 85–95.

Laschinger, H. K. S., Finegan, J., & Wilk, P. (2009). Context matters: The impact of unit leadership and empowerment on nurses' organizational commitment. *Journal of Nursing Administration*, *39*(5), 228–235.

Lee, H., Kim, M., & Yoom, J. (2011). Role of internal marketing, organizational commitment, and job stress in discerning the turnover intention of Korean nurses. *Japan Journal of Nursing Science*, *8*, 87–94.

Liou, S. (2008). An analysis of the concept of organizational commitment. *Nursing Form*, *43*(3), 116–125.

Locke, E. A. (1976). The nature and causes of job satisfaction. In M. D. Dunnette (Ed.), *Handbook of industrial and organizational psychology* (pp. 1297–1349). Chicago, IL: Rand-McNally.

Manion, J. (2004). Strengthening organizational commitment. Understanding the concept as a basis for creating effective workforce retention strategies. *Health Care Manager*, *23*(2), 167–176.

McNeese-Smith, D. (1995). Job satisfaction, productivity, and organizational commitment: The result of leadership. *Journal of Nursing Administration*, *25*(9), 17–26.

McNeese-Smith, D. K. (2001). A nursing shortage: Building organizational commitment among nurses. *Journal of Healthcare Management*, *46*(3), 173–186.

Meyer, J. P., Stanley, D. J., Herscovitch, L., & Topolnytsky, L. (2002). Affective, continuance, and normative commitment to the organization: A meta-analysis of antecedents, correlates, and consequences. *Journal of Vocational Behavior*, *61*(1), 20–52.

Meyers, J., Allen, N., & Smith, C. (1993). Commitment to organization and occupations: Extension and test of a three-component conceptualization. *Journal of Applied Psychology*, *78*(4), 538–551.

Mowday, R. T., Porter, L. W., & Steers R. M. (1979). The measurement of organizational commitment. *Journal of Vocational Behavior*, *14*, 224–247.

Porter, L. W., Steers, R. M., Mowday, R. T., & Boulian, P. V. (1974). Organizational commitment, job satisfaction, and turnover among psychiatric technicians. *Journal of Applied Psychology*, *59*, 603–609.

Yang, J., Liu, Y., Chen, Y., & Pan, X. (2014). The effect of structural empowerment and organizational commitment on Chinese nurses' job satisfaction. *Applied Nursing Research*, *27*(3), 186–191. Retrieved from www.elsevier.com/locate/apnr

Yurumezoglu, H. A., & Gulseren, G. (2012). Pilot study for evidence-based nursing management: Improving the levels of job satisfaction, organizational commitment, and intent to leave among nurses in Turkey. *Nursing and Health Sciences*, *14*, 221–228.

Zangaro, G. (2001). Organizational commitment. *Nursing Forum*, *36*(2), 14–22.

SIOBHAN SUNDEL AND SAPINA KIRPALANI

32

TEAMWORK

The concept of teamwork in health care has received increased attention from researchers and policy makers alike over the past two decades. Several studies (Adobamen & Egbage, 2014; Neily et al., 2010) and policy papers (Mitchell et al., 2012; Oandasan et al., 2006) have promoted teamwork as a cost-effective way to reduce errors, improve patient outcomes, enhance provider job satisfaction, and raise productivity. Accordingly, the concept of teamwork has become a cornerstone of policy recommendations to improve the health care system, establishing core competencies in medical and nursing school curricula (Institute of Medicine, 2001; Interprofessional Education Collaborative, 2011). Research has thus focused on what creates teamwork and how to produce better teamwork. However, while various tools have been developed to identify and assess factors driving team performance in the health care setting, a clear statement of what teamwork is has remained elusive.

In their concept analysis, Xyrichis and Ream (2008) described teamwork as a dynamic process in which team members with complementary backgrounds and skills engage in interdependent collaboration, characterized by open communication and shared decision making, in the pursuit of common goals. Other researchers have identified specific activities, such as mutual performance monitoring and adaptive back-up behaviors by team members, as being critical to effective team performance, by correcting deficiencies and increasing the efficiency of all team members in completing the task (Baker, Day, & Salas, 2006; Salas, Sims, & Burke, 2005). These behaviors directly reflect and support the process of open communication that Xyrichis and Ream see as integral to the process of interdependent collaboration.

DEFINING ATTRIBUTES

Defining attributes of teamwork are shared decision making, mutual performance monitoring, and adaptive back-up behaviors *in the context of interdependent effort* by team members.

Shared decision making is the first defining attribute of teamwork. Xyrichis and Ream (2008) observed that teams whose actions were directed rather than coordinated by the team leader lacked the attribute of shared decision making by members of the team. In contrast, the process of shared decision making was seen to be facilitated when all team members understood the specific procedures and objectives of the team enterprise (Morrison, Goldfarb, & Lanken, 2010).

Mutual performance monitoring occurs when team members understand how each other's roles fit together to achieve the team objective (Salas, Sims, & Klein, 2004; Salas et al., 2005). Mutual performance monitoring allows team members to identify workload distribution problems in the team and redistribute that workload to team members who are being underutilized (Porter et al., 2003).

Adaptive back-up behaviors describes the process of redistribution of workload that allows the team to effectively adapt to a changing environment (Salas et al., 2005). Marks, Mathieu, and Zaccaro (2001) identify three ways in which team members provide back-up behavior: feedback and coaching, assisting with task completion, or completing the task when another team member is unable to. Once the team is able to identify when a team member's ability is surpassed by the workload, these responsibilities can then be shifted to other team members who may be underutilized.

The context of interdependent effort by team members is another defining attribute of teamwork. Xyrichis and Ream (2008), investigating the unique attributes of teamwork, considered the interdependent effort of the team to be a key feature of teamwork, distinguishing it from mere cooperative or collaborative work. Enderby (2002) identified team member interdependence and interaction as being important for a team. In the research literature, the concept of teamwork is seen as a dynamic process reflecting the quality of interaction between team members, while remaining heavily dependent on team structures and team member competencies for its occurrence (Salas, Cooke, & Rosen, 2008; Valentine, Nembhard, & Edmondson, 2014; Xyrichis & Ream, 2008). Indeed, Salas et al. (2008) note that teamwork is embedded within team performance and is characterized by a set of interrelated perceptions, attitudes, and behaviors that contribute to the dynamic process of performance.

Because mutual performance monitoring and adaptive back-up behaviors directly reflect the quality of interactions between team members working interdependently, they are included in this concept analysis as defining attributes of teamwork, along with the context of interdependent effort by team members and shared decision making.

DEFINITION

Teamwork is defined as a dynamic process characterized by shared decision making, mutual performance monitoring, and adaptive back-up behaviors among team members in the context of their interdependent effort.

MODEL CASE

Mrs. G is an elderly female patient with multiple comorbidities who has been hospitalized for pneumonia and treated with intravenous antibiotics. Her symptoms have resolved and her condition is improving. A team meeting was held to discuss discharge planning. Team members included a staff nurse, a social worker, a geriatric fellow, the attending physician, and a nurse practitioner. All team members have worked closely with patient and family to prepare the patient for discharge (context of interdependent effort), and team members agreed with the decision to send the patient home (shared decision making). The geriatric fellow initiated the discharge paperwork but was paged for an emergency, so the paperwork was completed by the nurse practitioner (adaptive back-up behavior). The staff nurse reviewed all prescriptions and noted that one of the medication doses was incorrect; she contacted the nurse practitioner, who rewrote the prescription (mutual performance monitoring).

RELATED CASE

The nurse practitioner is contacted by the social worker covering the area where the patient lives. The social worker has a question about the medication and the patient is very anxious about the medication regimen. The nurse practitioner speaks to the social worker and agrees to review all the medication with the homecare nurse (context of interdependent effort and shared decision making). The nurse practitioner calls the homecare nurse, but the homecare nurse is unable to speak with her. The nurse practitioner is off the next day. The patient returns to the emergency room that night (failed mutual performance monitoring and adaptive back-up behavior).

BORDERLINE CASE

Mrs. G is back in the emergency room. Team members including the geriatric fellow, nurse practitioner, and social worker meet to discuss the patient's care (context of interdependent effort and shared decision making). The nurse practitioner presents the case to the team and team members discuss how to facilitate a smooth transition back to home this time, including communication with the homecare nurse and the patient regarding all discharge medications and follow-up care. Team members recognize that the patient returned to the emergency room due to her inability to contact the homecare nurse (mutual performance monitoring). The patient was readmitted to the hospital because of a medication-related adverse event caused by confusion over discharge medications and lack of a follow-up phone call (failed adaptive back-up behavior).

CONTRARY CASE

Mrs. G is scheduled for discharge. The social worker contacts the geriatric fellow, who is unable to speak with her (failed interdependent effort and shared decision making). The nurse practitioner is on vacation and the covering nurse practitioner is not familiar with the case (failed adaptive back-up behavior). Team members are unable to speak with Mrs. G's daughter, who is very upset about the patient being discharged home (failed mutual performance monitoring).

ANTECEDENTS

The antecedents to teamwork are *positive leadership, clearly defined roles, shared mental models,* and *mutual trust and respect.*

One of the most commonly cited antecedents of effective teams is positive leadership (Baker et al., 2006; Fernandez, Kozlowski, Shapiro, & Salas, 2008). Team leaders help to guide team members to identify goals and define roles, monitor team members' performance, intervene when needed, and help team members to reflect on deficiencies through the process of debriefing (Fernandez et al., 2008). By identifying deficiencies, team leaders can redistribute workload and responsibilities when necessary.

Clearly defined roles (Clements, Dault, & Priest, 2007; Mitchell et al., 2012) are commonly cited as an important antecedent of teamwork. Team members must understand each other's roles in order to function effectively within the team. Mitchell et al. (2012) state that there are clear expectations for each team member's responsibilities and accountabilities and that this expectation promotes the team's efficiency and division of labor. This in turn allows the team to accomplish more together than it would apart. Role responsibility can create a supportive team climate where team members carry out their roles and protect each other's interests, leading to greater opportunities for shared achievement (Baker et al., 2006; Mitchell et al., 2012).

Shared mental model refers to shared awareness and understanding by and between all team members of the team's processes and procedures, and each member's role and responsibility within that context. Salas et al. (2005) viewed shared mental models as an organizing knowledge structure which looks at the relationships between the task the team needs to complete and how team members will interact to complete the task. It is dependent on team members foreseeing each other's needs, identifying changes in the team, and adjusting strategies as needed.

Mutual trust and respect together are the fourth antecedent of teamwork. Salas et al. (2005) identified mutual trust as a shared belief that team members will perform their roles and be aware of the complementary roles of other team members. Mutual trust and respect imply information sharing and the ability of team members to admit to mistakes and accept feedback when needed. Team members are respectful of each others' contributions and this fosters an environment of mutual trust (Baker et al., 2006).

The occurrence of teamwork thus depends on a number of antecedent factors. It requires a team with positive leadership, clearly defined roles, and a supportive team environment based on mutual trust and respect. Team members demonstrate a shared knowledge and understanding of team processes and goals, otherwise known as a shared mental model, which allow team members to coordinate their activities to accomplish the goal.

CONSEQUENCES

There are several consequences associated with effective teamwork: increased satisfaction with working conditions; reduced staff turnover; increased efficiency and productivity; and improved patient outcomes, including lower mortality.

Effective teamwork has been generally considered in the literature to be associated with improved task performance (Baker et al., 2006; Salas et al., 2008). In the context of team-based health care, improved performance has been linked to positive outcomes for patients, providers, and health care organizations (Xyrichis & Ream, 2008).

A number of studies have pointed to increased patient safety, better patient outcomes, and improved patient satisfaction as consequences of teamwork (Adobamen & Egbage, 2014; Neily et al., 2010; Pucher, Aggarwal, Batrick, Jenkins, & Darzi, 2014). Under the Patient Protection and Affordable Care Act (2010), positive patient outcomes and improved patient satisfaction influence rates of value-based incentive payments for health care organizations.

Several studies have noted improved staff satisfaction as a consequence of teamwork (Chang, Ma, Chiu, Lin, & Lee, 2009; Mitchell et al., 2012), along with lower rates of provider burnout. Kalisch, Curley, and Stefanov (2007) investigated staff turnover rates on a 41-bed oncology unit in a community hospital. The purpose of the study was to determine the impact of an intervention that enhanced teamwork and promoted staff engagement. Kalisch et al. (2007) found a statistically significant drop in staff turnover rates after the intervention. Effective teamwork has been associated with greater operational cost-effectiveness and lower staff turnover for health care organizations (Catchpole et al., 2007; Forse, Bramble, & McQuillan, 2011).

EMPIRICAL REFERENTS

Empirical referents for teamwork consist of the observable aspects of the concept's defining attributes, taken together. The central observed phenomenon would be a dynamic process of interdependent collaboration between team members working toward a common goal. The joint occurrence in this collaborative activity of shared decision making, mutual performance monitoring, and adaptive back-up behaviors by team members would indicate the occurrence of teamwork. It is this combination of attributes that is associated with enhanced team performance. The concept of teamwork is defined here as a dynamic process of interactions linking a set of antecedent conditions to a set of desired outcomes by enhancing team performance.

However, in the literature reporting on survey instruments for assessing teamwork, the term *teamwork* is often used interchangeably with a vague idea of "team effectiveness" or "team performance," leaving the concept of teamwork itself undefined. Consequently, tools purporting to evaluate teamwork in multidisciplinary health care collaborations tend to rely on observations of team attributes defined in this chapter as antecedents to teamwork, such as leadership and clearly defined roles. These are sometimes combined with select attributes that are similar to those of teamwork, such as team monitoring or decision making, but removed from the matrix of interrelated attributes defining the dynamic interactive quality of teamwork.

Nonetheless, several such survey tools have been used in recent years to assess teamwork in the health care setting. They have generally been adapted from other non-health care team training models, such as the airline industry's crew resource management (CRM) curriculum (Sundar et al., 2007). The Observational Teamwork Assessment for Surgery (OTAS) tool looks at teamwork in the operating room. It assesses communication, leadership, cooperation, coordination, and team monitoring (Hull, Arora, Kassab, Kneebone, & Sevdalis, 2010). The Mayo High Performance Teamwork Scale (MHPTS) assesses communication, leadership, cooperation, situational awareness, and decision making (Malec et al., 2007). These tools help to measure several of the defining attributes and antecedents of teamwork identified in this chapter (Figure 32.1).

SUMMARY

Teamwork is a dynamic process of interaction between members of a team, comprised of a set of behaviors and attitudes leading to successful team performance. In practice, it is characterized by shared decision making, mutual performance monitoring, and adaptive back-up behaviors in the context of interdependent effort by team members. Antecedents to teamwork are positive leadership, clearly defined roles, shared mental models, and mutual trust and respect. As discussed in this chapter, the consequences of effective teamwork include increased satisfaction with working conditions, reduced staff turnover, increased efficiency and productivity, and improved patient outcomes, including lower mortality.

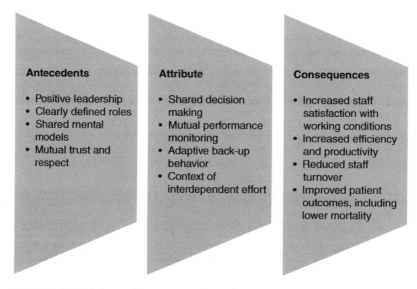

FIGURE 32.1 Schematic representation of concept analysis of teamwork.

An increased focus on teamwork in the literature has accompanied a shift in practice, from health care providers working in individual silos to working within a team. This transition from individual to team-based care is facilitated by adequate team training. Several authors (Morrison et al., 2010; Salas & Rosen, 2013; Weaver, Dy, & Rosen, 2014) emphasize the importance of developing interdisciplinary team training to promote teamwork in health care. The implementation of team-training programs in nursing and medical schools is advocated to orient both in the clinical setting as well as in nursing and medical education (Interprofessional Education Collaborative, 2011). Interdisciplinary team training programs could lead to improved patient outcomes and staff satisfaction.

REFERENCES

Adobamen, P. R., & Egbage, E. E. (2014). Ear, nose, throat, head and neck surgery department functioning as a team in Nigeria: Any benefit? *Indian Journal Otolaryngology and Head and Neck Surgery, 66*(Suppl. 1), 299–302. doi:10.1007/s12070-012-0498-5

Baker, D. P., Day, R., & Salas, E. (2006). Teamwork as an essential component of high-reliability organizations. *Health Services Research, 41*(4), 1576–1598. doi:10.111/j.1475-6773.2006.00566.x

Catchpole, K. R., Giddings, A. E., Wilkinson, M., Hirst, G., Dale, T., & de Leval, M. R. (2007). Improving patient safety by identifying latent failures in successful operations. *Surgery, 142*(1), 102–110.

Chang, W. Y., Ma, J. C., Chiu, H. T., Lin, K. C., & Lee, P. H. (2009). Job satisfaction and perceptions of quality of patient care, collaboration and teamwork in acute care hospitals. *Journal of Advanced Nursing, 65*(9), 1946–1955. doi:10.1111/j.1365-2648.2009.05085.x

Clements, D., Dault, M., & Priest, A. (2007). Effective teamwork in healthcare: Research and reality. *Healthcare Papers, 7*(SP), 26–34. doi:10.12927/hcpap.2013.18669

Enderby, P. (2002). Teamworking in community rehabilitation. *Journal of Clinical Nursing, 11*(3), 409–411. doi:10.1046/j.1365-2702.2002.00633.x

Fernandez, R., Kozlowski, S. W. J., Shapiro, M. J., & Salas, E. (2008). Toward a definition of teamwork in emergency medicine. *Academic Emergency Medicine, 15*(11), 1104–1112. doi:10.1111/j.1553-2712.2008.00250.x

Forse, A., Bramble, J. D., & McQuillan, R. (2011). Team training can improve operating room performance. *Surgery, 150*(4), 771–778. doi:10.1016/j.surg.2011.07.076

Hull, L., Arora, S., Kassab, E., Kneebone, R., & Sevdalis, N. (2010). Observational teamwork assessment for surgery: Content validation and tool refinement. *Journal of American College of Surgeons, 212*(2), 234–243. doi:10.1016/j.jamcollsurg.2010.11.001

Institute of Medicine (IOM). (2001). *Crossing the quality chasm: A new health system for the 21st century.* Washington, DC: National Academy Press. Retrieved from http://www.nap.edu/books/0309072808/html/

Interprofessional Education Collaborative Expert Panel. (2011). *Core competencies for interprofessional collaborative practice: Report of an expert panel.* Retrieved from Interprofessional Education Collaborative website: https://ipecollaborative.org/

Kalisch, B. J., Curley, M., & Stefanov, S. (2007). An intervention to enhance nursing staff teamwork and engagement. *Journal of Nursing Administration, 37*(2), 77–84.

Malec, J. F., Torsher, L. C., Dunn, W. F., Wiegmann, D. A., Arnold, J. J., Brown, D. A., & Phatak, V. (2007). The Mayo High Performance Teamwork Scale: Reliability and validity for evaluating key crew resource management skills. *Simulation in Healthcare, 2*(1), 4–10.

Marks, M. A., Mathieu, J. E., & Zaccaro, S. J. (2001). A temporally based framework and taxonomy of team process. *Academy of Management Review, 26*(3), 356–376.

Mitchell, P., Wynia, M., Golden, R., McNellis, B., Okun, S., Webb, C. E., ... Von Kohorn, I. (2012). *Core principles and values of effective team-based health care* (Discussion Paper). Retrieved from Institute of Medicine website: www.iom.edu/tbc

Morrison, G., Goldfarb, S., & Lanken, P. N. (2010). Team training of medical students in the 21st century: Would Flexner approve? *Academic Medicine, 85*(2), 254–259. doi:10.1097/ACM.0b013e3181c8845e

Neily, J., Mills, P. D., Young-Xu, Y., Carney, B. T., West, P., Berger, D. H., ... Bagian, J. P. (2010). Association between implementation of a medical team training program and surgical mortality. *Journal of the American Medical Association, 304*(15): 1693–1700. doi:10.1001/jama.2010.1506

Oandasan, I., Baker, G. R., Barker, K., Bosco, C., D'Amour, D., Jones, L., ... Way, D. (2006). *Teamwork in healthcare: Promoting effective teamwork in healthcare in Canada.* Retrieved from Canadian Health Services Research Foundation website: http://www.chsrf.ca

Patient Protection and Affordable Care Act. (2010). Retrieved from http://www.hhs.gov/healthcare/rights/

Porter, C., Hollenbeck, J. R., Illgen, D. R., Ellis, A. P. J., West, B. J., & Moon, H. (2003). Backup behaviors in teams: The role of personality and legitimacy of need. *Journal of Applied Psychology, 88*(3), 391–403. doi:10.1037/0021-9010.88.3.391

Pucher, P. H., Aggarwal, R., Batrick, N., Jenkins, M., & Darzi, A. (2014). Nontechnical skills performance and care processes in the management of the acute trauma patient. *Surgery, 155*(5), 902–909. doi:10.1016/j.surg.2013.12.029

Salas, E., Cooke, N. J., & Rosen, M. A. (2008). On teams, teamwork and team performance: Discoveries and developments. *Journal of Human Factors and Ergonomics Society, 50*, 540–547. doi:10.1518/001872008X288457

Salas, E., & Rosen, M. A. (2013). Building high reliability teams: Progress and some reflections on teamwork training. *BMJ Quality & Safety, 22*, 369–373. doi:10.1136/bmjqs-2013-002015

Salas, E., Sims, D. E., & Burke, C. S. (2005). Is there a "big five" in teamwork? *Small Group Research, 36*(5), 555–599. doi:10.1177/1046496405277134

Salas, E., Sims, D. E., & Klein, C. (2004). Cooperation and teamwork at work. In C. D. Spielberger (Ed.), *Encyclopedia of applied psychology* (pp. 497–505). San Diego, CA: Academic Press.

Sundar, E., Sundar, S., Pawlowski, J., Blum, R., Feinstein, D., & Pratt, S. (2007). Crew resource management and team training. *Anesthesiology Clinics, 25*(2007), 283–300. doi:10.1016/j.anclin.2007.03.011

Valentine, M. A., Nembhard, I. M., & Edmondson, A. C. (2014). Measuring teamwork in health care settings: A review of survey instruments. *Medical Care.* Advance online publication. doi:10.1097/MLR.0b013e31827feef6

Weaver, S. J., Dy, S. M., & Rosen, M. A. (2014). Team-training in healthcare: A narrative synthesis of the literature. *BMJ Quality & Safety, 23*(5), 359–372. doi:10.1136/bmjqs-2013-001848

Xyrichis, A., & Ream, E. (2008). Teamwork: A concept analysis. *Journal of Advanced Nursing, 61*(2), 232–241. doi:10.1111/j.1365-2648.2007.04496.x

33

TRANSFORMATIONAL LEADERSHIP

The term *transformational leadership* was first mentioned in 1973 by James V. Downton in his book *Rebel Leadership: Commitment and Charisma in the Revolutionary Process* (Bass, 1995). In 1978, in his book *Leadership*, the political historian James MacGregor Burns further described transformational leadership (Schwartz, Spencer, Wilson, & Wood, 2011). In that book, Burns described transformational and transactional leadership styles based on his study of political leaders. Bernard Bass continued the study of leadership to further define the attributes of transformational leadership and to be able to measure them (Bass, 1995). His work led to the development of four components of transformational leadership: idealized influence, inspirational motivation, intellectual stimulation, and individual consideration (Schwartz et al., 2011). *Idealized influence* described leaders who developed trust and conviction, emphasized purpose, demonstrated confidence, and shared purpose (Bass, 1997). *Inspirational motivation* described the ability to create a vision for the future, inspire followers with high standards to perform even better, and provide encouragement to accomplish the work (Bass, 1997). *Intellectual stimulation* described the ability to challenge the status quo and come up with new ideas to resolve challenges (Bass, 1997). *Individualized consideration* described the ability to treat each person individually, understanding his or her strengths and areas of development, and providing the appropriate coaching (Bass, 1997).

Transformational leadership is also defined as the ability to inspire others to achieve higher levels of productivity by appealing to their personal values (Schwartz et al., 2011). This type of leadership provides a model that is clearly defined and has been proven to support organizational and personal change (Gabel, 2012). *Transactional leadership* is defined as motivating others by rewarding them for the services they provide (Bass, 1995).

Since the introduction of transformational leadership in 1978, there have been many articles written and research studies completed to demonstrate the qualities of transformational and transactional leaders. Transformational leadership has also been compared to charismatic leadership. These two types of leadership are often considered the same (Bass & Riggio, 2006). However, transformational leadership is thought to be broader because of the leader's concern for the follower's intellectual stimulation and professional growth (Bass & Riggio, 2006). Another difference found in some of the literature about charismatic leadership is the ability of this type of leader to use his or her power to influence people for his or her own self-interest (Bass & Riggio, 2006; Dorian, Dunbar, Frayn, & Garfinkel, 2000).

It is also important to define transactional leadership as transformational leadership is explored. A transactional leader is one who leads by quid pro quo (Bass & Riggio, 2006). In other words, the followers are rewarded when the goals are achieved. According to Bass and Riggio (2006), transformational leadership is an expansion of transactional leadership. The transformational leader inspires the follower to work toward a shared vision for the organization, encourages creativity in problem solving, and coaches for departmental or organizational success (Bass & Riggio, 2006). Today's leaders are faced with many changes, and these changes require transformational leaders (Feinberg, Ostroff, & Burke, 2005).

The transformational leader is able to inspire staff to become actively engaged in their work environment. These leaders are seen as authentic, visionary, flexible, charismatic, confident, and experts in their field (Ward, 2002). They develop their staff professionally and create an environment where staff are able to work together to achieve the organizational goals.

According to the American Nurses Credentialing Center (ANCC), transformational leaders stimulate and inspire followers to achieve improved outcomes and increase their leadership abilities (ANCC, 2014). These transformational leaders empower staff to be part of the solution to the challenges they face every day as they care for their patients. They are collaborative and engaging and promote an environment where the voices of the staff are heard and listened to.

DEFINING ATTRIBUTES

The defining attributes of transformational leadership are *inspiration, influence,* and *motivation.*

Inspiration is the first defining attribute of transformational leadership. This type of leader has a strong sense of vision and is able to inspire employees to work toward that common vision. People feel committed to organizational goals and want to work toward that future state (Abu-Tineh, Khasawneh, & Omary, 2009). Transformational leaders communicate the goals of the organization with excitement, enthusiasm, and confidence. These leadership characteristics inspire the followers to focus on the organizational goals rather than their own self-interests (Hutchinson & Jackson, 2013). They are excited to partner with their leader and achieve success.

Influence is the second defining attribute of transformational leadership. This type of leader is able to influence the behaviors and work ethic of followers. The followers also have a higher degree of trust and job satisfaction (Yang, 2014). Staff perceive more commitment to the organization and experience less alienation from leaders with a transformational leadership style (Schwartz et al., 2011). Those with this style of leadership have high standards and model behaviors that their teams are able to emulate. Followers are clear on what is expected of them and how they contribute to the organizational goals. They develop loyalty to the leader and work toward mutual success.

Motivation is the third defining attribute of transformational leadership. With this type of leadership, staff are motivated to perform at a higher level. They feel intellectually stimulated and work toward achieving their full potential (Abu-Tineh et al., 2009). Followers of this type of leader are rewarded and recognized for their performance. The transformational leader pays attention to individual and group recognition. This type of recognition enables followers to feel part of something important, and they are thus motivated to work even harder (Abu-Tineh et al., 2009). They feel at ease asking questions about the work and are comfortable seeking clarification. The leader develops their potential and assists them to develop confidence and competence (Herman, Gish, & Rosenblum, 2015).

DEFINITION

Transformational leadership is a relationship that exists between a leader and followers where the leader demonstrates the characteristics of inspiration, influence, and motivation.

MODEL CASE

The nurse manager of the intensive care unit (ICU) is having a staff meeting with her team. This team is highly satisfied according to their last satisfaction survey scores. In the meeting, the manager is discussing the organization's and the ICU's goals related to quality and safety. She connects these goals to quality patient care (inspiration). She shows the team a graph with the ICU's performance in relationship to the national benchmark. They are outperforming the benchmark in some areas but have opportunities for improvement in others. She challenges them to develop strategies that will assist the group to outperform in all areas (influence). The manager praises the team for the hard work they have done to improve the scores in some areas and seeks their input on strategies for improvement in the other areas (motivation). All defining attributes are present in this case.

RELATED CASE

A nurse manager of the ICU is having a staff meeting with her team. This team is highly satisfied, according to their last satisfaction survey scores. In the meeting, the manager is discussing the organization's and the ICU's goals related to quality and safety. She connects these goals to quality patient care (inspiration). She shows the team a graph with the ICU's performance in relationship to the national benchmark. They are outperforming the benchmark in some areas but have opportunities for improvement in others. She praises the group for having excellent clinical skills. She also then challenges them to develop strategies that will assist the group to outperform in all areas (influence). The nurse manager discusses an extra weekend off for members of the team who assist in improving the metrics (failed motivation). In this case, the nurse manager was inspirational and continued to have influence over the team's performance, but failed to motivate them in developing strategies for success as a transformational leader would. Instead, she used the attribute of a transactional leader who rewards for the services provided.

BORDERLINE CASE

The nurse manager of the ICU is having a staff meeting with her team. This team is highly satisfied, according to their last satisfaction survey scores. In the meeting, the manager is discussing the organization's and the ICU's goals related to quality and safety. She relates these goals to quality patient care (inspiration). She shows the team a graph with the ICU's performance in relationship to the national benchmark. They are outperforming the benchmark in some areas but have opportunities for improvement in others. She praises the group for having excellent clinical skills. She also challenges them to develop strategies that will assist the group to outperform in all areas (influence). The nurse manager does not recognize the team for the areas in which they are outperforming. Instead, she focuses on the areas of opportunity and outlines the process to work on in order to improve the other metrics (failed motivation).

CONTRARY CASE

In this case, the nurse manager is meeting with her team to discuss the organization's and the ICU's quality and safety goals and metrics. She makes no connection between the goals and the patients. She simply informs the team that they are expected to improve their performance in the necessary areas (failed inspiration). The nurse manager is not clinically strong and is therefore unable to identify strategies for improvement (failed influence). She focuses on the area in need of improvement and does not recognize the area in which the team is outperforming. She informs the staff that they must improve their performance but gives no recommendations or opportunities for discussion (failed motivation).

ANTECEDENTS

In order for transformational leadership to exist, a number of antecedents must be present: develop the potential of followers, develop relationships with followers, self-confidence, emotional intelligence, and visibility. Transformational leaders are focused on developing the potential of others and developing relationships with their teams (Herman et al., 2015). This allows them to be very influential. These leaders possess self-confidence and emotional intelligence (Hutchinson & Jackson, 2013). They are seen as visible leaders

(Abu-Tineh et al., 2009). This allows them to build relationships and develop their teams while focusing on the organizational goals.

CONSEQUENCES

There are consequences of transformational leadership. Followers of this type of leadership experience a higher degree of job satisfaction and trust (Yang, 2014). Staff productivity ultimately increases as a result of this satisfaction. These leaders provide feedback, listen to opinions, and consider solutions from their followers, all of which result in trust of the leader (Yang, 2014). Transformational leaders are able to achieve positive quality outcomes while developing their followers (ANCC, 2014). Followers become more focused on achieving the organizational goals and a culture of quality and patient safety is created.

EMPIRICAL REFERENTS

Each of the defining attributes of transformational leadership requires an empirical referent. Based on the author's review of the pertinent literature, the Leadership Practice Inventory (LPI), which was developed to measure leadership qualities (Abu-Tineh et al., 2009), fills this need. This tool consists of two components: the LPI-Self and the LPI-Observer. This tool can measure the attributes of inspiration, influence, and motivation either as a leader self-assessment or as an observer assessment.

SUMMARY

Transformational leadership is well documented in the literature as a style that is essential in today's changing health care environment. In this concept analysis, the attributes of transformational leadership are the ability to develop others, the ability to develop relationships, the possession of self-confidence and emotional intelligence, and leadership visibility. The attributes of transformational leadership are the ability to inspire, influence, and motivate followers. These attributes have empirical referents, which ensure that they can be measured. The consequences are increased job satisfaction, trust, productivity, and quality. Figure 33.1 is provided to facilitate comprehension of the concept.

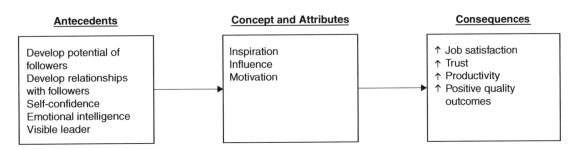

FIGURE 33.1 Transformational leadership.

REFERENCES

Abu-Tineh, A. M., Khasawneh, S. A., & Omary, A. A. (2009, Winter). Kouzes and Posner's transformational leadership model in practice: The case of Jordanian schools. *Journal of Leadership Education, 7*(3), 265–283.

American Nurses Credentialing Center. (2014). *2014 Magnet® application manual.* Silver Spring, MD: Author.

Bass, B. M. (1995). Theory of transformational leadership redux. *Leadership Quarterly, 6*(4), 463–478.

Bass, B. M. (1997, February). Does the transactional-transformational leadership paradigm transcend organizational and national boundaries? *American Psychologist, 52*, 130–139.

Bass, B. M., & Riggio, R. E. (2006). *Transformational leadership* (2nd ed.). Mahwah, NJ: Lawrence Erlbaum Associates.

Dorian, B. J., Dunbar, C., Frayn, D., & Garfinkel, P. (2000). Charismatic leadership, boundary issues, and collusion. *American Journal of Psychotherapy, 54*, 216–225.

Feinberg, B. J., Ostroff, C., & Burke, W. W. (2005). The role of within-group agreement in understanding transformational leadership. *Journal of Occupational and Organizational Psychology, 78*, 471–488. doi:10.1348/096317905X26156

Gabel, S. (2012, October–December). Transformational leadership in medical practice: Capturing and influencing principles-driven work. *Journal of Ambulatory Care Management, 35*, 304–310. doi:10.1097/JAC.0b013e3182606e66

Herman, S., Gish, M., & Rosenblum, R. (2015, February). Effects of nursing position on transformational leadership practices. *Journal of Nursing Administration, 45*(2), 113–119. doi:10.1097/NNA.0000000000000165

Hutchinson, M., & Jackson, D. (2013, January). Transformational leadership in nursing: Towards a more critical interpretation. *Nursing Inquiry, 20*(1), 11–22. doi:10.1111/nin.12006

Schwartz, D. B., Spencer, T., Wilson, B., & Wood, K. (2011). Transformational leadership: Implications for nursing leaders in facilities seeking magnet designation. *AORN Journal, 93*(737), 737–748.

Ward, K. (2002). A vision for tomorrow: Transformational nursing leaders. *Nursing Outlook, 3*, 121–126.

Yang, Y. (2014, June). Studies of transformational leadership: Evaluating two alternative models of trust and satisfaction. *Psychological Reports, 114*, 740–757. doi:10.2466/01.04.PR0.114k27w2

34

WORK ENGAGEMENT

The concept of work engagement can be applied to all occupations. Work engagement has been studied in various disciplines, including business, nursing, education, and psychology. Leiter and Bakker (2010) describe work engagement as a motivational concept which reflects the personal energy that employees enthusiastically apply to their work. Kahn (1990) describes persons who are personally engaged as people who simultaneously employ and express "their 'preferred self' in task behaviors that promote connections to work and others, personal presence (physical, cognitive, and emotional), and active, full role performances" (p. 700). Kahn (1990) refers to personal disengagement as withdrawing oneself physically, cognitively, and emotionally from one's work roles. Kahn (1990) also explains that the presence of three psychological conditions—meaningfulness, safety, and availability—results in personal engagement. Meaningfulness is described as experiencing a feeling of having worth or value for the physical, cognitive, and emotional energy one invests in one's work; feeling safe is described as having the ability to employ and express one's self without fear of negative consequences; and availability describes having adequate physical, emotional, or psychological resources to personally engage in one's work (Kahn, 1990).

Building on Kahn's work May, Gilson, and Harter (2004) explored the influence and effects of meaningfulness, safety, and availability on employee work engagement. All three psychological conditions were found to have a positive effect on engagement, with safety having a significant effect and meaningfulness having the strongest effect (May et al., 2004). May et al. (2004) distinguished job involvement from work engagement. Job involvement results from realization of the necessity to fulfill the skills required by the job (May et al., 2004). In contrast, engagement requires the active use of emotions, behaviors, and cognitions during work role performances and is concerned with how a person utilizes himself or herself during these performances (May et al., 2004).

Work engagement has also been identified as the opposite of burnout (Schaufeli & Bakker, 2004a). Malasch and Leiter (1997) identified energy, involvement, and efficacy as the three dimensions of work engagement which they believe are the direct opposites of the three dimensions of burnout, identified as exhaustion, cynicism, and ineffectiveness. The relationship between job demands, job resources, and work engagement and burnout has also been examined in the literature (Schaufeli & Bakker, 2004a). Schaufeli and Bakker (2004a) found that engagement and burnout are negatively related, that work engagement is predicted by available job resources, and that burnout is predicted by job demands and lack of resources.

Work engagement in nursing has been linked to a decrease in burnout (Demerouti, Bakker, Nachreiner, & Schaufeli, 2000; Mason et al., 2014; Schaufeli & Bakker, 2004a), a decrease in job turnover (Sawatzky & Enns, 2012), and an increase in well-being (Kanste, 2011). Bargagliotti (2012) explains that the concept of work engagement in nursing "contributes to a distinctive body of nursing knowledge because it theoretically underpins the actions of nurses and nurse managers as they create a practice environment that either supports safe and effective care or does not" (p. 1415).

DEFINING ATTRIBUTES

Vigor, dedication, and *absorption* are the three defining attributes of work engagement that have been repeatedly found in the literature (Bakker, Schaufeli, Leiter, & Taris, 2008; Bargagliotti, 2012; Halbesleben & Wheeler, 2008; Jenero, Flores, Orgaz, & Cruz, 2010; Laschinger, Wilk, Cho, & Greco, 2009; Simpson, 2009; Wonder, 2012).

Vigor is characterized as high levels of energy, mental resilience, and willingness to invest oneself in one's work; dedication is characterized by a feeling of significance, pride, and inspiration in one's work; and absorption is characterized by being fully engrossed in one's work and having difficulty detaching oneself from one's work (Schaufeli & Bakker, 2004b).

DEFINITION

Work engagement is defined as an optimistic, fulfilling, enthusiastic approach to one's work that is characterized by vigor, dedication, and absorption.

MODEL CASE

Daniela, BSN, RN, is a staff nurse in a busy emergency department. She worked the past 2 days and today is her day off. Her manager calls her and asks her to come in to help out because there were two sick calls which left the unit short-staffed. Daniela does not mind coming in on her day off because she understands how hard it is to work in a busy ED without sufficient staffing. Even though she is tired, Daniela comes into work energetic and with a smile (vigor) and is ready to start her work. As the day goes on, the ED gets busier, and before she realizes it the time is now

3 o'clock (absorption) and her charge nurse has sent someone to relieve her for her lunch break. During her lunch hour Daniela sends an email to her co-worker to set up a meeting for the community outreach committee that she is co-chairing (dedication). The committee is planning the hospital's next health fair and they need to meet to finalize some of the details for the event. Later that day, at the end of her shift, Daniela leaves work tired but fulfilled because it was a good day in the ED. This case demonstrates vigor exhibited by Daniella when she came to work, her ability to become absorbed in her work, and her dedication to her hospital and committee that she co-chairs.

RELATED CASE

Marie, BSN, RN, has been a nurse in the coronary care unit for 7 years. She has great leadership and clinical abilities and is often put in charge. Marie likes to be in charge because it gives her an opportunity to get involved with all of the patients on the unit and help her co-workers. When she is in charge, she feels more energized (vigor) while at work and the day always goes by quickly (absorption). Morale among the staff nurses has been low and Marie has considered applying for the vacant assistant nurse manager position on her unit, with the thought that she could try to make some positive changes for her colleagues. But, because she does not like her clinical nurse manager, Marie has decided not to pursue the role. Because she would like to develop her skills in leadership, Marie has decided to interview for an assistant nurse manager position another hospital (failed dedication). In this case, Marie's enthusiasm and feeling that time flies by when she is in charge exhibit her feelings of vigor and absorption when she is the charge nurse. However, her plans to pursue a leadership position at another hospital demonstrate her lack of dedication to her current job.

BORDERLINE CASE

Jessica, BSN, RN, is a new graduate nurse on a busy telemetry unit. She has been off orientation for 6 months. She is finally starting to feel comfortable in her new role as a staff nurse. Jessica is cautious when she is administrating medications and takes the time to perform full physical assessments on her patients when she starts her shift. She takes extra time to educate her patients when she is discharging them home. She will often become so concentrated on her work and what needs to get done that the day seems to fly by when she is working (absorption). She likes her job but she does not feel as if she fits in on the unit. This has made it difficult for Jessica to come in to work and lately she has begun to feel less energized and is not enthusiastic while she is working (failed vigor). She has already decided that she will stay on this unit for another 6 months and then look for a new job when she has more experience (failed dedication). Even though Jessica becomes absorbed in her work, she does not exhibit vigor while she is working, resulting in a lack of dedication for her job.

CONTRARY CASE

Michelle, RN, has been a nurse on a medical/surgical unit for all of the 7 years that she has been at the hospital where she is employed. Lately, she has been arriving to work late and finds her job draining (failed vigor). When she is working, the day seems to drag on (failed absorption) and she cannot wait until the end of her shift. Michelle is not interested in participating in any of the committees on her unit or in the hospital. She prefers to work her three required shifts a week and does not commit to anything that involves extra work (failed dedication). In this case, none of the attributes of work engagement are present. Michelle's lack of vigor is exemplified by her arriving to work late; she does not become absorbed in her work and therefore her day drags along. Her lack of participation in work-related committees displays her lack of dedication for her job.

ANTECEDENTS

The antecedents of work engagement are meaningfulness, empowerment, and job resources. With regard to work engagement in staff nurses and Schaufeli and Bakker's definition of work engagement, the literature includes empowerment (McDermott, Spence, & Shamian, 1996; Laschinger et al., 2009) and adequate job resources (Bakker et al., 2008; Schaufeli & Bakker, 2004a; Demerouti et al., 2000). Bjarnadottir (2011) also identified meaningfulness as an antecedent to work engagement.

Kahn (1990) identifies meaningfulness as one of the three psychological conditions that influence people to be engaged. People experience psychological meaningfulness when they feel valuable, and this experience results in feelings of physical, cognitive, or emotional energy (Kahn, 1990). Kahn (1990) found that higher levels of meaningfulness were linked to higher levels of engagement. May et al. (2004) define *meaningfulness* as the relationship of an individual's standards with the value of the individual's work objectives. The more meaningful individuals find their roles at work, the more motivated they become to invest themselves into their profession (May et al., 2004).

Many nurses enter the profession because of the holistic nature of nursing. Nurses facilitate healing and provide comfort. These are some of the aspects of the nursing profession that bring a sense of meaningfulness to nurses' roles. Bjarnadottir (2011) found that nurses' feelings of meaningfulness in their jobs contributed to the creation of resilience when dealing with the demands of their work, which resulted in increased work engagement. The nurses in Bjarnadottir's (2011) study expressed that they felt that their jobs were meaningful and reflected their personal values. These feelings of meaningfulness enabled the nurses to remain engaged in their jobs despite the demands and difficulties that they faced at times (Bjarnadottir, 2011).

Bakker et al. (2008) posit that work engagement is predicted by adequate job resources. These are described as the physical, social, or organizational aspects of a job that enhance learning and opportunity; decrease the physiological and psychological demands of a job; and are effective in achieving work-related goals (Bakker et al., 2008). Leiter and Bakker (2010) explain that job resources have both an intrinsic and an extrinsic motivational role in promoting work engagement. Job resources have an intrinsic motivational role because they both promote employees' learning and development and an extrinsic motivational role because they support the achievement of work goals (Leiter & Bakker, 2010). Supportive nurse managers and colleagues facilitate engaging work environments. McDermott et al. (1996) found a strong correlation between staff nurses' perceptions of nurse manager power and access to support. This finding "emphasizes the importance of positive feedback recognizing achievement, celebrating successes, fostering pride in one's work and backing new ideas and innovations" (McDermott et al., 1996, p. 46). Bjarnadottir (2011) found that nurses' support from their colleagues and managers helped them maintain engagement by adapting positively to change and the demands at work. To further support the impact of managerial support on job resources, Rivera, Fitzpatrick, and Boyle (2011) found that staff nurses considered manager action one of the most influential drivers of their level of work engagement. In addition, having adequate physical resources to perform their jobs can facilitate work engagement in nurses. When nurses have the supplies and materials that they need readily available, their jobs become less stressful and they have more time to dedicate to performing their roles.

Empowerment has been found to be linked to work engagement (Laschinger & Finegan, 2005; Laschinger, Wong, & Greco, 2006; Laschinger et al., 2009; McDermott et al., 1996). Empowerment has been found to affect the six areas of work life (work load, community, control, reward/recognition, fairness, values congruence) in nurses that result in greater work engagement (Laschinger & Finegan, 2005). Organizational structures that support nurse empowerment have been found to result in greater work engagement through enhancement of perceived fit in work life in staff nurses (Laschinger et al., 2006). In addition, empowerment has been found to have a significant positive relationship with work engagement regardless of years of nursing experience (Laschinger et al., 2009). Creating and supporting an environment where nurses perceive that they are empowered may increase work engagement.

CONSEQUENCES

Job retention, enhanced well-being, and decreased burnout are consequences of work engagement in nursing. Work engagement can have personal as well as organizational consequences. Work engagement in health care employees leads to greater job retention (Lowe, 2012). Specifically, engaged nurses are less likely to leave their jobs. Simpson (2009) found that as thoughts of quitting increased, work engagement decreased in medical/surgical staff nurses. Sawatzky and Enns (2012) found that work engagement in

ED nurses was a strong predictor of intent to leave. Increased feelings of work engagement may promote well-being in nurses. Work engagement has been found to be moderately positively correlated with personal well-being (Kanste, 2011). Engagement also leads to decreased burnout (Schaufeli & Bakker, 2004a). In nurses, burnout has been found to decrease as levels of work engagement increase (Demerouti et al., 2000; Mason et al., 2014).

EMPIRICAL REFERENTS

The Utrecht Work Engagement Scale (UWES), developed by Schaufeli and Bakker in 1999 (2004b), is a self-report questionnaire designed to measure the three core attributes of work engagement: vigor, dedication, and absorption. The UWES is a 17-item questionnaire with three subscales to measure vigor, dedication, and absorption. Six items measure vigor, five items measure dedication, and six items measure absorption. Psychometric analysis confirmed the factorial validity of the UWES (Schaufeli & Bakker, 2004b). The UWES is also available as a 9- and 15-item survey. It can be used to measure work engagement in all occupations. The key components can be found in Figure 34.1.

SUMMARY

This chapter analyzed the concept of work engagement. Three attributes—vigor, dedication, and absorption—were identified. The antecedents and consequences were detailed and sample cases given.

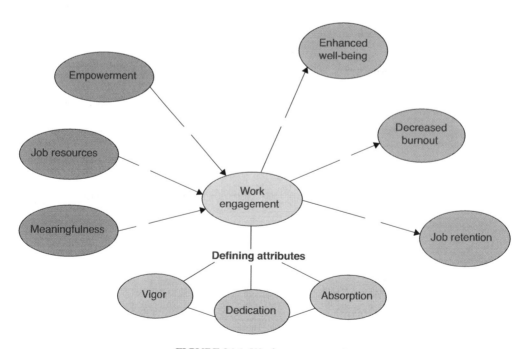

FIGURE 34.1 Work engagement.

REFERENCES

Bakker, A. B., Schaufeli, W. B., Leiter, M. P., & Taris, T. W. (2008). Work engagement: An emerging concept in occupational health psychology. *Work & Stress, 22*(3), 187–200.

Bargagliotti, L. A. (2012). Work engagement in nursing: A concept analysis. *Journal of Advanced Nursing, 68*(6), 1414–1428.

Bjarnadottir, A. (2011). Work engagement among nurses in relatively demanding jobs in the hospital sector. *Nursing Science, 31*(3), 30–34.

Demerouti, E., Bakker, A. B., Nachreiner, F., & Schaufeli, W. B. (2000). A model of burnout and life satisfaction amongst nurses. *Journal of Advanced Nursing, 32*(2), 454–464.

Halbesleben, J. R. B., & Wheeler, A. R. (2008). The relative roles of engagement and embeddedness in predicting job performance and intention to leave. *Work & Stress, 22*(3), 242–256.

Jenero, C., Flores, N., Orgaz, M. B., & Cruz, M. (2010). Vigour and dedication in nursing professionals: Towards a better understanding of work engagement. *Journal of Advanced Nursing, 67*(4), 865–875.

Kahn, W. A. (1990). Psychological conditions of personal engagement and disengagement at work. *Academy of Management, 33*(4), 692–724. Retrieved from http://www.jstor.org/stable/256287

Kanste, O. (2011). Work engagement, work commitment and their association with well-being in health care. *Scandinavian Journal of Caring Sciences, 25,* 754–761.

Laschinger, H. K. S., & Finegan, J. (2005). Empowering nurses for work engagement and health in hospital settings. *Journal of Nursing Administration, 35*(10), 439–449.

Laschinger, H. K. S, Wilk, P., Cho, J., & Greco, P. (2009). Empowerment, engagement and perceived effectiveness in nursing work environments: Does experience matter? *Journal of Nursing Management, 17,* 636–646.

Laschinger, H. K. S., Wong, C. A., & Greco, P. (2006). The impact of staff nurse empowerment on person-job fit and work engagement/burnout. *Nursing Administration Quarterly, 30*(4), 358–367.

Leiter, M. P., & Bakker, A. B. (2010). Work engagement: Introduction. In A. B. Bakker & M. P. Leiter (Eds.), *Work engagement: A handbook of essential theory and research* (pp. 1–9). East Sussex, UK: Psychology Press.

Lowe, G. (2012). How employee engagement matters for hospital performance. *Healthcare Quarterly, 15*(2), 29–39.

Malasch, C., & Leiter, M. P. (1997). *The truth about burnout: How organizations cause personal stress and what to do about it.* San Francisco, CA: Jossey-Bass.

Mason, V. M., Leslie, G., Clark, K., Lyons, P., Walke, E., Butler, C., & Griffin, M. (2014). Compassion fatigue, moral distress, and work engagement in surgical intensive care unit trauma nurses. *Dimensions of Critical Care Nursing, 33*(4), 215–225.

May, D. R., Gilson, R. L., & Harter, L. M. (2004). The psychological conditions of meaningfulness, safety, and availability and the engagement of the human spirit at work. *Journal of Occupational and Organizational Psychology, 77,* 11–37.

McDermott, K., Spence, L. H. K., & Shamian, J. (1996). Work empowerment and organizational commitment. *Nursing Management, 27*(5), 44–47.

Rivera, R. R., Fitzpatrick, J. J., & Boyle, S. M. (2011). Closing the RN engagement gap. Which drivers of engagement matter? *Journal of Nursing Administration, 41*(6), 265–272.

Sawatzky, J. V., & Enns, C. L. (2012). Exploring the key predictors of retention in emergency nurses. *Journal of Nursing Management, 20,* 696–707.

Schaufeli, W., & Bakker, A. (2004a). Job demands, job resources, and their relationship with burnout and engagement: A multi-sample study. *Journal of Organizational Behavior, 25,* 293–315.

Schaufeli, W., & Bakker, A. (2004b). *Utrecht work engagement scale.* Retrieved from http://www.wilmarschaufeli.nl

Simpson, M. R. (2009). Predictors of work engagement among medical-surgical registered nurses. *Western Journal of Nursing Research, 31*(1), 44–65.

Wonder, A. H. (2012). Engagement in RNs working in Magnet®-designated hospitals: Exploring the significance of work experience. *Journal of Nursing Administration, 42*(12), 575–579.

SUMMARY AND CONCLUSIONS

In this chapter, we summarize content throughout the concept analysis chapters and draw conclusions based on an evaluation of the content of those chapters. The concept analysis chapters have been organized broadly within three sections: Part I: Patient/Client-Focused Concepts, comprising 15 chapters; Part II: Caregiver-Focused Concepts, which consists of 14 chapters; and Part III: Organization-Focused Concepts, which has five chapters. All analyses are supported by a literature review and, where appropriate, previously published specific or broadly related concept analyses are examined and referenced. In the evaluation of the concept analyses within the groupings, evident interrelationships are described. Subclusters of like concepts are formed and similarities and differences presented. Yet, all concepts stand alone with little relationship to other concepts, thus fulfilling the requirement that each analysis be rigorous and precise in defining attributes, antecedents, and consequences. Thus, the contribution of this book is to promote understanding about the specific phenomena explored, independent of other related concepts.

PATIENT/CLIENT-FOCUSED CONCEPTS

Four chapters in Part I are related to the personal characteristics of patients/clients experiencing health/illness; all are important in influencing positive health outcomes. These concepts include hardiness (Chapter 4), hope (Chapter 6), motivation (Chapter 9), and self-motivation (Chapter 14). Hartigan wrote of hardiness in stroke, which enables individuals to deal with stressful life events rather than using avoidance or denial. The positive influence of hardiness is emphasized and the defining attributes of perception of the changed situation as stressful, the individual's ability to find meaning and a sense of purpose, and the ability to influence the situation are described. Murphy and O'Donovan write of hope in mental illness provoked by a challenging life event and uncertainty and with attributes of attribution of meaning, enabling the possible, and cognitive goal-directed processes.

Common antecedents in both hardiness and hope are stressful life events and common attributes relate to finding meaning in the situation.

Wills identifies motivation as a driving force within individuals, with the attributes of self-determination, self-efficacy, and readiness to change. Ben-Zacharia examined the concept of self-motivation for attaining success in personal and social life. Included in the attributes are an inner drive and external drive to achieve a goal or to do an action or behavior. Although these two concepts might be conceived as similar, the only attribute that is common is that related to determination or drive.

Six chapters in Part I of the book are related to health behavior, including exercise adherence (Chapter 3); help seeking for breast cancer symptoms (Chapter 5); meaning in life (Chapter 7), medication habits (Chapter 8), patient engagement (Chapter 11), and self-care strategies (Chapter 13). The health behavior-related characteristics that are reflected could prevent or ameliorate illness or ill health. Gali wrote of exercise adherence and its physical and mental benefits. The defining attributes of self-efficacy promotion, active voluntary involvement, and relapse prevention are described. Help seeking for breast cancer symptoms is examined by O'Mahony, with attributes of a response to a self-discovered breast symptom, symptom interpretation, and decision making identified. Weathers identifies meaning of life as a subjective experience, a sense of coherence, and connections or relationships. Defining attributes are creative, experiential, and attitudinal values. Fitzgerald and Lehane examine the concept of medication habits, indicating that habit is an undervalued construct in health and adherence research. Habitual automaticity, cues in the environment, behavior reutilization, and volitional control are attributes. Ventura analyzes the concept of patient engagement and develops a definition including the attributes, of empowerment, collaboration, health information, and patient activation. Landers investigated self-care strategies. Included in the attributes are self-care behaviors, trial and error, self-taught, and learned over time.

Taken together, these six analyses provide a wealth of information on the concepts themselves, together with their attributes, antecedents, and consequences. There is no overlap in attributes, and an examination of both the text and the associated figures reveals that while knowledge is the only common antecedent for the concepts of patient engagement and help-seeking behavior, the only consequence common to all of these concepts is improved outcomes for patients/clients.

Other chapters in Part I are related to concepts concerning a response to a health issue, such as elder self-neglect (Chapter 2), parental concerns (Chapter 10), quality of life (Chapter 12), stigmatization (Chapter 15), and caregiver burden (Chapter 17). Day identifies self-neglect as a complex multidimensional concept comprising environmental neglect, cumulative behaviors, and deficits. Antecedents are multiple comorbidities, mental health issues, and absence of social networks. Consequences are increased use of health resources, lower health, caregiver neglect, and mortality. This chapter is enhanced by the integration of recently published research conducted on the concept. Parental concern is the focus of work by Mulcahy. This chapter offers clarity of meaning, as previously parental concern has lacked precision and definitions in its use in both research and professional practice. Attributes are parental/health care professional interaction, parental uncertainty, child well-being, and verbal expression. The consequences are increasing or decreasing parental anxiety and positive or negative child well-being. This analysis is enhanced with the integration of research conducted by Mulcahy.

A very different yet pertinent subject for analysis was quality of life, investigated by Cajulis and colleagues. Here attributes identified were satisfaction with one's life, perception of well-being, and autonomy, with consequences being happiness, self-esteem, and self-worth. In analyzing the concept of stigmatization, Gardenier identifies the concept as a social phenomenon that affects the provision and utilization of health care. Attributes identified are separation, labelling, and misunderstanding.

A variety of concepts were analyzed in Part I. Although the concepts can be clustered broadly under categories and subcategories, there is little overlap in the attributes or in the antecedents or consequences identified.

CAREGIVER-FOCUSED CONCEPTS

Part II includes caregiver-focused concepts: anxiety (Chapter 16), caregiver burden (Chapter 17), clinical autonomy (Chapter 18), compassion fatigue (Chapter 19), cultural competence (Chapter 20), decision making (Chapter 21), emotional intelligence (Chapter 22), empathy (Chapter 23), inter professional collaboration (Chapter 24), mindfulness (Chapter 25), social support for new mothers (Chapter 27), resilience (Chapter 28), and triage nurse expertise (Chapter 29). For caregivers, if one or more of these characteristics exist, then their ability to provide care may be enhanced or impeded, with concomitant effects on quality of care.

For the purpose of drawing conclusions, the concepts anxiety, caregiver burden, empathy, emotional intelligence, compassion fatigue, resilience, and mindfulness are clustered together for evaluation purposes; these can be viewed as inherent characteristics of the individual carer yet can be accentuated in stressful encounters or situations. Based on the literature reviewed, Heffernan asserts that anxiety, is a global health problem with prevalent rates varying across the world, predisposing individuals to physical and mental illnesses. While there is an abundance of literature investigating the sources of anxiety, there is a paucity of published papers examining anxiety itself. In her analysis of the concept, the attributes identified were a subjective unpleasant experience or an unknown source and an emotional response; consequences were both positive (personal growth) or negative (physical, illness). In Mulad's analysis of caregiver burden in mental health, the attribute of caregivers' subjective experience is again emphasized, as well as hardship and change over time provoked by unexpected events with morbidity or coping and adjustment consequences.

Empathy was investigated by Ku, who concluded that empathy is the ability to communicate a sensing of other individuals' feelings without losing a sense of self. It serves as an integral part of the nurse–patient relationship and can significantly influence this relationship. The attributes identified are emotional intelligence, past experiences, and the ability to understand and effectively communicate. Consequences include enhanced communication and compassion. In a separate yet linked analysis, Prufeta examined emotional intelligence and identified attributes as empathy, self-regulation, awareness, and motivation; consequences were shown to be positive outcomes such as success or happiness and leadership effectiveness. Compassion fatigue is present when restorative processes are less than the compassionate energy used by the carer. In the analysis of this concept, Quinn Griffin and Mir identify attributes of exhaustion, erosion of coping capacities, and a decline in work performance. Continuing exposure to stress and overuse of emotional reserve are antecedents and the consequences are both physical and emotional.

Though all of these concepts are related to the carer's ability to care, they are distinctly different. They share only a few dimensions such as those just discussed. Thus, this demonstrates the differentiating aspect of the concept analysis methodology.

The following two analyses are focused on entities which if enhanced would help in stressful carer situations. Garcia-Dia and O'Flaherty focus on resilience, emphasizing its necessity for nurse effectiveness in diverse situations. Attributes that emerged from the analysis are self-efficacy, coping, and hope. The primary antecedent is an adverse event and the consequences are personal control and growth and psychological adjustment. In the literature reviewed by Matthes, mindfulness was conceived of as a mental quality and a self-regulation of attention, the practice of which has been shown to reduce stress, pain, anxiety, and depression. Noticing, nonjudgmental, and awareness of the present moment are attributes. Antecedents include openness to change and consequences include increased overall well-being and coping.

Concepts of cultural competence, clinical autonomy, decision making, interprofessional collaboration, and triage nurse expertise are clustered, as it is perceived that these are a concern for carers/nurses when working or dealing with a health care organization. Cultural competence is examined by Bauce from an organizational perspective, where it is necessary to be knowledgeable about cultural variations, particularly health beliefs and practices. The attributes are cultural awareness, sensitivity, knowledge, and skills. Antecedents are cultural encounter and commitment and there are consequences for both the patient and the provider.

Cotter examines clinical autonomy and differentiates clinical autonomy from organizational autonomy. Attributes that emerged for clinical autonomy are the professional practice context, clinical judgment, decision-making authority, and interdisciplinary collaboration. Antecedents are knowledge, ability, and desire for autonomy and the consequences are job satisfaction and nurse retention.

Decision making by nurse managers was investigated by Quinn Griffin, Stilgenbauer, and Nelson, who stated that it is a key aspect of leadership and implementing a course of action in the organization. Attributes are information gathering, critical thinking, and use of defined process. Antecedents include identification of a problem, and consequences include elimination or acceptance of the problem. Inter professional collaboration was the focus of Bell's analysis; she maintains that the lack of this collaboration is fragmented delivery of health care services. However, the literature demonstrates little evidence of collaboration in practice, nor is there clarity of meaning regarding the concept. Attributes that emerged from the analysis are shared care goals and decision making, power sharing, and nonhierarchical relationships. Antecedents include trust, respect, and professional confidence and consequences include improved patient care and enhanced staff morale. Quinn and Quinn Griffin identify antecedents of nurse manager accountability as commitment, openness, answerability, and resilience. Antecedents are self-awareness, motivation, and eagerness and consequences are empowerment and job satisfaction. Corbett and Quinn Griffin examine triage nurse experience, which is so necessary to increasing access to health care. Attributes are triage skill and knowledge. Antecedents are education and experience and consequences are decision making and appropriate action.

In conclusion, while all of these concepts relate to carers within the health care organization, an examination of the related text and the associated chapter figures representing the attributes, antecedents, and consequences show minimal overlap in dimensions. The only similarity is in the consequences, where better outcomes for carers themselves and potentially for the care recipients are detailed.

ORGANIZATION-FOCUSED CONCEPTS

Part III presents analysis of concepts pertinent to nurse workaround (Chapter 30), commitment (Chapter 31), teamwork (Chapter 32), transformational leadership (Chapter 33), work engagement (Chapter 34), and nurse manager accountability (Chapter 26). Nurse workarounds are described as nurses devising an alternative work procedure to address a block in the workforce, even though these alternatives are deviations from policies, procedures, and work processes. For Harris, the attributes are modification or circumvention of standard care or protocol, patient care directed to increase efficiency, and the issue temporarily addressed but not solved. Consequences are identified as destabilization of the workforce, error, or evolution of the system. Sundel and Kirpalani assert that teamwork has received considerable attention from policy makers and researchers over the years, yet a clear statement of its meaning is still elusive. Attributes identified within the concept analysis are shared decision making, mutual performance monitoring, and adaptive back-up behaviors in the context of independent effort by team members. Antecedents are positive leadership and mutual trust and consequences include increase in staff satisfaction and reduced staff turnover. Khan identifies transformational leadership as including the attributes of inspiration, influence, and motivation. Antecedents include visible leaders and consequences include job satisfaction and trust. Siller, in presenting a concept analysis of work engagement, identified the attributes as vigor, dedication, and absorption. Empowerment is identified as an attribute and well-being, decreased burnout, and job retention are consequences. Positive leadership and being a visible leader emerged as antecedents for both teamwork and transformational leadership. Staff/job satisfaction and reduced staff turnover were consequences of both transformational leadership and work engagement. As can be seen in the above evaluation similarities in attributes, antecedents, and consequences are few and each analysis stands alone with little overlap.

In conclusion, this text presents 34 concept analyses, including a wide range of concepts relevant to the discipline of nursing. These are underpinned by literature reviews, including a review of any pertinent previously published concept analysis. The concept analyses follow a specific method, with defining attributes, antecedents, and consequences given. These are illustrated in the figures associated with each chapter, from which it can be clearly seen that each of the concepts stands alone with specific attributes, antecedents, and consequences articulated.

Definitions based on attributes identified give the clarity of meaning that is necessary for research to be undertaken. Some of the authors have completed research on the concepts. For example, Day references her work on self-neglect, O'Mahony her research on help-seeking behavior for breast cancer, Fitzgerald and Lehane research on medication habits, Mulcahy research on parental concern, and Landers research on self-care strategies. This research is integrated into the case descriptions. The references to research undertaken by the authors will prove valuable insights to neophyte researchers as they seek clarity on a research topic. More experienced researchers will find the analyses useful in building theory, particularly using the antecedents as determinants of behavior and consequences as relevant outcomes. Antecedents and consequences of various concepts also will help in determining variables or relationships for future research. The listing of empirical referents within each chapter provides researchers with information regarding instruments and measurements for consideration in future research. We expect that all readers will find the text informative and that many research projects will emerge as a result of this work.

INDEX